THE
PLANT-BASED
baby & toddler

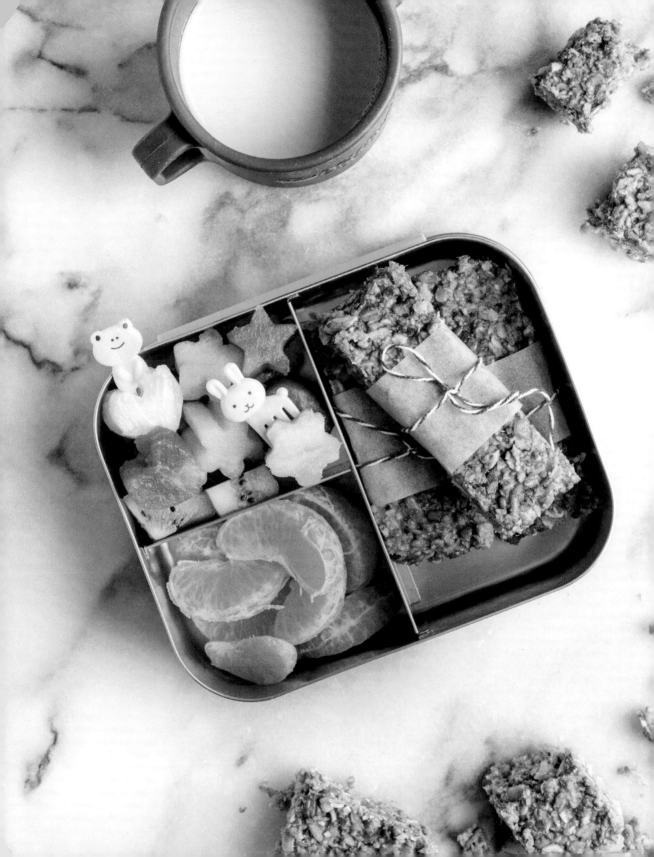

THE
PLANT-BASED
baby & toddler

YOUR COMPLETE FEEDING GUIDE
FOR THE FIRST 3 YEARS

Whitney English, MS, RDN, &
Alexandra Caspero, MA, RDN

AVERY
AN IMPRINT OF PENGUIN RANDOM HOUSE
NEW YORK

AVERY

An imprint of Penguin Random House LLC
penguinrandomhouse.com

Most Avery books are available at special quantity discounts for bulk purchase
for sales promotions, premiums, fund-raising, and educational needs.
Special books or book excerpts also can be created to fit specific needs.
For details, write SpecialMarkets@penguinrandomhouse.com.

Library of Congress Cataloging-in-Publication Data

Names: Caspero, Alexandra, author. | English, Whitney, author.
Title: The plant-based baby and toddler: your complete feeding guide
for the first three years / by Alexandra Caspero, MA, RDN and Whitney English, MS, RDN.
Description: New York: Avery, [2021] | Includes index.
Identifiers: LCCN 2020030485 (print) | LCCN 2020030486 (ebook) |
ISBN 9780593192115 (paperback) | ISBN 9780593192122 (ebook)
Subjects: LCSH: Infants—Nutrition. | Toddlers—Nutrition. |
Baby foods—Nutrition. | LCGFT: Cookbooks.
Classification: LCC RJ216 .C343 2021 (print) | LCC RJ216 (ebook) |
DDC 641.5/6222—dc23
LC record available at https://lccn.loc.gov/2020030485
LC ebook record available at https://lccn.loc.gov/2020030486

Printed in the United States of America
2nd Printing

Book design by Laura K. Corless

Graphics © Elle Om and Darrick Hays
Lifestyle photos © Lani Ohye and Whitney English
Food photos © Alexandra Caspero

To Vander, Caleb, Emery, and Ella.

Getting to be your moms is the greatest honor of our lives.

We love you so much.

Contents

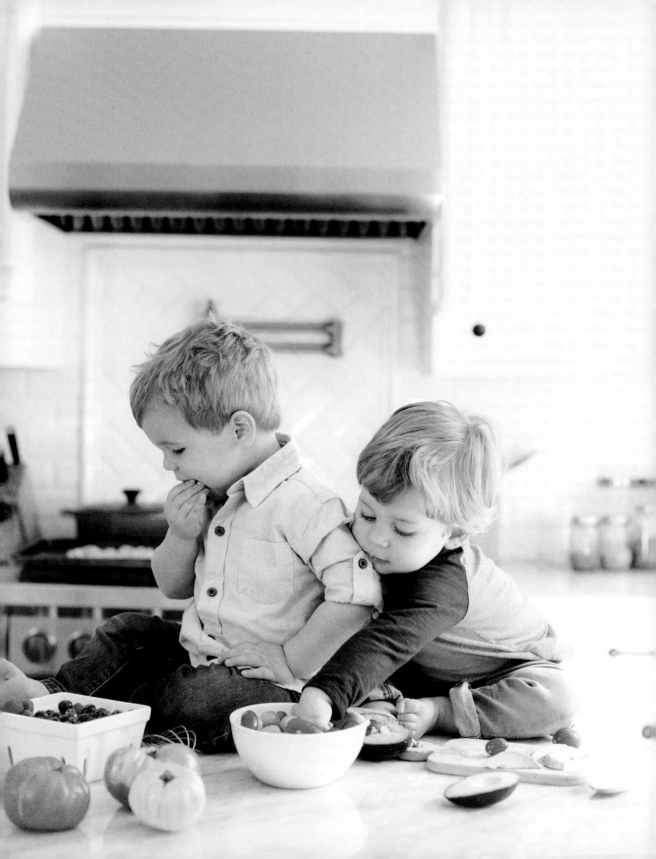

THE
PLANT-BASED
baby & toddler

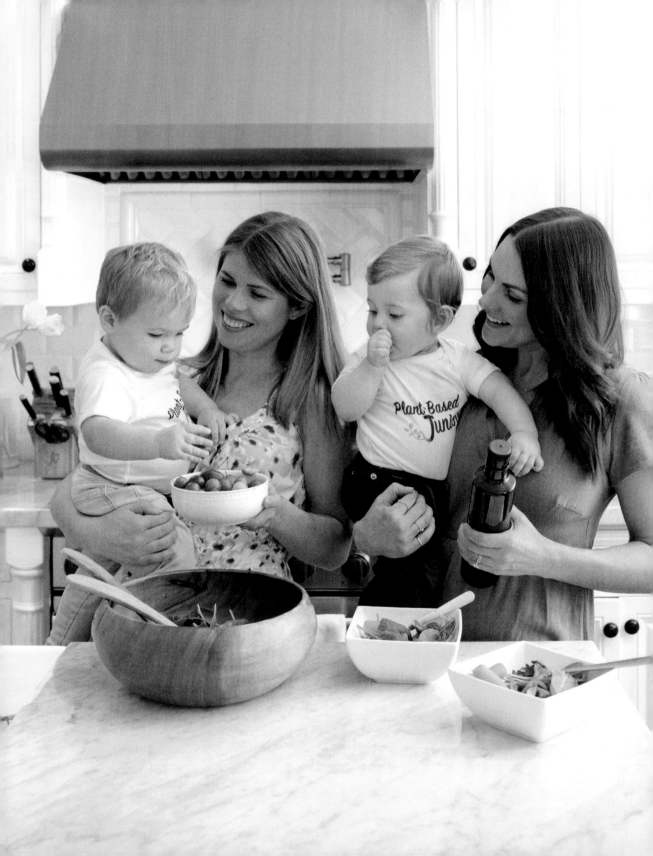

Introduction

Hi, friends. We're Alex and Whitney, registered dietitian nutritionists, mamas to predominantly plant-based babes, and the creators of Plant-Based Juniors (PBJs), an online community for parents interested in raising healthy, conscientious children.

We've been "predominantly plant-based" for a while now (more on that soon). Alex dabbled with vegetarianism throughout high school and fully stopped eating meat in college after a breakup with a protein-obsessed meathead. Whitney's journey began during her graduate nutrition program, when after taking a class in Italy on diet and disease taught by world-renowned longevity expert Dr. Valter Longo, she ditched her chicken breast-based diet and never looked back.

When we each learned we were going to become parents, our initial reaction was utter joy. But this bliss was quickly followed by that not-so-pleasant feeling all parents-to-be can relate to: uncertainty. There are just so many things to *consider*, and as parents we are compelled to do everything in our power to ensure that our children are set up for a lifetime of success. From choosing the safest car seat to the best pediatrician, we spend countless hours researching, talking to friends, and seeking expert opinions on every detail of our child's care. There are decisions to make and countless opportunities to "get it wrong."

Nutrition is one area that can be both confusing and emotionally charged. Although the scientific consensus is clear that "appropriately planned" plant-based diets are safe—and likely beneficial—for both adults and children, we still frequently hear criticisms and concerns from skeptical parents and medical practitioners.

For decades, the medical community has insisted that the only way to raise a healthy child is on the standard American diet, rooted in meat and dairy. We're told milk "does a body good," and that growing tots should be drinking three glasses a day. We're advised by pediatricians that meat is an essential first food, and that without it our babes won't get enough protein or iron. Meanwhile, media outlets using fear-mongering headlines warn that plant-based diets are dangerous for children. Naturally, these messages would lead any conscientious parent to question raising their baby plant-based.

Even as dietitians, with master's degrees in nutrition and years of hands-on experience, we both felt natural anxiety in response. The overwhelmingly pro-animal-product agenda in our society instills fear in plant-based parents, especially when coupled with a lack of accessible, evidence-based, and expert-delivered resources informing parents of how to properly implement a plant-based diet.

But in the face of fear, we decided to look for facts. We scoured the medical literature and consulted experts across the globe in plant-based, prenatal, and pediatric nutrition. And we ultimately came to the decision we knew in our hearts to be true: Plant-based diets are safe and nutritionally adequate. Relieved and rejuvenated, we wanted to share what we'd learned with other parents to remove the stigma around plant-based diets for infants and toddlers and help you simply and confidently feed your child a diet that is *scientifically proven* to achieve optimal health.

The Current State of Children's Health

It's pretty absurd that in the face of rising obesity rates and chronic diseases in children, many use a standard American diet (SAD diet) as a benchmark for what proper nutrition should look like.

One in three children in the US is overweight and one in six is considered obese, with the most recent studies showing that obesity affects 13.9% of preschool-aged children.

Globally, obesity in our youngest demographic (preschoolers younger than 5 years of age) has also skyrocketed, increasing by about 60% since 1990. Many attribute this increase to a shift in developing countries away from primarily plant-based diets to diets heavy in meat and processed foods.

We've also witnessed an increase in "lifestyle diseases" in children, such as heart disease and diabetes, that were previously thought to affect only adults. Unlike type 1 diabetes, an autoimmune disease typically diagnosed in early childhood, type 2 diabetes usually occurs in adulthood and is linked to factors such as poor diet and a lack of exercise. However, type 2 diabetes in children has been rising rapidly. From 2001 to 2008, it increased by over 30%, and children as young as 10 years old are now commonly afflicted. Experts estimate that if this trend continues, we'll see a 2-to-4-fold rise in cases by 2050.

Something is seriously wrong with the way we're feeding our kids.

Research on Plant-Based Diets for Children

The American Academy of Pediatrics, the Academy of Nutrition and Dietetics, and the Canadian Paediatric Society all agree that well-planned vegan and vegetarian diets are safe and healthy for breastfeeding moms, infants, toddlers, and throughout all stages of life.

If you were already eating plant-based prior to becoming a parent, we're guessing you're well aware of the health benefits for adults—a reduced risk of chronic diseases like diabetes, heart disease, and some cancers, and a potentially greater life span. And while we could certainly use more research, the studies we do have suggest that many benefits of a plant-based diet extend to children.

One of the biggest benefits is a reduced risk of obesity. Studies show that vegan and vegetarian children typically weigh less than omnivorous children, while still attaining normal height. One study of 404 mainly vegan children showed that the majority fell between the 25th and 75th percentiles for weight and height on US growth charts and were only slightly below the median of the reference population.

Studies also show that plant-based children have lower levels of inflammatory signaling molecules linked to obesity and insulin resistance and higher levels of anti-inflammatory messengers compared to omnivorous children.

Another benefit is that plant-based children typically eat more fruits, vegetables, fiber, and important micronutrients like vitamin C and folate, while eating fewer

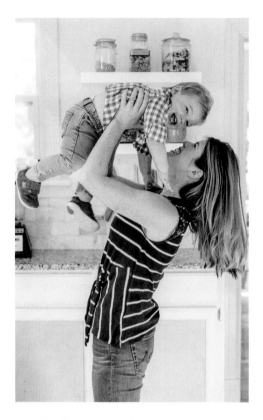

unhealthy items like sweets, salty snacks, and saturated fat-rich foods. As we will discuss in Chapters 4–6, taste preferences are shaped early in life, so helping kids learn to love fruits and vegetables at an early age sets them up for a lifetime of positive eating habits.

Plant-based children are also exposed to fewer environmental contaminants. This is because toxins bioaccumulate in animal tissue and build up the higher you get up the food chain. For example, one study found that the breast milk of vegetarian moms had just 1%–2% the amount of pollutants compared to omnivorous women. Another showed that children with a high intake of fish, meat, poultry, and dairy products had higher levels of both human and veterinary antibiotics present in their bloodstream.

Finally, a plant-rich diet may even be beneficial for children's cognition. A study of American vegetarian preschool children found that their IQ scores corresponded with a mental age more than a year higher than their chronological age. Although parental educational status likely played a role in this outcome, at the very least, this suggests that a plant-based diet supports normal brain and cognitive development.

PBJ BOTTOM LINE: While there isn't as much research on children as there is on adults in regard to plant-based diets, the studies we have suggest similar benefits: Plant-based kids typically eat more nutritious foods and less junk food, have healthier body weights and lower cholesterol levels, and have a reduced exposure to harmful environmental compounds. Plus, eating more fruits and veggies sets kids up for a lifetime of positive dietary habits!

Risks of a Meat-and-Dairy-Heavy Diet

As plant-based parents, we frequently find ourselves on the defensive—having to justify our choices and provide evidence for the benefits of our diet. But rather than letting the burden of proof fall in our court, we ask, where is the evidence showing that a meat-heavy diet is advantageous? Search the medical literature and you will not find a single study showing that meat provides benefits to already well-nourished children. Instead we find a plethora of research revealing the risks of a diet rich in meat and animal products.

Several studies have linked a high intake of cow's milk with an increased risk of childhood obesity. There are two proposed explanations for this: (1) hormonal factors and (2) the high protein content. While protein is important for growing kids, too much protein is never a good thing at any age, and very high protein intake (more than 15% total calories) in the first two years of life is associated with an increased risk of obesity later in life. As cow's milk is typically the major contributing source of protein in a toddler's diet, many experts have recommended a reduction in milk consumption to avoid the harms of excessive intake.

We often hear critics proclaiming that iron intake is low on a plant-based diet (which you'll learn shortly is untrue), but the reality is that consuming large amounts of cow's milk is actually a major cause of iron deficiency in toddlers. Cow's milk is both low in iron and reduces iron absorption due to a high content of absorption inhibitors like calcium and casein. In addition, while iron is a critical nutrient for growing babes, meat is not the ideal source. Iron in animals, known as heme iron, is linked to an increased risk of type 2 diabetes, heart disease, and some cancers, while iron found in plants, non-heme iron, does not have the same associations. Low iron status is harmful, but too much iron can be equally detrimental. And while the body has the ability to self-regulate non-heme iron absorption from plants, it does not have a mechanism to slow heme iron absorption from meat. This can lead to excessive absorption of heme iron.

A diet heavy in animal products is also associated with an increased risk of early menstruation, which has been linked to breast cancer, endometriosis, type 2 diabetes, metabolic syndrome, and cardiovascular disease. One study found that girls between the ages of 4 and 12 with a high intake of milk had more than double the risk of early menstruation, while another found that girls between the ages of 3 and 7 with a high intake of animal protein or meat had a 14% and 75% increased risk, respectively.

Finally, consuming a diet heavy in meat and animal products means consuming fewer plants. It's simple—the more you eat of one food, the less room you have to eat other foods. Plants are our only source of fiber, a nutrient essential to fuel a healthy gut microbiome. Our microbes use fiber for fuel and in turn produce short-chain fatty acids, which benefit our health and metabolism. Children who consume diets rich in plants have been shown to have a more favorable microbial composition and more short-chain-fatty-acid-producing bacteria compared to children eating a Western diet, high in animal-based foods. One study showed that adolescents with a high intake of whole grains, legumes, and folate (found in leafy greens) were more likely to have a higher proportion of *Bacteroides* and *Bifidobacterium* (short-chain-fatty-acid-producing bacteria) compared to participants eating a Western, meat-heavy diet. Those in the Western group were also more likely to be obese.

 PBJ Bottom Line: Children who consume diets rich in meat and animal products may be at a higher risk of obesity and chronic disease.

Fears and Misconceptions about Plant-Based Diets

Hopefully the research we've rattled off has reassured you that a plant-based diet is safe and beneficial for your child. But it's natural to still have some hesitations. There are just so many critics out there (family and friends often the loudest) that make it easy for us to veer away from the facts. We'll explore many of these in depth, but we'd like to address a few common misconceptions right away.

1. A vegan diet is dangerous for children.

Headlines like "Baby Dies of Vegan Diet" (not an exact quote, but close) would induce fear in any parent. We see tragic stories like this pop up every few years, and the resulting media blitz often leads to the rampant spread of misinformation. The reality is, in all these cases, the children sadly died of malnutrition. When one reads past the headlines, it's apparent that the parents were feeding infants almond milk instead of formula or providing toddlers with *only* fruits and vegetables. These are cases of starvation—the children suffered from a lack of calories and nutrients overall, not from a lack of animal products. Research shows that plant-based children are at an increased risk of nutrient deficiencies only when their diet is not properly supplemented or is severely restricted, such as with raw or macrobiotic diets (which we do not recommend for children). There is not a single case of an appropriately fed vegan or vegetarian child dying or suffering from serious nutrient deficiencies. When plant-based diets—vegan, vegetarian, or predominantly plant-based—are properly administered and all essential nutrients are provided, children are not only healthy, they thrive.

2. Toddlers need [meat, milk—fill in the blank] to thrive.

The first 1,000 days of life—from conception through age 2—is a critical period for nutrition. Though a child's brain continues to develop and change throughout their life span, growth occurs more rapidly during this window than at any other stage.

Nutrients like protein, polyunsaturated fatty acids, iron, zinc, iodine, choline, and vitamins A and B12 are particularly critical for development. But your child doesn't need to eat animals to get them. In fact, plants may be a superior source for a number of reasons. When you choose plant-based sources of important nutrients, they come with tons of other benefits. For example, when you use whole grains and legumes to meet your child's zinc needs, you're also giving them microbiome-supporting fiber instead of the harmful components of red meat, like the carcinogenic compounds formed during cooking. Similarly, when you provide sweet potatoes and butternut squash for vitamin A, you're also giving your babe disease-fighting antioxidants instead of the environmental toxins found in vitamin A-rich animal foods like liver (which we've never seen a toddler enjoy anyway!).

3. A plant-based diet isn't "natural."

We're "food first" dietitians. We advocate obtaining nutrients from whole foods as much as possible before turning to supplements. So we understand the popular argument that if you need supplements to achieve a proper plant-based diet, it must not be what nature intended. But the fact is that all diets are supplemented in one way or another. Yes, plant-based children should receive a vitamin D supplement, but where do omnivorous children (and most adults) get their vitamin D? *Fortified* cow's milk. Cow's milk is not naturally high in vitamin D—it's added to it.

Iodine is another important supplement for vegans. Plants contain varying amounts of iodine, and this is likely where our ancestors got theirs, but soil degradation makes obtaining iodine solely from plants an unreliable option. So where do most people get their iodine? Dairy products. This is because cows' udders and dairy manufacturing equipment are cleaned with iodine-based solutions—not because iodine is "naturally" found in milk. Many governments have recognized this widespread iodine deficiency and mandated that it's added to table salt. So, just like vegans and vegetarians, most omnivores are getting iodine from supplements too.

In fact, B12 is the *only* nutrient in the human diet that simply must come from animal products. Omnivores always point to B12 as the best evidence that a plant-based diet is not innate.

Did our ancestors derive B12 from meat? Yes. That can't be disputed. However, we probably didn't eat as much meat as people often think, and the quantity was largely determined by geographical location. For example, in Okinawa, Japan—home to one of the world's longest-lived populations—only about 2% of their diet came from meat and animal products. Whereas, in the Arctic, the majority of their diet came from animals.

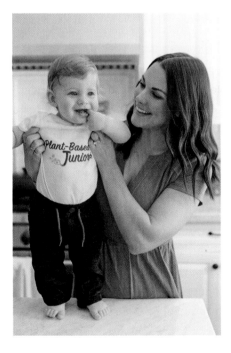

Additionally, researchers debate whether meat has always been the only dietary source of B12. Bacteria are responsible for creating B12, and microbes in our colon even produce it, but this happens too far down in the digestive tract for us to absorb. (Primates also produce B12, but unlike us, they're able to absorb it, which is why they can survive on herbivorous diets.) Some theorize that as humans evolved to eat meat, it was no longer necessary to produce or absorb our own B12. Others hypothesize that humans may have met at least some of their B12 needs from bacteria found naturally in soil and untreated water. Unlike us, cave dwellers drank straight from streams and didn't obsessively scrub their veggies with soap and water.

It's impossible to verify these theories, but what we do know is that B12 deficiency is common in certain populations, like in about 20% of older adults in the US. Some common food products like breakfast cereal are fortified with B12, and research shows that people who consume a lot of fortified foods have a lower risk of B12 deficiency compared to those who eat a lot of meat. This is because B12 is more readily absorbed from supplements than from foods.

Regardless of whether or not humans were intended to eat strict plant-based diets, the point is that we no longer *need* to eat animals to survive—and it may be more beneficial to our health to get these nutrients elsewhere. For most of human existence, meat provided a dense source of nutrients when food scarcity was one of the greatest perils. Today, the opposite is true. We are taking in more food than we need at the expense of health span and longevity. Additionally, we have many other factors to consider now that our ancestors did not—polluted oceans, depleted soil, hormones and environmental contaminants, overpopulation, climate change, and the horrific conditions of animal agriculture. Thanks to modern innovations and an unlimited supply of nutrient-dense, easily accessible plant foods, kids can get everything they need without meat.

Every Bit of Plant-Based Eating Is Beneficial

We recognize that, for many reasons, some people just can't cut animal products entirely out. The good news is that the decision to raise a plant-based child does not have to be black and white. Research shows that all forms of plant-based diets—vegan, vegetarian, pescatarian, flexitarian, reducetarian, *greensandtheoccasionalgoatcheese*-atarian—show major health benefits over a traditional omnivorous diet.

We call ourselves "predominantly plant-based." We eat a lot of plants but allow for the occasional consumption of animal products. The exact breakdown changes from week to week, but about 95% of our diet is plant-based. That means it is composed of animal-free foods like whole grains, nuts, seeds, legumes, fruits, and vegetables. We share this to be completely transparent about our diets. Our eating philosophy is based on science, not on personal agenda or dogma. The fact is that populations with exceptional health and longevity eat minimal animal products. Does that mean we think your family *should* eat some animal products? Absolutely not. We fully support veganism. It means we acknowledge that whether you're strictly plant-based or mostly plant-based, you'll get massive health benefits, and we want you to use that knowledge to determine what makes the most sense for your family.

Bottom line: We want more kids eating more plants and less meat as early and often as possible.

More families eating more plants is not only good for human health, it's essential for the health of our planet. The recent EAT-*Lancet* Commission on Healthy Diets from Sustainable Food Systems determined that we need a global shift in meat and animal product consumption by 2050 in order to reduce climate change and feed our growing population. One study out of Oxford estimated that a global shift toward a plant-based diet by 2050 could save about 8 million lives, reduce food-related greenhouse gas emissions by about two-thirds, and save approximately $1.5 trillion in health-care and climate-damage costs.

We like this message because it makes plant-based eating more approachable and sustainable for the majority of families. And if you can stick to a healthy eating pattern indefinitely, that is the key to good health. Let us guide you in raising your little one with the healthiest, scientifically supported eating pattern: a predominantly plant-based diet.

1

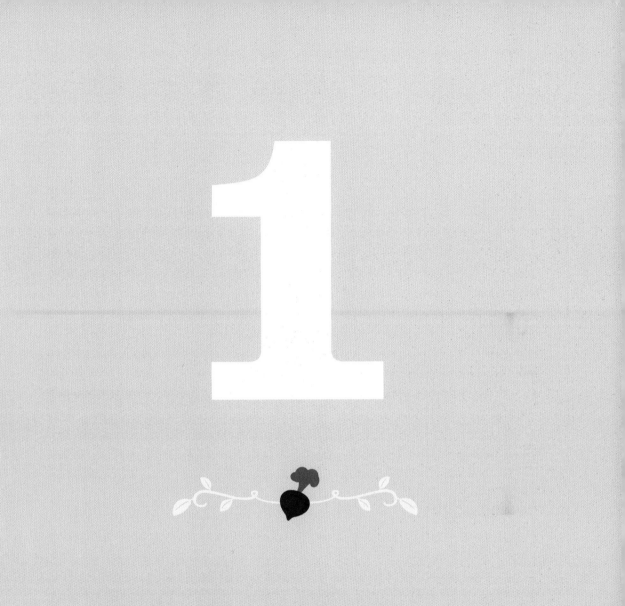

Plant-Based Nutrition for Plant-Based Babies and Toddlers

Y our son's iron is low," our pediatrician informed my husband and me at our son's 8-month checkup. He had done an early iron screening at my request despite the standard protocol to wait until a baby's first birthday. My son had a few risk factors for iron deficiency (exclusive breastfeeding, rapid early growth, no delayed cord clamping), and the ever-vigilant dietitian in me knew that if anything was awry, I wanted to catch it early on. After all, iron deficiency in childhood can lead to long-term developmental problems.

"Wow, that's really upsetting to hear," I responded, shocked. "I guess I should have given him iron drops when he was younger."

"No, that's only necessary for some babies—premature, low birth weight, that sort of thing," he rattled back.

Wrong. The American Academy of Pediatrics (AAP) recommends iron supplementation for *all* exclusively breastfed babies from 4 to 6 months, regardless of risk factors.

"You should get your iron levels checked too," he continued. "You're probably anemic, since babies get iron from breast milk."

Wrong again. Breast milk is extremely low in iron (hence the AAP recommendation), and iron levels in breast milk are not reflective of mother's iron status. Spoiler alert: I was not anemic.

"Oh, and I know you're 'plant-based,'" he persisted with a not-so-subtle eye roll, "but do you think you could at least give him an egg every day? They're a good source of iron."

Wrong again. Eggs do contain 1 mg of iron each (babies 6–12 months need 11 mg per day—as you'll learn shortly), but they also contain a protein known as phosvitin that inhibits iron absorption. One study found that only 3.7% of the iron found in an egg yolk gets absorbed. In addition, phosvitin can decrease the absorption of other iron-rich foods in a meal.

I left that doctor's appointment feeling scared, frustrated, and ashamed for failing my son, even more so as a nutrition expert who should have been able to prevent this from happening. I questioned his plant-based diet and my feeding abilities, and I was determined to rectify the issue as quickly as possible and find out how we'd gotten into this situation in the first place.

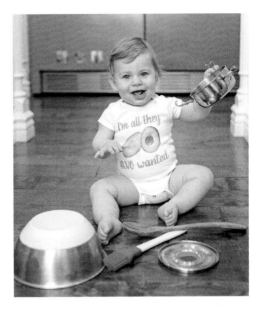

I scoured the literature and learned more about iron than any person, nutrition expert or otherwise, would ever care to know. I learned that it would have been very easy to prevent this issue had I been armed with complete, accurate information to begin with—namely the AAP recommendation.

But there was no comprehensive guide to feeding infants, much less plant-based infants, and this information wasn't common knowledge. I hadn't read it in my baby books, heard about it from other parents or dietitians I'd talked to, or been alerted to it by my own pediatrician.

Time and again we have heard from our clients, or experienced firsthand, that the nutrition information provided by pediatricians is inaccurate, especially when it comes to plant-based diets. The average doctor takes just one nutrition course during their entire medical training. ONE. This means that practitioners often turn to the same unreliable sources for guidance as a layperson—the media, the internet, or outdated practice guidelines. Yet they are often the primary providers of nutrition advice.

As you'll see in the following section, there is a lot to learn about proper plant-based nutrition—but we break it down for you in an easy-to-digest fashion so that you can feel confident you're covering all of your bases. In this section, you'll find a thorough explanation of each of the essential nutrients your baby needs to thrive. We know being a new parent can be overwhelming, so if you don't have the time (or desire) to learn the nuances, feel free to skip to the bottom of each section and read the PBJ Bottom Line to get the fast facts on feeding. Don't worry about memorizing it; we'll bring it together with easy meal-planning strategies in Chapter 2.

We encourage you to flip to the back of the book and grab the Create Your Own Supplement Regimen handout so you can fill in the blanks with the nutrients you'll need to supplement at each age/stage to meet your baby's unique needs.

Calories

Most healthy babies will double their weight in the first 6 months and triple it in the first 12. This rapid growth requires a lot of energy, aka calories. The proportion of calories per pound of body weight that a baby needs is higher during infancy than any other point in life. Energy needs decrease as growth slows after the first year. For example, the average 1-year-old needs about 900 calories per day while a 2-to-3-year-old needs about 1000—that's only a difference of 100 calories despite several pounds' difference in weight.

Every baby's energy needs are different due to genetics, body size, activity level, sex, and medical conditions, therefore it's hard to pinpoint exactly how many calories you should be offering each day. Luckily, you don't need to do that! Instead, focus on feeding on demand during infancy and providing structured, energy-dense meals as your babe gets older.

Letting babies regulate their own food intake is key, and fortunately, babies are very good at telling us when they're hungry. Trying to force or limit a baby's intake is never a good idea. Research shows that babies who are pressured to eat more end up eating less, and those who are restricted end up eating more. Manipulation always backfires. We'll dive deeper into this in the age-specific chapters, but for now remember this: Your job as a parent is to simply make nourishment available and allow your baby to regulate their intake.*

One thing to keep in mind is that plant-based diets tend to be lower in calories than a typical Western diet. This is because fruits, vegetables, grains, and legumes are naturally lower in fat than animal products are. This is one reason of several that we advise against raw and macrobiotic diets for babies; they simply cannot get enough calories on these restrictive diets. To ensure babies meet their needs, it's important for

PBJ Bottom Line: Babies and toddlers need a lot of calories to grow optimally; however, you don't need to obsessively measure their intake. Simply offer age-appropriate, balanced nourishment and allow your child to self-regulate. *Failure to thrive is a different story; talk to your physician if you are concerned about your child's growth.

parents to include plenty of energy-dense foods, which pack a lot of calories in a small amount of space. We'll talk more about how to do that in the next chapter.

Macronutrients

Macronutrients are the three major molecules that provide our bodies with energy in the form of calories—carbohydrates, protein, and fat (alcohol also technically qualifies as a macronutrient, but baby will have no use for that for many years to come).

While some trendy diets focus on eliminating or reducing certain macronutrients or obsessively "counting macros," the key to good health and optimal growth for babies and toddlers (and really people of all ages) is making sure to get a balance of all three. This is easy on a plant-based diet, as all whole plants contain all three macronutrients in varying amounts. For example, nuts contain a large amount of both protein and fat with a small amount of carbohydrates. Beans contain a good deal of protein and carbohydrates with minimal amounts of fat. Because plants don't fit nicely into one macronutrient group (unlike most animal products; e.g., butter is almost exclusively fat and chicken breast is mostly protein), we prefer to categorize foods by food groups instead of by macronutrients.

TERMS TO KNOW		
RDA	Recommended Daily Allowance	The amount of a nutrient needed to prevent deficiency in the majority of adults or children.
AI	Adequate Intake	The recommended amount when an RDA cannot be established.
UL	Upper Tolerable Limit	The maximum amount of a nutrient that is safe to consume.

Carbohydrates (RDA)
- 0–6 months: 60 g
- 7–12 months: 90 g
- 1–3 years: 130 g (45%–65% daily intake)
- Breastfeeding moms: 210 g (45%–65% daily intake)

Carbohydrates are the body's preferred source of energy, and they're needed to fuel everything from your baby's first blink to their lightning-speed neural connections. Providing your babe with plenty of carbohydrates for energy ensures that protein and fat are free to do their job supporting their rapid growth.

Carbohydrates are widespread in a plant-based diet, making up the bulk of nutrients in foods like vegetables, fruits, grains, and starches. The main source of carbohydrates for most infants is the milk-derived sugar lactose, which is found in breast milk and formula. Lactose in human milk is higher than that of any other species due to the enormous nutritional demand of the human brain, which reflects just how essential carbohydrates are to development.

PBJ BOTTOM LINE: Carbs are your baby's major life source, starting from milk all the way to full meals. Babies and toddlers should receive 45%–65% of their calories from carbohydrates.

Protein (RDA)
- 0–6 months: 9 g
- 7–12 months: 1.2 g/kg or 11 g
- 1–3 years: 1 g/kg or 13 g
- Breastfeeding moms: 71 g

While carbohydrates are the fuel that babies need, proteins are the building blocks. Proteins are made up of single units known as amino acids, which provide the materials to build, maintain, and repair your baby's growing cells and organs and create important molecules, including hormones and antibodies that keep everything running properly.

If you've been plant-based for a while, you've likely encountered the litany of questions us herbivores get about protein. *Do plants even have protein? How do you get enough of it? Are vegans one veggie burger away from withering away?*

Yes, babies need protein. But, like adults, their protein needs

PBJ Quick Bite

Did you know that a slice of bread has about 4 grams of protein? That's a third of the protein a toddler needs in a day!

can easily be met with grains, legumes, nuts, and seeds, all rich sources of protein and easy to incorporate into baby's diet in appealing, age-appropriate ways. Protein from plants is not inferior to protein from animals, and the requirements for plant-based dieters and omnivores are the same, provided plant-based dieters are eating a varied diet. You may have heard some experts suggest that protein requirements for young vegan children are slightly increased due to lower digestibility of unprocessed plant proteins, and propose that vegan children 1–2 years of age should consume 30%–35% more protein, putting their daily average at about 17 grams versus 13 grams. However, studies show that both vegan and omnivorous children typically eat way more protein than they need—almost double, in fact! For reference, 2 cups of soy milk provide 14 grams of protein and an additional 5 grams can be found in 2 tablespoons of black beans or an ounce of chia seeds. We recommend that you avoid stressing about numbers and focus on providing regular, varied, protein-rich foods.

The Incomplete Protein Myth

PBJ Quick Bite

Legumes (beans, soy foods) are a major source of the amino acid lysine. Include them 2–3 times a day!

You may have heard the claim that, unlike animal products, plant proteins are "incomplete" and that you need to combine different plants at each meal to get all the amino acids your body needs to function. This persisting myth, while not entirely inaccurate, is itself incomplete.

All whole plants contain all nine of the essential amino acids our bodies need. There is no difference in the structure or function of amino acids derived from plants and those derived from animals. They all work exactly the same in our bodies. However, some plants have a lower amount of one amino acid compared to others. For example, beans are typically low in the essential amino acid methionine but high in lysine, while grains are the opposite. It was previously thought that in order to get enough of each amino acid, plant-based dieters needed to combine different protein sources at each meal. But more recent research has shown that as long as *enough* protein and *varied sources* are consumed *throughout the day*, the body will figure out how to put it all together.

You don't need to meticulously combine proteins to meet your child's needs. As long as you provide your child with varied sources of plant protein throughout the day—

beans, soy foods, grains, nuts, and seeds—they will have no trouble getting all the building blocks their bodies need to thrive. If your baby cannot eat legumes (beans, soy, peas), we recommend you speak with a registered dietitian nutritionist to figure out an individualized plan.

PBJ BOTTOM LINE: Offer protein-rich plants at each meal, starting at six months. Strictly vegan children may need slightly more protein—about 4 grams a day, which can be found in ¼ cup of lentils or a slice of bread. However, most children eat more protein than they need. Therefore, instead of worrying about a number, focus on providing varied sources like beans, soy foods, nuts, seeds, and grains throughout the day.

Fat (RDA)

- 0–6 months: 30 g
- 7–12 months: 31 g
- 1–2 years: 30%–40% daily intake
- Breastfeeding moms: 20%–35% daily intake

One of the biggest differences between plant-based diets for adults and for babies is the importance of fat. While a low-fat, plant-based diet can be beneficial for supporting weight loss and reversing heart disease in adults, this approach is extremely dangerous for babies and toddlers. Babies need fat—lots of it!

Not only does fat provide life-sustaining calories; it is critical to the development of the brain, eyes, and other major organs. Fat creates padding to protect babies' organs, prevents heat loss, allows for the absorption of essential vitamins, and makes molecules used to fight infection and disease. In fact, fat makes up 44% of breast milk, and toddlers should get 30%–40% of their daily calories from it.

Fat is an "energy-dense" nutrient. One gram of fat contains nine calories, while one gram of protein or carbohydrate contains only four. This is why a small portion of fat-rich nuts or seeds is so much higher in calories than a larger, low-fat food like a potato—the fat adds energy density.

PBJ Quick Bite

Include fat with every meal—we love avocados, nut butter, and vegetables cooked in olive oil.

Energy density is important for babies and toddlers who need these calories to thrive.

In the next chapter, we'll discuss many ways to easily work fat into your baby's diet.

Types of Fat

There are many different types of dietary fat, but only two are considered "essential"—linoleic acid (LA) and alpha-linolenic acid (ALA). This means that unlike other types of fat, humans cannot make them and need to obtain them from their diet.

LA is an omega-6 polyunsaturated fatty acid that is used to make molecules involved in immune functioning. The body converts LA to arachidonic acid (AA), a major fatty acid found in babies' brains and in breast milk. LA is abundant in most diets (plant-based and not) because it is found in so many foods including nuts, seeds, and plant oils.

ALA is a "long-chain" omega-3 fatty acid found in foods like walnuts, soy products, chia seeds, and flaxseed/flaxseed oil. It is vital to the production of anti-inflammatory molecules. Additionally, ALA is used to make two other very important fats for infant development, the "very long-chain" omega-3 fatty acids, eicosapentaenoic acid (EPA) and docosahexaenoic acid (DHA).

DHA

While both EPA and DHA are important for overall health, DHA specifically is vital for visual and cognitive development. It is the main omega-3 fatty acid in the brain and eyes, and it plays a major role in neurological, physical, and behavioral functioning. DHA is rich in the prefrontal cortex, the area of the brain responsible for higher-level activities such as planning, problem solving, and focused attention. In fact, anthropologists believe that the evolution of humans and the expansion of the brain can be traced back to when man first migrated toward the water and began consuming omega-3-rich seafood.

DHA consumption during pregnancy has been shown to increase birth weight and reduce preterm birth, and supplementation in preterm infants has been shown to reduce the risk of mental delays. High levels of DHA in breast milk have been associ-

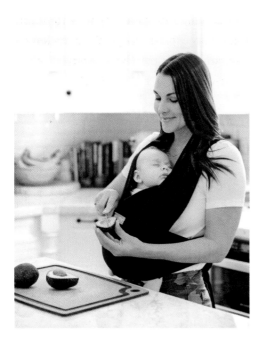

ated with better mental development, increased motor skills, enhanced attention, and better memory scores later in life. Meanwhile, low blood levels of DHA have been reported in children with developmental and behavioral disorders, such as ADHD, dyslexia, and dyspraxia (a coordination disorder). Many studies have shown benefits to learning, memory, and cognition with omega-3 fatty acid supplementation in these groups.

DHA is not considered an "essential" fatty acid because we can make it from ALA, but the conversion rate of ALA to DHA is very low—1%–10%. And while we make this conversion in our tissues, eating ALA does not increase the amount of DHA found in blood or breast milk. Only "preformed" DHA, found in fish and algae oil, raises the level of DHA in breast milk and reaches babies in utero. Therefore, breast milk from vegan mothers has the lowest amount of DHA. For this reason, it is essential to obtain DHA through diet or supplementation.

Seafood provides the majority of DHA in many people's diet, but there's an easy solution for plant-based eaters—algae oil. Microalgae is the original source of DHA, and studies have shown that it is just as effective at raising blood levels of DHA as fish oil. Fish consume this microscopic seaweed and accumulate the fatty acids in their tissues. So basically, supplementing algae oil cuts out the middleman (or middle animal, we should say).

Even better, giving algae oil instead of fish helps to minimize baby's exposure to toxins found in seafood such as mercury, polychlorinated biphenyls, polybrominated diphenyl ethers, dioxins, and

PBJ Quick Bite

Although our bodies convert ALA to DHA, consuming ALA-rich foods does not raise the amount of DHA in breast milk. Plant-based breastfeeding mamas must supplement DHA to ensure babies receive adequate amounts.

chlorinated pesticides, which accumulate in our oceans and waterways due to runoff from agricultural and industrial practices. Infants are more susceptible to the harmful effects of these toxins because their nervous systems are still developing; therefore, supplementing with microalgae may be a safer option for meeting DHA requirements.

DHA NEEDS	
0–6 months	20 mg/kg DHA
7–12 months	15–20 mg/kg DHA + EPA
1–3 years	15–20 mg/kg DHA + EPA (~170–230 mg for a 25-lb. toddler)
Breastfeeding moms	minimum of 300 mg

DHA accumulation in the brain ramps up in the third trimester of pregnancy and continues throughout the first two years of life. Most infant formulas contain adequate amounts of DHA, but as mentioned above, the DHA content of breast milk depends on mom's intake. Therefore, experts advise breastfeeding moms who do not eat fish to supplement with 200–300 mg of DHA per day.

Once babies switch from breast milk or formula to dairy or plant-based milk (usually sometime in the second year), their DHA intake typically declines substantially. Dairy contains minimal amounts of DHA and most plant milks contain none. Given the demonstrated negative effects of suboptimal intake, we think it's prudent to recommend DHA supplementation for any children who do not consume fish as soon as breast/bottle-feeding ends.

Unfortunately, there's no firm consensus on how much DHA is advised for toddlers or older children. The World Health Organization recommends that children 2–4 years old receive 100–150 mg per day of EPA and DHA combined. Meanwhile, the Health Council of the Netherlands recommends that children 6 months to 2 years receive 15–20 mg/kg per day of EPA and DHA combined from fish. To figure out how much your child needs, simply divide their weight in pounds by 2.2 to get their weight in kilograms (kg). Then multiply that amount by 15 or 20.

We recommend a daily liquid algae oil supplement. You can add this to water or milk or drop it directly in their mouth. Strangely, both of our sons eagerly slurp up their daily dose, despite its fishy taste and smell!

Saturated Fat

Saturated fats are not considered essential because our bodies make them from unsaturated fat. Decades of research have pointed to the potentially harmful effects of these types of fatty acids, found primarily in animals and animal products, as they have been shown to raise levels of so-called bad cholesterol. However, recent research has called into question this association and raised further questions—like what about the saturated fat found in plants? Is it harmful too?

Some studies have shown that the length of the saturated fatty acid chain may determine its effect on health and suggested that shorter-chain saturated fats (primarily found in plants and dairy) may be healthier than longer-chain fatty acids (found mainly in meat).

We typically associate saturated fat with meat and dairy, but 50% of the fatty acids found in breast milk are saturated. This suggests that infants have a biological need for dietary saturated fat. Infant formulas mimic this fat content with the addition of coconut oil, palm oil, or dairy fat.

Many plant-based parents ask us whether we think saturated fat-rich plant foods such as coconut, coconut oil, peanut butter, and chocolate are healthy for children. Our answer: in moderation (with the exception of chocolate because of the caffeine). The jury is still out on the health effects of dietary saturated fat, but we'd venture to guess that as with most things in life, the answer is not black and white. In our homes, we regularly serve plant-based sources of saturated fat but mainly focus on unsaturated fats from avocado, nuts, seeds, and olive oil.

PBJ BOTTOM LINE: Babies need a lot of fat. Breast milk and formula will provide the majority of fat during your child's first year, but once food is introduced, it should be prioritized in the diet. The fatty acid DHA is specifically important for brain and eye development. Plant-based breastfeeding moms and toddlers who do not consume fish should supplement with algae oil. As algae oil supplements can be expensive, we support parents who choose to provide a more affordable fish oil supplement.

Micronutrients

Vitamins and minerals are known as "micronutrients" because we need only a small amount of them compared to the bigger macronutrients. Despite their small contribution to the diet, they play a major role in babies' health and development.

While macronutrient needs are pretty straightforward, micronutrients can be a bit trickier. For the first 4–6 months, your baby will get all the macronutrients and many of the micronutrients they need from breast milk or formula. However, there are a few vitamins and minerals that can be low or, in the case of B12, completely absent in a plant-based diet. In order to prevent deficiencies, it's extremely important that parents learn which essential nutrients they need to watch out for and which to supplement. This will depend on several factors—your baby's age, whether they're breastfed or formula fed, and the type of diet they follow (vegan, vegetarian, flexitarian, etc.). Make sure to have your Create Your Own Supplement Regimen tear-out on page 287 handy as you read this section.

Iron (RDA)
- 0–6 months: 0.27 mg
- 7–12 months: 11 mg
- 1–3 years: 7 mg
- Breastfeeding moms: 9 mg

Crack open a pediatric nutrition book and you're likely to find meat recommended as a first food. Why? Iron. Red meat is high in an easily absorbable form of iron, an important nutrient for babies' red blood cell production and brain development. Iron deficiency is the most common nutrient deficiency in both children and adults and can lead to long-lasting detrimental effects on health.

While meat is a good source of iron, it's not the only (or even best) source. Plants have plenty of iron too, and unlike meat, they come packaged with tons of other health-promoting nutrients. You might be surprised to learn that vegans typically consume more iron than vegetarians or meat eaters.

Plant Iron versus Meat Iron

Foods contain two types of iron: heme and non-heme. Heme iron, found only in animal foods, is much more readily absorbed and not affected by other factors in the diet. The body continues to absorb it even if it has enough or too much. Non-heme iron on the other hand, found in both animal and plant foods, is less absorbable and is affected by other components of the diet. The body regulates non-heme iron by increasing absorption when iron is low and decreasing it when it has enough. This is important, as too much iron can be toxic.

The reduced absorption of non-heme iron is the reason people make a big deal about the iron in meat versus plants. But don't worry! We've got a few absorption-increasing tricks to ensure your baby maximizes their intake.

Increasing Absorption

Arguments that plant-based iron is harder to absorb are not unwarranted. Many plant foods are high in compounds called phytates, or phytic acid. These bind to iron and other minerals and prevent their absorption. However, since phytates are found in some of the most nutrient-dense foods, like whole grains and legumes, the answer isn't to avoid them. Instead, adding in a source of vitamin C to phytate-containing, iron-rich foods can increase the absorption of iron by 2–4 times. Wow, right? Research shows that the more vitamin C added, the more iron is absorbed. The most marked effects are seen with between 50 and 100 mg—the amount in 5–10 large strawberries.

PBJ Quick Bite
Adding just five strawberries to a meal can double iron absorption!

The fermentation process used to make sourdough bread can also help increase absorption, as can sprouting, soaking, and cooking grains and legumes.

Finally, calcium competes with iron for absorption. Therefore, it's best to serve high-calcium foods like fortified plant milk or fortified yogurt separately from your child's most iron-rich meals. We accomplish this by offering fortified milk as a snack between meals.

The Popeye Myth

We have some potentially upsetting information to share—Popeye got it wrong. You know Popeye, the spinach-pounding sailor with superhuman strength? Turns out, the iron in that can of greens he kept stashed in his back pocket is mostly unavailable. Despite the fact that the majority of nutrition experts will tell you that spinach is an excellent source of iron, regurgitating widely believed but inaccurate information, research actually shows it's a poor source due to its extremely low bioavailability (the amount of the nutrient that is absorbed from food).

Unlike the other iron sources listed in the table on p. 25, spinach absorption isn't improved by the addition of vitamin C. This is because phytic acid isn't the problem with spinach—a cocktail of calcium, polyphenols (typically beneficial phytochemicals), and oxalates (another type of iron inhibitor) is what prevents these greens from doing good. Now, this is not to say that spinach doesn't have other awesome properties. It's packed full of plenty of great nutrients—just don't count on it to meet your babe's iron needs.

IRON-RICH FOODS	
Iron-fortified baby cereal, ¼ cup	6.75 mg
White beans (cooked), ¼ cup	2 mg
Tofu, ¼ cup	1.5 mg
Lentils (cooked), ¼ cup	1.5 mg
Tempeh, ¼ cup	1.12 mg

IRON-RICH FOODS	
Canned tomatoes, ¼ cup	1 mg
Kidney beans (cooked), ¼ cup	1 mg
Almond butter, 1 tablespoon	0.6 mg
Bread, 1 slice	1 mg
Legume pasta, ½ cup	3 mg

Iron Needs

Babies are born with a reserve of iron accumulated in utero. This store lasts 4–6 months, at which point babies need to start getting iron from their diet. As discussed previously, breast milk is low in iron, and because it is recommended to wait until 6 months to start solids (you'll learn more about this later), there is a short period from 4 to 6 months in which some babies are at a high risk of becoming iron deficient, like Whitney's did. For this reason, the AAP recommends that all predominantly and exclusively breastfed babies receive an iron supplement of 1 mg per kg per day from 4 to 6 months of age until they can get enough iron from their diet. This does not apply to

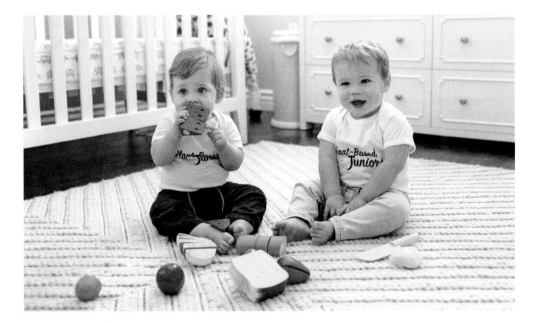

formula-fed babies, who get all the iron they need from fortified formula. However, if your baby was born prematurely, you'll want to chat with your doctor to make sure your formula provides enough. Many preemie babies will receive an iron supplement from 8 weeks until 1 year old.

At 6 months of age, iron needs skyrocket to 11 mg per day. For reference, an ounce of steak (or about 2 tablespoons if you tossed it in a food processor) has 0.8 mg, while peas have about 0.9 mg of iron per ounce. The average 6-month-old is not eating much more than an ounce at a meal and usually only one meal a day. You can see the conundrum. We recommend filling the gap with iron-fortified products such as iron-fortified baby cereal (more on that in Chapter 2) and continuing to supplement if your child has a small appetite or you are having trouble meeting their needs through diet. Again, formula-fed babes will get enough iron without supplementation.

From 12 months to 3 years, iron needs decrease to 7 mg per day, making it much easier to meet toddlers' needs through food alone.

PBJ BOTTOM LINE: Iron is one of the most important nutrients for babies, and dwindling iron stores is one of the main reasons they need to begin eating solids at 6 months of age. Exclusively and predominantly breast-fed babies should receive an iron supplement of 1 mg per kg of body weight per day from 4 to 6 months. After 6 months, offer iron-rich foods at each meal and always pair with a source of vitamin C.

Zinc (RDA)
- 0–6 months: 2 mg
- 7–12 months: 3 mg
- 1–3 years: 3 mg
- Breastfeeding moms: 12 mg

Similar to iron, zinc is a mineral that is widespread in plant-based diets yet slightly harder to absorb from plant foods. It is essential for normal growth and development and plays an important role in immune functioning and DNA synthesis. Additionally, zinc is necessary for normal taste processing. And every parent knows we need all the help we can get in that department!

Zinc Needs

Like iron, there is relatively little zinc in breast milk, and needs increase around 6 months of age. Because of reduced absorption, some experts estimate that plant-based dieters need about 50% more zinc than omnivores. However, routine zinc supplementation isn't recommended for babies and toddlers, and increased needs can easily be met by consuming plenty of zinc-rich foods. Luckily, the same foods that are high in iron are also high in zinc—legumes, grains, nuts, and seeds—and many of the same tactics that help increase iron absorption work for zinc too, including sprouting and soaking.

Like iron, zinc is also inhibited by high-calcium foods, so it's best to avoid serving calcium-fortified products like soy or pea milk with your toddler's high iron and zinc meals.

ZINC-RICH FOODS	
Wheat germ, 1 tablespoon	1.4 mg
Bran flakes, ½ cup	1 mg
Tahini, 1 tablespoon	0.7 mg
Chickpeas, ¼ cup	0.6 mg
Lentils, ¼ cup	0.6 mg
Peanut butter, 1 tablespoon	0.6 mg
Quinoa, ¼ cup	0.5 mg
Pumpkin seeds, 2 teaspoons	0.4 mg

PBJ BOTTOM LINE: Zinc has many of the same nutritional considerations for babies as iron. So if you focus on optimizing your babe's iron intake, you'll likely knock out their zinc needs too. Double whammy!

Calcium (RDA)
- 0–6 months: 200 mg (AI)
- 7–12 months: 260 mg (AI)
- 1–3 years: 700 mg
- Breastfeeding moms: 1000 mg

Most of us are familiar with calcium's role in helping form strong, healthy bones. It's also necessary for normal nerve and muscle functioning. Calcium deposition in the bone occurs at a higher rate during the first year than at any other time in life. This deposition continues throughout childhood until peak bone mass is achieved during puberty. Therefore, it's incredibly important to ensure that your child's calcium needs are met early on.

What many people are less familiar with are sources of calcium other than dairy. Calcium is abundant in a plant-based diet and is twice as bioavailable from plants as from dairy, in foods like cruciferous vegetables, fruit, beans, and soy. Many of these foods are also a good source of the bone health–promoting nutrient vitamin K.

CALCIUM-RICH FOODS	
Fortified soy/pea milk, 1 cup	300–450 mg
Tofu, ¼ cup	213 mg
Figs (dried and pureed), ¼ cup	61 mg
Orange, medium	60 mg
White beans (cooked), ¼ cup	40 mg
Bok choy (cooked), ¼ cup	40 mg
Kale (cooked), ¼ cup	24 mg
Pinto beans (cooked) ¼ cup	20 mg
Broccoli (cooked), ¼ cup	16 mg
Red beans (cooked), ½ cup	13 mg

Absorption Inhibitors

Some calcium-rich plants are actually bad sources of calcium due to a high content of the absorption inhibitor oxalic acid. Like phytic acid found in beans and grains, oxalic acid is a naturally occurring compound that prevents calcium from being absorbed into the body. It's found in spinach, rhubarb, and beet greens, to name a few. This does not mean that your child should avoid these foods—just don't count them toward your babe's daily calcium intake.

Calcium Needs

Breast milk and formula provide all the calcium your little one needs until they start eating solid food exclusively. At 12 months, your baby's calcium needs triple. At this time, many pediatricians will recommend that your child start drinking two glasses of whole milk a day, but despite what the Dairy Board would have you believe, your tot doesn't need cow's milk to do a body good. As long as you provide calcium and other important nutrients for bone health from plant-based sources, your babe will be just fine. (We'll discuss cow's milk in depth in Chapter 5.)

While calcium needs can theoretically be met with food alone, this is difficult due to babies' and toddlers' low intake. The easiest way is by providing calcium-fortified foods like dairy-free yogurt and fortified pea/soy milk 2 to 3 times a day in addition to calcium-rich whole foods. Note: You should always shake plant milk before serving to ensure added vitamins and minerals that have settled on the bottom are evenly dispersed.

> **PBJ BOTTOM LINE:** Babies need calcium to form strong, healthy bones— but they don't need cow's milk to get it. Provide several servings of calcium-rich foods like cruciferous vegetables, beans, and soy every day in addition to fortified foods like nondairy yogurt and fortified pea or soy milk. In order to avoid inhibiting iron and zinc absorption, offer calcium-fortified foods and beverages as a snack between meals.

Iodine (RDA)
- 0–6 months: 110 mcg (AI)
- 7–12 months: 130 mcg (AI)
- 1–3 years: 90 mcg
- Breastfeeding moms: 290 mcg

Iodine is one of the lesser-known nutrients of importance for plant-based babies but deserves equal attention as the more well-known players. It is essential for normal brain, metabolism, and thyroid functioning. Iodine deficiency is one of the most common nutrient deficiencies worldwide and considered the most prevalent and preventable cause of mental impairment. Mild iodine deficiency in young children has been linked to lower than average IQ and negative performance on cognitive tasks. Additionally, it can lead to the enlargement of the thyroid gland, known as goiter.

PBJ Quick Bite

To combat widespread iodine deficiency, many countries add iodine to salt. But the rise in popularity of specialty products like pink Himalayan salt or sea salt, which do not contain iodine, has led to a decrease in the use of iodized table salt. Additionally, the salt found in processed and packaged foods is not iodized.

Plant-based babes have to be especially careful of iodine deficiency because the main sources of iodine in the diet are dairy and seafood. Most of the planet's iodine is found in the ocean, which is why seafood is a good source, but many people are surprised to learn that dairy products are not naturally high in iodine. Iodine ends up in cow's milk and yogurt because iodine-based chemicals (iodophors) are used to disinfect cows' udders during the production process. Yummy.

Iodine *is* naturally found in soil, but plants are not a reliable source because amounts vary considerably, and reports suggest that soil erosion and water runoff have depleted the natural iodine content of soil worldwide.

Sea vegetables are commonly cited as a good source of iodine, and while it is true that many contain large amounts, they may be *too* high. Excessive iodine can be just as harmful as too little iodine and cause goiter or harm to brain functioning.

The amount varies widely depending on the species and country of origin. Nori and wakame tend to be lower in iodine, while kombu is significantly higher. We recommend using sea vegetables in moderation and abiding by serving sizes.

PBJ Quick Bite

Sea vegetables are often too high in iodine. We recommend limiting your kid's intake.

Goitrogens

Some foods contain compounds known as goitrogens, which can interfere with the body's production of thyroid hormones. These include foods such as cruciferous vegetables, soy, millet, and cassava. However, goitrogens do not cause problems when iodine intake is adequate. As long as your baby is receiving enough iodine, they can freely eat these foods without concern.

Iodine Needs

Babies will get all the iodine they need from formula or breast milk (provided mom's diet is adequate) during the first year. Once breast milk or formula is discontinued, babies need to obtain iodine through their diet. Plant milks are not fortified with iodine, so if your child does not consume dairy, you'll want to supplement.

The "upper tolerable limit" for total iodine intake (meaning the most a baby can safely consume from both food and supplements) is 200 mcg per day. Considering the RDA is 90 mcg, this is a very small window of optimal intake. We recommend offering a daily supplement containing half of the RDA of iodine (45 mcg per day) for toddlers if you use iodized salt at home. If you choose not to use iodized salt, we recommend providing the full RDA of 90 mcg per day. We don't recommend trying to meet needs with iodized salt alone because you would need to provide a large amount of salt to get enough, and we want to limit salt for our under 2s.

PBJ BOTTOM LINE: Infants receive all the iodine they need from formula or breast milk (as long as mom gets enough). Toddlers need to get iodine from their diet, and since plants are not a reliable source, all vegan toddlers who are no longer breastfeeding and those who do not consume dairy should receive a daily supplement with 45–90 mcg of iodine, depending on whether or not you use iodized salt at home.

Selenium (RDA)

- 0–6 months: 15 mcg (AI)
- 7–12 months: 20 mcg (AI)
- 1–3 years: 20 mcg
- Breastfeeding moms: 70 mcg

Like iodine, selenium is a trace mineral that is important for thyroid hormone metabolism. It's also required for DNA synthesis and the production of antioxidant enzymes.

While selenium is naturally found in soil, and therefore in plants, amounts vary widely depending on soil conditions. The main dietary sources of selenium are meat and seafood, but it is also found in whole grains, soy products, and beans.

SOURCES OF SELENIUM	
Whole wheat pasta, ½ cup	21 mcg
Sunflower seed butter, 1 tablespoon	16 mcg
Wheat germ, 1 tablespoon	9 mcg
Chia seed, 1 tablespoon	8 mcg
Oatmeal, ½ cup	6.5 mcg
Firm tofu, ¼ cup	6 mcg
Soy milk, 1 cup	6 mcg

Selenium Needs

Some studies have shown that vegans and vegetarians have lower intakes of selenium compared to omnivores, but this varies by country. In some areas, like rural China, where people eat mostly plants grown in selenium-poor soil, selenium intake may be a concern. However, in the US, vegans typically meet the recommendations for selenium intake.

Excessive selenium can be harmful, and routine supplementation is not recommended.

B12 (RDA)

- 0–6 months: 0.4 mcg
- 7–12 months: 0.5 mcg
- 1–3 years: 0.9 mcg*
- Breastfeeding moms: 2.8 mcg*

Supplementation recommendations far exceed the RDA due to bioavailability factors.

While some earnest (but incorrect) vegans argue that everything we need as humans to survive and thrive can be obtained from plants, there is one nutrient that simply cannot be found in reliable amounts or in the proper form in plants—B12. Animals and animal products are the only reliable dietary sources.

B12 is a critical nutrient for infants, necessary for producing the myelin sheath around brain cells, a protective layering that guards against cellular damage. We cannot stress the point enough—inadequate B12 intake in infancy and early childhood may result in psychomotor and cognitive delays and potentially cause long-term damage to your baby's brain. Studies have reported brain shrinkage in infants of vegetarian breastfeeding mothers who do not supplement B12. And one study reported that in about 40%–50% of cases, damage was irreversible. Additionally, B12 is needed to make healthy red blood cells in rapidly growing babes, and deficiency produces a condition known as megaloblastic anemia.

Luckily, there's a very easy (and kind) alternative to eating animals—taking a B12 supplement.

All vegans, vegetarians, and predominantly plant-based children should receive a B12 supplement from the time they are weaned. A common mistake vegetarians make is assuming they get enough from B12-containing

PBJ Quick Bite

All vegans, vegetarians, and predominantly plant-based children should receive a B12 supplement from the time they are weaned.

animal products. However, research shows that despite eating milk and eggs, vegetarians are still at a high risk of deficiency. Fortified foods are helpful but not as reliable as a daily supplement because the amounts vary and fortification processes may change. The safest way to ensure your babe gets this vital nutrient is with a supplement.

B12 Needs

B12 is water soluble, meaning it does not accumulate in fat tissue. We store a small amount in our liver and kidneys, but generally, we can consume large amounts of B12 and the excess will simply be excreted in urine.

B12 absorption is a bit of a complicated process. Before it can be absorbed, it must bind to a protein that our bodies make known as intrinsic factor (IF). IF can only handle about 1.5–2 mcg of B12 at a time before it becomes "saturated." Therefore, amounts far greater than the RDA are needed to absorb enough B12 through a supplement in a single dose.

There is no scientific consensus on the proper amount, form, or type (oral versus intravenous) of B12 to supplement plant-based children and breastfeeding moms, so we've developed recommendations based on current research and our discussions with experts in plant-based nutrition and on B12 metabolism.

We recommend that breastfeeding moms supplement with at least 150 mcg per day. If your pre/postnatal vitamin does not contain at least 150 mcg, you should take an additional B12 supplement.

Toddlers who have been weaned should receive at least 5 mcg per day. We say "at least" because as we said before, higher amounts are considered safe and some experts recommend up to 40 mcg per day for toddlers. We would advise against giving massive doses to children who are not deficient. Though there are no reports of ill effects, we don't have research on long-term high-dose supplementation for children.

Supplements can be provided via liquid drops into milk or water or as part of a multivitamin. It can be difficult to find an individual B12 supplement in such a low amount for toddlers, so one option is to titrate the dose by using a small mL dropper. Another option, if you can only find supplements that are less than 5 mcg, is to provide two daily doses of at least 1 mcg each, which would be absorbed at a higher rate than a single dose. Many multivitamins on the market provide ~2 mcg of B12; therefore, you could split the supplement and offer half in the morning and half at night to maximize absorption.

Though milk should continue to provide the majority of calories throughout the first year, if your child significantly reduces their breast milk intake before 12 months, you may want to begin supplementation sooner.

Forms of B12

Cyanocobalamin is the most common, affordable, and stable form of B12 with the most clinical testing. Methylcobalamin and adenosylcobalamin are the two "active" forms of B12, meaning they are the form our body uses in chemical reactions. Our bodies make these forms from cyanocobalamin, but recent research has shown that some people have trouble with this conversion process, so many companies now offer supplements in the methyl and adeno forms. Hydroxocobalamin is another biologically produced form, but it too must be converted to the active form. We prefer the cyanocobalamin form because of its stability and history of efficacy, but at this time there is no strong evidence to suggest one form is better able than another to raise B12 levels.

> **PBJ Bottom Line:** B12 supplements are a nonnegotiable. All vegan, vegetarian, and predominantly plant-based babies should receive a supplement after weaning. We recommend a daily supplement with at least 5 mcg for toddlers 1–3 years or a 1 mcg dose taken twice daily. Breastfeeding moms should supplement with at least 150 mcg of B12 per day to ensure proper amounts are transferred via breast milk.

Vitamin D (RDA)
- 0–6 months: 400 IU
- 7–12 months: 400 IU
- 1–3 years: 600 IU
- Breastfeeding moms: 600 IU

Vitamin D is unique from other micronutrients in that our bodies actually make it from sunlight, when UVB light aids in the conversion of cholesterol to vitamin D in our skin.

Vitamin D helps regulate the body's absorption and use of calcium and therefore plays an important role in forming and maintaining strong, healthy bones. Vitamin D deficiency in children results in the softening and weakening of the bones, a condition known as rickets.

Theoretically, we could all meet our needs for this fat-soluble vitamin through sun exposure alone; however, given the risk of skin cancer from excessive sun exposure, the increase in sunscreen use, and the differing rates of synthesis based on age, skin color (people with darker pigmentation synthesize less vitamin D), and health status, most people need to get vitamin D from the diet. Additionally, it is advised that infants are to be kept out of the sun as much as possible.

The main dietary sources of vitamin D are fatty fish, some eggs (although only in small amounts), and fortified cow's milk. Specialized UV-treated mushrooms are also able to synthesize large amounts of vitamin D, though they are hard to find in normal grocery stores. (Also, we don't know about your babes, but ours won't touch mushrooms.)

PBJ Quick Bite

Our bodies make vitamin D from the sun, but it is advised that babies are to avoid sun exposure, so supplementation is the safest option!

Vitamin D Needs

Breast milk is low in vitamin D, regardless of mom's intake. Therefore, the AAP recommends that all breastfed babies receive a daily supplement with 400 IU vitamin D, starting at birth. Formula contains vitamin D, so babies who receive it do not need extra supplementation.

Once a baby is weaned, they may be able to meet their vitamin D needs with fortified soy or pea milk, which often contains the same amount of vitamin D as dairy milk (~30% of the RDA per cup). However, not all products are fortified, so it is important to read the nutrition label. If your child is fair-skinned and/or you live in a very sunny climate, this may be enough to meet their needs, as they will also generate vitamin D from the sun. If you live in a cold climate, however, your child has darker pigmentation, or they do not consistently drink 2-3 cups of fortified milk a day, you should continue to supplement.

Forms of Vitamin D

Vitamin D supplements come in two forms—D2 and D3. D2 is synthesized from fungi, while D3 has traditionally been synthesized from lanolin, found in sheepskin. Some studies have found that D3 is more effective at raising blood levels of active vitamin D. Luckily, there is now a vegan form of D3 produced by a plantlike organism known as lichen.

> **PBJ Bottom Line:** Vitamin D is important for building strong, healthy bones. All breastfed babies should receive a 400 IU supplement of vitamin D at birth until they are weaned to vitamin D-containing foods or a fortified plant milk. If your child does not consume 2-3 cups of fortified milk a day, has dark skin, or you live in a high-latitude, cold location, you should continue supplementation. We recommend the widely available vegan D3.

Vitamin A (RDA—RAE)
- 0-6 months: 400 mcg (AI)
- 7-12 months: 500 mcg (AI)
- 1-3 years: 300 mcg
- Breastfeeding moms: 1330 mcg

Vitamin A, also known as "retinoic acid," is a fat-soluble vitamin necessary for normal vision, growth, and immune function. Severe vitamin A deficiency may cause blindness or thyroid dysfunction, while mild vitamin A deficiency puts children at risk of respiratory infections and diarrhea. Fortunately, it is easily preventable and uncommon in the developed world.

Vitamin A is found in two forms—"preformed vitamin A," found in meat and animal products, and "provitamin A," found in dark-colored fruits and vegetables such as carrots, mangoes, kale, sweet potato, spinach, and butternut squash. Our bodies convert provitamins to the active form of vitamin A in the digestive tract.

The vitamin A content of cow's milk is significantly lower than that of breast milk, and because vitamin A is found in the fat portion of milk, low-fat and skim milk must be fortified with vitamin A in the US.

VITAMIN A (BETA-CAROTENE) SOURCES (RAE)	
Sweet potato, cooked, ¼ cup	481 mcg
Pumpkin, cooked, ¼ cup	477 mcg
Butternut squash, cooked, ¼ cup	286 mcg
Spinach, cooked, ¼ cup	236 mcg
Kale, cooked, ¼ cup	222 mcg
Carrots, cooked, ¼ cup	213 mcg
Cantaloupe, ⅛ of medium melon	117 mcg
Mango, ¼ fruit	45 mcg

Vitamin A Needs

There is no biological need for vitamin A from animal products. Arguments that plants are poor sources are incorrect. The daily values listed for vitamin A in plant foods reflect absorption rates, so as long as your child eats enough provitamin A from plant sources, which includes the phytochemical beta-carotene, their bodies will make enough active vitamin A.

During infancy, your child will get all the vitamin A they need from breast milk or formula. Studies show that regardless of the type of vitamin A mom consumes (preformed versus provitamin), the body ensures that mom's milk contains adequate amounts of the active form. After baby discontinues breast milk or formula, they'll need to obtain vitamin A through their diet.

As you can see from the foods list, vitamin A is abundant

PBJ Quick Bite
Just ¼ cup of sweet potato fries is enough to meet your babe's total daily dose of vitamin A!

in plants, and a single ¼ cup serving of sweet potato or pumpkin can provide your baby's total daily requirement. Because vitamin A is fat soluble, these foods should be provided with a good source of fat for the best absorption.

To note—ripe fruits and cooked vegetables are more easily converted to the active form of vitamin A than raw. An awesome example of a vitamin A–optimized snack is baked sweet potato fries made with olive oil!

PBJ BOTTOM LINE: Vitamin A is an important nutrient for immune functioning and development. Breast milk and formula contain enough active vitamin A to meet babies' needs. Your toddler should be able to obtain enough by consuming brightly colored fruits and vegetables and green leafy vegetables, and pairing them with a fat source to increase absorption. If vitamin A is included in a multivitamin, make sure it has less than 100 percent of the RDA or is found in the beta-carotene form versus retinol, as too much active vitamin A can be toxic.

Choline (AI)

- 0–6 months: 125 mg
- 7–12 months: 150 mg
- 1–3 years: 200 mg
- Breastfeeding moms: 550 mg

Choline, a B vitamin–like compound, may be one of the most hotly debated nutrients on the block these days. "Ancestral diet" advocates claim that our requirement for choline is a major reason we need to eat animals, while plant-based eaters point to studies showing that choline creates a molecule known as TMAO that has been associated with heart disease. The truth is, there's a lot we don't know about choline.

Here's what is certain—choline is an important nutrient for the development of the brain and healthy functioning of the liver. Emerging research in animals suggests that proper intake of choline during pregnancy may help protect against neurocognitive and developmental disorders such as autism, down syndrome, epilepsy, and Rett syndrome. Studies have shown that children born to mothers who consumed the recommended amount of choline during pregnancy had better scores on memory tests at 7 years of age. However, studies on choline supplementation during pregnancy and infant cognitive outcomes have been mixed, with some showing benefits from supplementation and others showing no benefit when pregnant women are already consuming moderate amounts.

We produce some choline in the liver, but not enough to meet the body's requirement. Though animal products contain the largest amount of choline in the diet, it is widespread in both animal and plant foods. Small amounts are found in most plants, which usually adds up to meet daily needs. Good sources include wheat germ, broccoli, beans, and quinoa, and soy foods like tofu and edamame are considered an excellent source of choline. As such, experts acknowledge that "a variety of diets can satisfy the need for this nutrient."

SOURCES OF CHOLINE	
Soymilk, 1 cup	58 mg
Soybeans (cooked), ¼ cup	50 mg
Wheat germ, 1 tablespoon	25 mg
Kidney beans, ¼ cup	23 mg
Quinoa, ¼ cup	11 mg
Peas, ¼ cup	11 mg
Broccoli (cooked), ¼ cup	8 mg

Choline Needs

Breastfeeding moms are advised to consume 550 mg of choline per day. While these needs can theoretically be met through diet, we think it's best for strict vegans to supplement to be sure you're getting enough. If your postnatal vitamin does not contain any choline, we'd recommend an additional supplement with about half of the RDA. Formula contains adequate choline to meet infants' needs.

Choline needs for toddlers have not been well established, as the bulk of research has been conducted on pregnant and lactating women. Therefore, we don't recommend routine supplementation. As discussed above, the daily requirement can be met by eating a wide variety of plants, especially soy foods. If you practice a predominantly plant-based diet, you may choose to include eggs, as they are an excellent source of choline (~150 mg/egg). However, we know this isn't an option for our strict plant-based families. Therefore, we've created a sample menu that meets choline needs solely with plants.

SAMPLE CHOLINE-RICH MENU FOR 1-TO-2-YEAR-OLD		
Morning Snack	8 ounces soy milk (58 mg), medium banana (12 mg)	70 mg
Breakfast	½ cup oatmeal (4 mg), 1 tablespoon wheat germ (24 mg), ¼ cup raspberries (4 mg), 1 teaspoon chia seeds	32 mg
Lunch	1 slice wheat bread (6 mg), 1 tablespoon peanut butter (11 mg), ¼ avocado (7 mg), 1 small shredded carrot (4 mg), ¼ cup sliced cherry tomatoes (4 mg)	32 mg
Snack	1 clementine (10 mg) + 8 ounces soy milk (58 mg)	68 mg
Dinner	½ cup navy beans (22 mg), ¼ cup cooked broccoli (9 mg), ¼ cup cooked cauliflower (10 mg), ½ small baked potato (13 mg), 1 teaspoon olive oil (none)	54 mg
TOTAL		256 mg choline

The two glasses of soy milk make up the bulk of choline in this meal plan—this is another reason we like soy milk as a cow's milk replacement.

PBJ Bottom Line: Choline is essential for baby's growing brain. While it is a good idea for pregnant and breastfeeding mamas to supplement choline, routine supplementation is not currently recommended for babies and toddlers. Because soy is such a rich source, we recommend including 2–3 servings a day. Predominantly plant-based families may choose to include eggs to help meet needs.

A Word on Supplements

As you can see, certain supplements are 100 percent necessary for plant-based babes. But not all supplements are created equally. Supplements are not regulated by the FDA, and companies do not have to provide evidence that their products are safe or contain the ingredients they claim to contain before they go to market. The FDA will only act retroactively to pull products from shelves after problems have been reported. Many supplements have been found to be contaminated or contain ingredients that are not listed on the label. This could be harmful to anyone, but especially children.

Most vitamins, minerals, and algae oil supplements are low risk, but other supplements or those that have several different ingredients, like multivitamins, may contain more questionable ingredients. We recommend sticking to single-ingredient supplements or multivitamins that contain exactly the micronutrients you're looking for. Babies and toddlers not only do not need a medicine cabinet's worth of obscure herbs, but also these untested additives may be harmful to them.

Another way to protect your babe is by looking for supplements with third-party testing verification. Some marks to look for on the bottle include NSF, USP, and ConsumerLab.com.

Whew! That was a lot. That's why we've provided our "PBJ Bottom Line" for each nutrient—so you can quickly reference the most pertinent facts anytime you need them. We've also provided our tear-out supplement sheet in the back so you can jot down the nutrients and amounts you'll need for each of your baby's stages for easy reference.

Now that you've got these nutrition facts down, the rest will be easy breezy. In the following chapters, we'll show you exactly how to apply all this information into fuss-free, nutrient-dense meals that your babe will love.

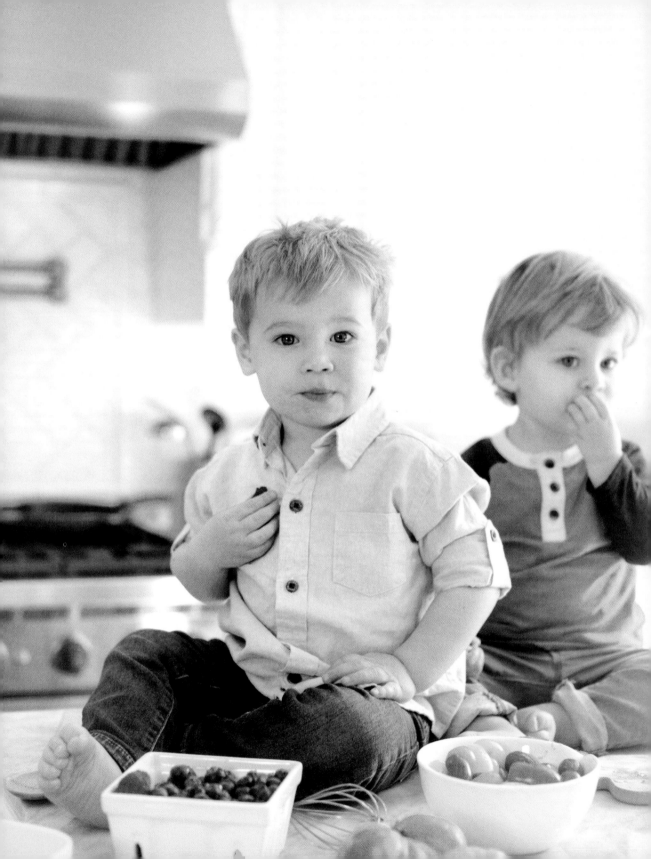

2

The PB3 Plate

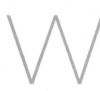

We get it. Nutrition can be overwhelming. Even as registered dietitians who can rattle off the nutritional composition of any vegetable upon request, we still find ourselves standing in front of the refrigerator at times wondering how we're going to put together a healthy meal our family will enjoy.

Our goal is to make feeding your baby as effortless as possible. Of course, we're also here to educate, but we hope we do it in a way that feels practical and not intimidating. There is a lot of confusion around plant-based eating, so we will walk you through the science, then show you how to apply the knowledge to your baby's plate.

Think of this section as your plant-based nutrition action plan. A crash course in how to take the information you learned in the previous chapter to fill your baby's plate with foods to help them thrive.

The PB3 Plate

Introducing our PB3 Plate! Isn't she cute? Our plate is broken into three main components: Fruits and Vegetables (F/V); Legumes, Nuts, and Seeds (L/N/S); and Grains and Starches (G/S). An easy way to remember these core groups is "Beans, Greens, and Grains!"

Unlike other models, these three components each take up one-third of the plate. Why don't we dedicate half of the plate to produce like the other models? Because of caloric density. While we want children to eat plenty of F/V, we don't want them to fill up so much that they don't have room for more high-calorie, nutrient-rich items from the other categories.

We want you to start thinking of your baby's plate this way, aiming to include each main category at meals and at least two of the three with snacks. You may not *always*

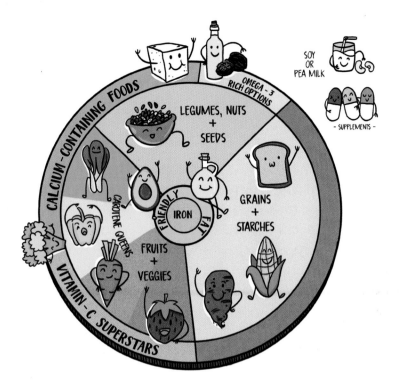

get them in at each meal, and that's OK. But as often as you can fill your babe's plate with fruits and vegetables, grains and starches, and nuts, seeds, and legumes, the better.

Breaking foods into groups is meant to be less confusing, not more. If your family has been plant-based for a while, you likely already eat this way. For example, a burrito bowl is filled with lettuce and roasted vegetables (F/V), brown rice (G/S), black beans (L/N/S), and maybe a scoop of guacamole for extra fat. A bowl of berry oatmeal contains fruit, grains, and perhaps a drizzle of peanut butter on top.

Now that you get the gist, let's dig a little deeper!

Fruits and Vegetables

The one thing that all experts agree upon, despite differing opinions on overall dietary patterns, is the importance of fruits and vegetables. Studies show that people with higher intakes of fruits and vegetables have lower rates of heart disease, cancer, obesity, dementia, osteoporosis, and respiratory disorders.

Unfortunately, about 60% of children consume fewer fruits than recommended, and 93% do not meet vegetable intake recommendations. And these numbers only decline as children get older. Introducing fruits and vegetables at an early age helps set up healthy eaters for life.

Fruits and vegetables are a major source of fiber in our diet, an indigestible carbohydrate that helps maintain a healthy digestive system and body weight and reduces the risk of chronic disease.

Fruits and vegetables are also a great source of vitamins and minerals. They all tend to be high in the antioxidant immune booster, vitamin C. Cruciferous vegetables like broccoli, Brussels sprouts, kale, and collard greens are great plant-based sources of calcium, essential for healthy bones and muscle functioning. Brightly colored fruits and vegetables like carrots, cantaloupe, and bell peppers are high in vitamin A, important for vision and cell growth.

Finally, plants (mainly fruits and vegetables) are the only source in our diet of powerful disease-fighting compounds known as phytochemicals.

Phytochemicals

Phytochemicals are compounds produced by plants that help them fight off predators and pathogens and have also been shown to be beneficial to human health. Phytochemicals possess anti-cancer, anti-inflammatory, antimicrobial, and antioxidant properties, which may help in preventing disease. Many are better absorbed when consumed with a source of fat, which is another reason we prioritize fat for infants and toddlers.

PBJ Quick Bite
Pairing fruits and veggies with a source of fat helps absorb disease-fighting phytochemicals! Think berries and cashew yogurt or veggies and hummus.

Phytochemicals come in all shapes and sizes but are often classified by color. This is why you may have heard the recommendation to "eat the rainbow," and why our fruits and vegetables section is bursting with color.

PBJ BOTTOM LINE: Include fruits and/or vegetables at every meal and offer a wide variety of produce in different colors to maximize their diverse benefits.

Forget what you've heard from the bread-bashing crowd—diets rich in whole grains are linked to immense health benefits, including lower rates of heart disease, diabetes, and cancer.

Grains and starches are also packed with energy that infants and toddlers need to thrive. While some people may classify grains and starches as mere "carbs," they have so many other important nutrients like protein, fiber, B vitamins, and minerals that help support metabolism, provide building blocks for muscles, and fuel a healthy microbiome.

In fact, about half of the protein in a plant-based diet comes from the grains and starches group, and grains also contain certain amino acids that are lower in other protein-rich plant foods. For example, most grains are high in the essential amino acid methionine, which is found in smaller amounts in beans. This is why we recommend offering multiple options from each food group to ensure your baby is eating enough of each essential amino acid.

> **PBJ Quick Bite**
>
> Grains are an important source of plant-based protein. Just one slice of sprouted whole grain bread contains 4 grams of protein (one-third of a toddler's daily needs).

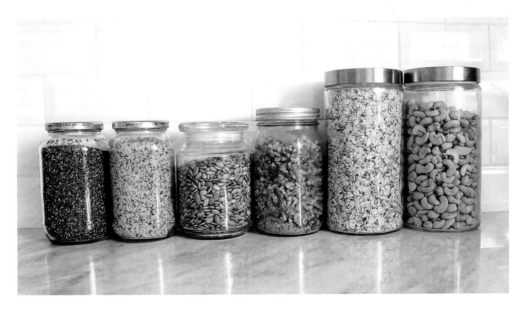

You may think of quinoa when we say high-protein grains, but quinoa is actually a seed, and in fact *all* grains contain a good amount of protein. Oats contain 5 grams of protein per half cup, while sprouted whole grain bread has about 4 grams of protein per slice.

This category also includes foods that are often categorized as vegetables but are better described as starches, such as potatoes and corn—both excellent choices to fill your baby's tummy.

PBJ'S FAVORITE GRAINS & STARCHES

Food	Serving Size for 6–9 months	Serving Size for 9–12 months	Serving Size for 1–3 year olds
Amaranth	1–2 tbsp cooked amaranth	2–4 tbsp cooked amaranth	½ cup cooked amaranth
Barley	1–2 tbsp cooked barley	2–4 tbsp cooked barley	½ cup cooked barley
Brown Rice and White Rice*	1–2 tbsp cooked rice	2–4 tbsp cooked rice	½ cup cooked rice
Buckwheat	1–2 tbsp cooked buckwheat	2–4 tbsp cooked buckwheat	½ cup cooked buckwheat
Corn	1–2 tbsp cooked corn	2–4 tbsp cooked corn	½ cup cooked corn or ½ corn-on-the-cob
Couscous	1–2 tbsp cooked couscous	2–4 tbsp cooked couscous	½ cup cooked couscous
Farro	1–2 tbsp cooked farro	2–4 tbsp cooked farro	½ cup cooked farro
Oats	1–2 tbsp cooked oats	2–4 tbsp cooked oats	½ cup cooked oats
Peas	1–2 tbsp peas	2–4 tbsp peas	½ cup peas
Potatoes and Sweet Potatoes	1–2 potato "sticks" or ⅛ cup cooked potatoes	3–4 potato "sticks" or ¼ cup cooked potatoes	4–6 potato "sticks" or ½ cup cooked potatoes
Quinoa	1–2 tbsp cooked quinoa	2–4 tbsp cooked quinoa	½ cup cooked quinoa
Whole Wheat and Enriched Bread, Pita, Pasta, and Tortillas	1–2 tbsp cooked pasta, ¼ slice bread	2–4 tbsp cooked pasta, ½ slice bread	½ cup cooked pasta, 1 slice bread

While brown rice is typically considered a healthy grain option, it may contain high levels of arsenic, a neurotoxic compound especially detrimental to children. Check out our FAQ section at the end of this chapter on minimizing arsenic exposure and for recommendations on the amount and type of brown rice that is safe for babies.

A "whole" grain contains all of the grain's natural components, including the bran and germ. Refined grain products, like your typical white bread, contain similar amounts of protein and carbohydrates to whole grains but with the bran and germ removed, losing important nutrients like phytochemicals, vitamins, minerals, and fiber. "Enriched" refined grains add back in certain vitamins and minerals.

Fiber is the non-digestible part of carbohydrates that supports proper digestion and feeds the healthy gut bacteria that make up our microbiome. Plants contain two types of fiber: fermentable and non-fermentable, and both have unique benefits. Fermentable fiber is digested by our gut bacteria and produces fuel for the cells of our digestive tract and creates compounds that help regulate food intake and prevent disease. Non-fermentable fiber creates bulk in our stool and helps maintain normal bowel movements and prevent constipation—helpful for our babies with tummy troubles.

Diets high in whole grains are associated with less chronic disease, while those high in refined grains have the opposite effect—increasing the risk of metabolic syndrome and type 2 diabetes. Studies show that children who eat whole grains have healthier body weights and a better intake of nutrients overall.

The RDA of fiber is 19 grams per day for 1–3 years. There is no set RDA for infants. This amount is easily achieved on a plant-based diet, as fruits, vegetables, beans, nuts, and seeds are all rich sources.

The Whole Grain Paradox:
Why Plant-Based Babies Should Eat White Bread

Despite what we know about the benefits of whole grains, plant-based babies and toddlers should limit their intake of them.

We know what you're thinking—didn't you *just* say that refined grains aren't healthy? Hear us out. This is another example of how adult, and even older kids', nutrition differs from that of babies/infants.

Little stomachs fill up easily, especially with fiber-rich foods. Fiber slows digestion and makes us feel fuller longer—great for weight management, not so great for babies with small appetites. And while fiber can prevent constipation, too much can cause it.

This is why for our under 2s we offer half whole grains and half refined grains. This way, babies still get the benefits of grains—protein and calories—without taking in too much fiber. If constipation, diarrhea, slow weight gain, or small appetites are a problem, then we recommend reducing whole grain intake further and providing only refined grains. Don't worry, your babe will still get plenty of micronutrients from the other fantastic stuff they're eating, and most refined products are enriched with essential nutrients. This recommendation can be adjusted based on your child's unique needs. If you have a 1-to-2-year-old with a big appetite and regular bowel movements, serving all whole grains may not be an issue.

PBJ BOTTOM LINE: Grains are great! They provide much-needed protein and carbohydrates for growing bodies and brains. Make sure to include them with every meal. While whole grains are the optimal option for adults and older kids, they can be overly filling for small stomachs. We recommend offering half whole grains and half refined grains for our under 2s, especially if they tend to have a smaller appetite.

Legumes, Nuts, and Seeds

Just in case you're still worrying, let us reiterate—plants have plenty of protein!

While all whole plant foods have some protein, the richest sources are from legumes, nuts, and seeds. Common foods in this category include beans (aka pulses), soy foods (tofu/tempeh), peanuts, tree nuts, and hemp, chia, flax, sunflower, pumpkin, and sesame seeds. They're not just protein packed, though; they also provide carbohydrates, fiber, healthy fat, and numerous important micronutrients like iron, zinc, calcium, selenium, folate, and vitamin E.

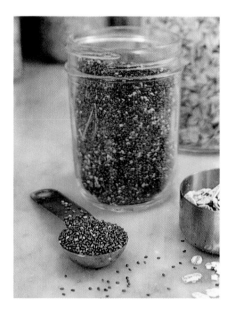

PBJ'S FAVORITE GRAINS & STARCHES

Food	Serving Size for 6–9 months	Serving Size for 9–12 months	Serving Size for 1–3 year olds
Lentils	1 tbsp mashed lentils	2–3 tbsp cooked lentils	⅓ cup cooked lentils
Black beans	1 tbsp mashed beans	2–3 tbsp cooked beans	⅓ cup cooked beans
Kidney beans	1 tbsp mashed beans	2–3 tbsp cooked beans	⅓ cup cooked beans
Chickpeas	1 tbsp mashed beans	2–3 tbsp cooked beans (halved)	⅓ cup cooked beans
Navy beans	1 tbsp mashed beans	2–3 tbsp cooked beans	⅓ cup cooked beans
Soybeans	1 tbsp mashed beans	2–3 tbsp cooked beans	⅓ cup cooked beans
Tofu	1 tofu stick	2 tbsp cubed tofu	⅓ cup cubed tofu
Tempeh	1 tempeh stick	2 tbsp cubed tempeh	⅓ cup cubed tempeh
Soy milk	n/a for under 12 months	n/a for under 12 months	½–1 cup
Almonds	1 tsp finely ground almonds in a recipe	2 tsp finely ground almonds in a recipe	1 tbsp finely ground almonds in a recipe
Cashews	1 tsp finely ground cashews in a recipe	2 tsp finely ground cashews in a recipe	1 tbsp finely ground cashews in a recipe
Pecans	1 tsp finely ground pecans in a recipe	2 tsp finely ground pecans in a recipe	1 tbsp finely ground pecans in a recipe
Walnuts	1 tsp finely ground walnuts in a recipe	2 tsp finely ground walnuts in a recipe	1 tbsp finely ground walnuts in a recipe
Peanut butter	½ tsp thinly spread peanut butter	1 tsp thinly spread peanut butter	2 tsp thinly spread peanut butter
Almond butter	½ tsp thinly spread almond butter	1 tsp thinly spread almond butter	2 tsp thinly spread almond butter
Chia seeds	½ tsp chia seeds	1 tsp chia seeds	1 tbsp chia seeds
Flax seeds	½ tsp ground flax seeds	1 tsp ground flax seeds	1 tbsp ground flax seeds
Hemp seeds	½ tsp hemp seeds	1 tsp hemp seeds	1 tbsp hemp seeds
Pumpkin seeds, aka "pepitas"	1 tsp finely ground pepitas in a recipe	2 tsp finely ground pepitas in a recipe	1 tbsp ground pepitas
Sunflower seeds	1 tsp finely ground sunflower seeds in a recipe	2 tsp finely ground sunflower seeds in a recipe	1 tbsp chopped sunflower seeds
Sesame seeds	½ tsp sesame seeds	1 tsp sesame seeds	2 tsp sesame seeds
Tahini	½ tsp thinly spread tahini	1 tsp thinly spread tahini	2 tsp thinly spread tahini

Improving Nutrient Bioavailability

One concern about these foods is so-called anti-nutrients, compounds found in legumes, nuts, seeds, and grains that bind to minerals and interfere with their absorption.

Anti-nutrients are generally not harmful, and some may even possess health benefits, but they can reduce the amount of minerals that make it into your babe's body.

Sprouting, Soaking, and Fermenting

There are several ways to decrease the amount of anti-nutrients in food and increase the bioavailability of essential micronutrients. One way is just by cooking food, one of many reasons we advise against raw plant-based diets for children.

Other options to improve bioavailability are soaking and sprouting. Soaking dry beans overnight before cooking can reduce the amount of phytates about 30% and increase the availability of iron and zinc. Simply add beans to a bowl or jar and cover with water. Store in the refrigerator for 12–24 hours before draining, rinsing, and cooking.

Sprouting also increases bioavailability and refers to letting the legume, grain, or seed sit out after soaking until it begins to germinate. Both of these practices can increase the risk of bacterial contamination, which is why it's important to practice proper food safety and cook food that has been soaked or sprouted before serving to infants and toddlers.

As busy moms, we know that sprouting grains is not practical for most families. Thankfully, many food companies sell sprouted products, and we choose to purchase these as part of our whole-grain options. See our list of preferred products in the Index.

Finally, ascorbic acid, also known as vitamin C, counteracts the effects of these inhibitors by increasing the absorption of iron found in plant-based food. This is why we recommend that all meals include a source of vitamin C, such as pairing beans with roasted bell peppers.

PBJ BOTTOM LINE: Legumes, nuts, and seeds provide babes protein, fiber, and essential nutrients like iron and zinc. Include them at every meal, or at least twice a day. Pairing iron-rich foods with a source of vitamin C helps increase iron absorption, which is why we highlight vitamin-C superstars on the PB3 Plate.

In addition to the "core 3" food groups, our PB3 Plate also calls out nutrients from each category—the ones you want to make sure to include regularly in your babe's diet. Let's take a closer look and talk about how to easily work them into meals.

Fat

Babies need a lot of fat (30%–40% of their diet). And while fat is not a main category in our PB3 Plate, that's not because it isn't important. Quite the opposite—we put it at the center of the plate because we want to see you incorporating fat into all aspects of the meal.

Avocados were a favorite first food for both of our sons, and they ate them daily. We also regularly offered nut butters on toast, in sauces, and drizzled on veggies. We included chia and hemp seeds in oatmeal, smoothies, and pasta dishes. And we used olive oil to roast veggies, make stir fries, and provide moisture to baked goods.

Here are a few of our favorite fat-rich meals and snacks:

- Sweet potatoes roasted in olive oil
- Avocado toast strips
- Banana slices with a dab of peanut butter
- Oatmeal with chia and hemp seeds
- Almond butter and berry smoothies
- Hummus sandwiches
- Cashew mac and cheese

But wait, isn't oil bad for you?

Oil is a nonessential food, but it's healthy in moderation and helpful in meeting baby's high energy and fat needs. Additionally, oil increases the absorption of fat-soluble vitamins, and olive oil has specifically been shown to be beneficial for brain and heart health.

Plant oils provide a good source of mono and polyunsaturated fat (LA and ALA—discussed in the previous chapter). While you can certainly get those fats from avocados, olives, nuts, and seeds, whole nuts and seeds or big globs of nut butter are a choking hazard. Therefore, we recommend cooking foods in olive, avocado, or coconut oil, especially phytochemical-rich vegetables, as fat helps absorb these beneficial compounds.

Iron

Iron is found in all three main categories of the PB3 Plate. In the L/N/S category, you have beans, soy foods, nuts, and seeds. Chia seeds are an especially rich source of iron, which is why we like to add them to smoothies, muffin mixes, or yogurt, or sprinkle them directly onto our babe's meals. They've got about 1.5 mg of iron per tablespoon. However, chia seeds are also high in fiber, so don't go overboard. We think ½ tablespoon for babies under 12 months and 1–2 tablespoons a day for babes 1–3 years is appropriate. We also love legume pastas like red lentil pasta or chickpea pasta—another awesome source of iron, with 3 mg per ½-cup serving.

Grains are another fantastic go-to. Both whole wheat and refined grains contain iron, though it is added to the latter. One slice of bread may contain anywhere from 1 to 2.5 mg. Opt for sprouted grain products when possible, as sprouting increases the bioavailability of iron and other minerals.

In the produce section, ½ cup of cooked broccoli or kale contains about ½ mg of iron each. As we discussed in the previous chapter, while spinach does contain a lot of iron, it's not very bioavailable.

As you can see, many foods have iron. However, as previously discussed, babies' iron needs are very high—11 mg per day from 6 to 12 months. This is why we're big fans of iron-fortified infant cereals, which contain about 7 mg of iron per serving. They get a bad rap from the whole-foods, plant-based crowd, as they are considered a processed food, but they serve an important purpose—filling the nutrient gap during a time of high iron needs and low food intake.

PBJ Quick Bite

Bean-based pastas are a great source of protein and iron and an easy-to-grasp food for our baby-led weaners.

After their initial iron scare, Whitney ensured her son Caleb met his iron needs by providing him with iron-fortified oatmeal every morning. She also added iron-fortified oat cereal to Caleb's batch of their favorite family waffle recipe. For our baby-led weaners, you can roll slices of avocado (a vitamin C source!) in fortified cereal to help baby grip the food.

Iron-Optimized Oatmeal

- ¼ cup rolled oats
- 1 teaspoon chia seeds
- 1 teaspoon hemp seeds
- ⅓ cup water
- ¼ cup iron-fortified baby oat cereal
- 1 ounce orange juice

Combine oats, chia, hemp, and water in a small bowl and microwave for 1½ minutes. Stir in baby cereal and orange juice. Serve to baby!

Vitamin C Superstars

Because vitamin C drastically increases the amount of iron our bodies can absorb, we like to include it as often as possible. Fortunately, it's found in pretty much all produce. Especially rich sources include citrus, strawberries, potatoes, leafy green vegetables, bell peppers, and cauliflower.

Combining iron and vitamin C is easy. Instinctively, we already do this with many foods—black beans and salsa, hummus made with lemon juice, or baked beans in a tomato sauce.

Here are some of our favorite ways to pair iron and vitamin C:

- Oatmeal + strawberries
- Black beans + tomatoes
- Legume pasta + marinara
- Tofu + orange marinade
- Broccoli + lemon juice

- Peanut butter sandwiches + strawberry chia jam
- Tempeh triangles + roasted bell peppers

Check out our recipe section for more iron-vitamin C combinations.

Calcium-Containing Foods

Most plant-based toddlers will meet their calcium needs through fortified soy/pea milk, but we still want to include natural sources of calcium. Many plants have a small amount, but the best sources include tofu, beans, sesame seeds, tahini, oranges, and cruciferous vegetables.

If you choose not to serve your child any type of milk, you will have to be extremely vigilant about providing enough of these sources on a daily basis, or consider a supplement.

Large amounts of calcium (usually from fortified foods or supplements) can interfere with iron absorption, so we recommend serving soy or pea milk separate from your child's most iron-rich meal. We do this by offering milk by itself first thing in the morning, right before bed, or as a snack paired with fruit midday.

PBJ Quick Bite
Offer fortified milk at snack time instead of with meals to prevent the calcium from inhibiting iron absorption from the meal.

Omega-3-Rich Options

ALA is the omega-3 fat found in plants—flip back to the previous chapter for a deep dive into this topic. While ALA intake doesn't replace the need for DHA—another critical fat for babies—it's still important for growth, and we want to include it as much as possible.

ALA is found in the L/N/S category in foods like walnuts, chia seeds, hemp seeds, flaxseed, flax oil, and soy. We work this into our babes' diets by regularly providing tofu and tempeh but mainly by incorporating lots of seeds!

Here's how we add ALA to our babes' plates:

- Add chia and hemp seeds to oatmeal and smoothies
- Use "flax eggs" in baked goods
- Roll avocado or banana in hemp seeds

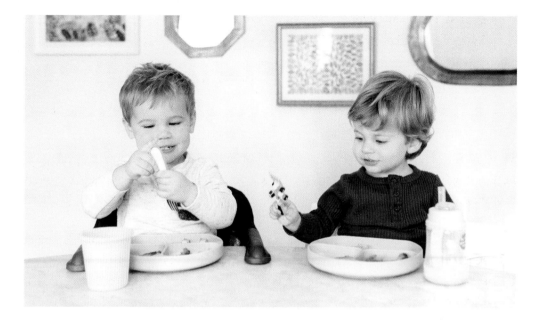

- Serve tofu or tempeh daily
- Spread toast strips with walnut butter
- Use walnuts as a meat replacement in meatball and burger recipes

Carotene Queens

Carotenes are a form of vitamin A found in plants. As discussed, our bodies convert these compounds to active vitamin A.

Rich sources include sweet potatoes, butternut squash, pumpkin, carrots, persimmon, mango, kale, and collard greens. To ensure your babe gets enough, offer 1–2 servings of these foods a day.

Lucky for parents, most kids (even veggie haters) seem to love sweet potato. Or if not, they like fruit! And as we'll discuss later, whole fruit is a nutrient-dense food to celebrate, not fear. Remember to always serve these foods with a source of fat to aid absorption.

Here are our favorite carotene-rich dishes:

- Mashed baked sweet potato combined with cashew yogurt
- Steamed baby carrots tossed with olive oil

- Finely diced kale sautéed with olive oil and mixed into a tofu scramble
- Mango slices served with soy milk for snack
- Pureed persimmon and peanut butter sandwich strips
- Pureed pumpkin stirred into oatmeal

Nondairy Milk

The only appropriate beverage for babies younger than 12 months is breast milk or formula and 1-2 ounces of water with meals starting at 6 months. After 1 year, toddlers may replace breast milk/formula with whole cow's milk or nondairy alternatives.

While there is nothing in milk that toddlers can't get elsewhere in the diet or from supplements, fortified nondairy milk is a convenient way to address baby's needs for essential nutrients like protein, vitamin D, vitamin B12, and calcium. We recommend offering them with snacks to your babe 2-3 times a day (8-16 ounces). Specifically, fortified soy and pea milk, which are the only nutritionally equivalent substitutes for cow's milk. Other nondairy milks (almond, cashew, coconut, oat, rice) are typically too low in protein or fat to be appropriate substitutes. However, soy and pea milk are also lower in fat than cow's milk, another reason that plant-based parents need to prioritize fat in the diet. Be sure to look for calcium and vitamin D on a product's ingredient label to make sure they're fortified.

While other milk alternatives do not provide a lot of added nutrition, they can be useful ingredients for baking, cooking, and adding flavor to meals.

For more information on milk, including the history of cow's milk consumption, the health risks and benefits of cow's milk, and an in-depth explanation of nondairy options, check out Chapter 5.

Supplements

We include supplements on the PB3 Plate as a reminder that no plant-based diet is complete without thoughtful supplementation. Children have unique needs, so we recommend that you use the handout we created in the back of the book to figure out the amount and types of supplements that are right for your babe. Make sure to review this list with your doctor or dietitian.

Sweets and Treats

One nutrient we haven't discussed yet—but that is crucial to a healthy diet—is vitamin P, for pleasure! While we want our kids to grow up appreciating whole foods and enjoying the natural sweetness of fruit or the savory flavor of roasted vegetables, we fully acknowledge that kids are going to (and should be able to) enjoy small amounts of less-nutrient-dense foods like cookies, cakes, chips, crackers, and candy. As these foods are not essential for proper growth and functioning, we haven't included them on the PB3 plate, but we cover them in depth in Chapter 6.

Meal Planning 101

OK, we've got the nutrients down. We've got the food categories down. Now you're probably wondering, *How do I put it all together?* Let's talk meal planning.

The biggest deterrent to getting a healthy, balanced meal on the table is a lack of preparation. Even as dietitians who literally wrote the book (hi!), we still have those weeks when we forget to prep and end up empty-handed in the kitchen. When you take the time to plan ahead and prepare a few staple items each week, you will be richly rewarded with less stress and a greater sense of control over your child's meals.

Here's how we do it.

We set aside 2–3 hours each week (this can be all at once or in increments, depending on your schedule) and cook a large batch of food from each of the core three PB3 Plate categories. Whitney likes to do this on Sunday after her trip to the farmer's market. Alex does it

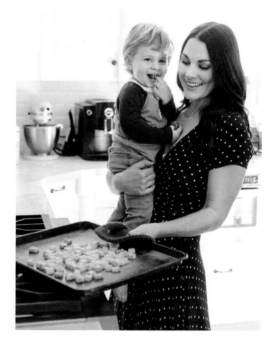

throughout the week, batch prepping a few items on the weekend, midweek, and at the end of the week for easy mix-and-match lunches and dinners.

Here's an example of a typical rundown:

Fruits + Vegetables

- Berries: Rinse with a water/vinegar mix and store in glass containers with paper towels to avoid molding.
- Baby carrots: Steam a bag's worth and store in a glass container.
- Broccoli: Wash florets, steam, and store in a glass container.

Grains + Starches

- Sweet potatoes: Cut two large sweet potatoes into fries, toss with olive oil, bake at 350°F for 20 minutes or air fry. Store in a glass container.
- Whole wheat pasta: Cook one box and store in a glass container.
- Farro: Cook 1–2 cups' worth and store in a glass container.

Legumes, Nuts + Seeds

- Tofu: Cube, toss with olive oil and Italian seasoning, bake at 350°F for 20 minutes. Store in a glass container.
- Beans: Rinse one can of beans and store in a glass container (lasts about 3 days) or pressure-cook dry beans.

In addition to prepping staples that can be mixed and matched for easy meals, we like to batch cook two full recipes. Batch cooking means doubling or tripling (even quadrupling) a recipe in order to have a large amount of leftovers to eat during the week or to freeze for later. It saves time on prep and cleanup and is a lifesaver on nights when you only have time to reheat a meal. You can make these two recipes on the same day that you do your meal prep or you can cook one recipe on Sunday night and another on Wednesday to cover your whole week and have an opportunity to enjoy at least one of the servings fresh. We suggest picking the recipes in advance so you can be sure to grab everything you need on your weekly grocery run.

We know it can be hard to find the time to do anything but brush your teeth when

PBJ Quick Bite

Set aside 2–3 hours once a week to meal prep food from the main PB3 Plate categories for easy assembly throughout the week.

you've got a baby, but trust us, planning pays off in the long run when you're able to throw together a meal or snack in less than ten minutes. So strap that baby to your chest, or commission your significant other/MIL/babysitter to watch them for a couple of hours while you get it done.

PBJ Quick Bite

Pick two recipes to batch cook during the week for family dinners and easy lunch leftovers.

Safe Food Storage

We avoid plastic as much as possible. Not only is it bad for the environment, but also plastic containers have been shown to leach endocrine-disrupting chemicals into food and beverages. The most researched chemical is BPA (bisphenol-A), which has been linked to developmental problems and an increased risk of chronic diseases. Leaching occurs more readily when plastic is heated or when it comes in contact with acidic substances, but it happens even under normal conditions. BPA-free plastics may seem like a better option, but these alternatives may contain compounds that are structurally similar to BPA, but just haven't been spotlighted yet. Therefore, we opt for plastic-free food storage: glass or stainless-steel containers and bottles for storing food, and silicone plates, cups, and bags for serving food or stashing snacks when traveling.

PB3 Plate Examples

Let's be real—not all meals and snacks will contain a perfect combo of the PB3 Plate nutrients. It's hard enough to physically balance your baby and all their feeding products (plate, cup, utensils, bib) while trying to set the table/tray. Again, as long as you aim to hit the three main categories (F/V, G/S, and L/N/S) at each meal, and include two out of three of each at most snacks, you're doing well.

We want to give you some concrete examples of what this looks like. The portion sizes shown here are just an example. Every child's appetite is different, and their intake can vary from day to day and meal to meal. Use this as a guide, but don't stress if your baby eats more or less than these examples show. We talk more about portion sizes in the individual chapters for each age group.

PB3 Southwest Plate

Iron, fat, omega-3s, calcium, carotenes, vitamin C

6–9 months: Tex-Mex Millet Meatballs (page 208) with a squirt of lemon, avocado rolled in hemp seeds, and baked sweet potato fingers

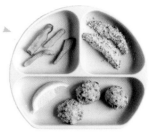

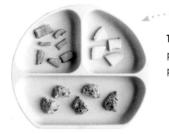

10–12 months: Tex-Mex Millet Meatballs (page 208) cut into pincer grasp–sized pieces, diced avocado, and diced sweet potato

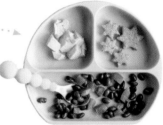

1–3 years: black beans and diced tomatoes served with a spoon, avocado chunks, and Sweet Potato Stars (page 212)

PB3 Italian Plate

Omega-3s, iron, vitamin C, calcium, carotenes, fat

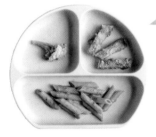

6–9 months: wheat penne pasta tossed with low-sodium marinara and olive oil, Tofu Marinara strips (page 218), and one Cheezy Broccoli Tree (page 215)

10–12 months: wheat spaghetti cut into pincer grasp–sized pieces, chopped Tofu Marinara (page 218), and chopped broccoli

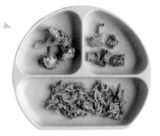

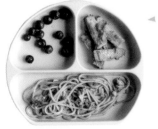

1–2 years: wheat spaghetti with marinara and broccoli bits, Tofu Marinara strips (page 218), and blueberries

Iron, omega-3s, fat, vitamin C

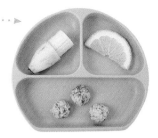

6–9 months: oatmeal with baby oat cereal and chia seeds rolled into balls, orange slice (for squeezing), and banana with a handle

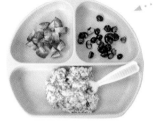

10–12 months: oatmeal with baby cereal and chia seeds served on a self-feeding baby spoon, chopped strawberries, and halved blueberries

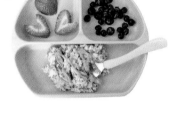

1–2 years: oatmeal with chia seeds and nut butter served with a spoon, whole blueberries, and sliced strawberries

PBJ-Approved Snack Combos

Think of snacks for toddlers and the first thing that comes to many parents' minds are puffs. We'll come right out with it—we're not big fans. They're glorified bites of air that lack protein, fiber, fat, and phytochemicals. Puffs are basically just stripped-down starch with vitamins and minerals added back in. Additionally, rice flour is the main ingredient in many of these products, and research has shown that rice-based baby products may contain potentially dangerous levels of the heavy metal arsenic (more in the Frequently Asked Feeding Questions on page 66). While puffs aren't the *worst* food out there, there are just so many other easy, nutrient-dense options.

We like to think of snacks as mini meals, another opportunity to provide our babes with essential nutrients to support their growth—not a time to just fill their bellies or pacify bad moods. We use the PB3 Plate to guide our snacks, just like we use it to guide meals.

Note—before age 1, most babes will be fine with three

PBJ Quick Bite

Snacks should be mini meals—not just snack food. Aim to include at least two of the three main PB3 Plate categories.

square meals a day, but around the 12-month mark, you'll want to start incorporating 1 or 2 snacks a day (more on this in Chapter 5). Here are a few examples:

- Banana rolled in hemp seeds (F/V + L/N/S)
- Avocado rolled in sesame seeds (F/V + L/N/S)
- PBJ's Blender Bean Muffins (page 206—all three!)
- Cashew yogurt + berries (F/V + L/N/S)
- Sweet potato fries drizzled in nut butter or tahini (G/S + L/N/S)
- Toast strips with peanut butter and chia jam (all three!)

Frequently Asked Feeding Questions

As pediatric plant-based dietitians, we've heard it all. There are so many claims about the right way to feed children, it's no wonder parents are confused! There are several questions that we hear frequently, so we decided to compile them into an easy reference FAQ section.

Q: Does organic matter?

A: The research on the benefits and risks of organic versus conventional produce is mixed. While most studies show they have similar amounts of vitamins and minerals, some studies show organic produce is higher in phytochemicals and lower in heavy metals and pesticide residues.

We buy organic produce the majority of the time. While the amount of pesticides used in conventional agriculture has been deemed safe for human consumption by the FDA, these same pesticides are toxic at higher amounts. The long-term effects from the bioaccumulation of pesticides and the potential synergistic effects of multiple types of pesticides on human health are still largely unknown. And some experts believe that the government limits set for pesticide use are based on outdated science and that new risk assessments need to be made in order to protect the public.

A handful of studies have shown that consumers who can't afford to buy organic end up eating less produce overall, and that is certainly not what we want. If the choice is between conventional produce or no produce at all, it's a no-brainer. The research on the benefits of fruits and vegetables is solid: increased intake of produce is associated with a reduced risk of chronic disease, regardless of how it's grown. Conventional produce will almost always be a superior choice to any other snack food, and we want you to feel confident in purchasing items that fit your budget and your family's needs.

If you can only afford to purchase a few organic items, we recommend the following:

1. Grains. Farmers use chemicals to dry out conventional grains prior to harvest. This helps speed up the production process. A 2018 study found that out of 28 samples of conventional oat-based products, mainly cereals marketed to children, every single one had detectable levels of the herbicide glyphosate and 26 exceeded the acceptable upper level recommended by the research group.

2. Soy. The majority of soy grown is genetically modified. While we don't want to get into a debate about the merits or harms of GMOs, we would like to point out that genetically modified plants are often sprayed with more chemicals than other conventional plants and therefore may contain higher pesticide residues. "Roundup Ready" soybeans are engineered to be resistant to the effects of the herbicide glyphosate. Therefore, farmers can spray fields with large amounts of the chemical without harming their crops. All organic foods are also non-GMO.

3. Fruits and vegetables without a removable outer layer. Though studies have shown that pesticides can seep into plants, the majority of residues are found on the outer peel. If you can't afford to buy all produce organic, save money by opting for conventional fruits and vegetables with removable skins like bananas, pineapple, cantaloupe, mango, pomegranate, honeydew, watermelon, onions, butternut squash, and spaghetti squash, or those that you peel, like potatoes, carrots, beets, and ginger.

PBJ BOTTOM LINE: The research on the benefits of organic food is mixed. If you have the means to buy organic, go for it. If not, don't skimp on beneficial fruits and veggies just because they're not organic.

Q: How should I clean my fruits and vegetables?

A: Plain old water and elbow grease (scrubbing) is all you need to properly clean your produce. Fancy vegetable washes are expensive and unnecessary.

Q: Is juice OK?

A: Get a handful of nutritional professionals in a room together and they likely all will have differing opinions on juice intake. We love that 100% fruit juice contains vitamins and phytochemicals, which makes it a superior choice to sweetened beverages like fruit punch and soda. But juice lacks protein, fat, and fiber, and given that it can be very filling, it may displace these other important nutrients in your babe's diet.

Additionally, studies show that fruit juice consumption increases weight gain in children who are overweight or at risk of being overweight/obese.

We agree with the American Academy of Pediatrics' recommendation to avoid fruit juice for children less than 1 year of age, and to limit its consumption to no more than 4 ounces per day for children 1–3 years of age. We think 100% juice is fine on occasion, but we would much rather you offer these same micronutrients in their whole fruit form. A whole apple (or pureed apple for our little ones), with its fiber and phytochemicals, is always a better choice over apple juice.

Children should not be given juice before bedtime or from sippy cups, which encourage constant consumption and may increase the risk of tooth decay.

PBJ Bottom Line: Kids don't need juice. Whole fruit is a much better option. That said, a small amount of juice in an otherwise balanced, whole foods–rich diet, is likely not a problem. It's certainly a better option than soda.

Q: When can kids have sugar?

A: Humans are biologically programmed to prefer the taste of sweet food and dislike bitter flavors in infancy and early childhood. You may have noticed this if your babe refuses vegetables but will gobble up any fruit you place in front of them. This is thought to be an evolutionary survival mechanism that drove humans to seek out high-calorie, energy-dense foods like breast milk and fruits and avoid bitter, poisonous plants.

Because children naturally prefer sweet flavors right from the start, we don't want to give them food at an early age that will modify their taste receptors to prefer *unnaturally* sweet food. When children are repeatedly exposed to sugar-sweetened foods and beverages, their preference for these foods increases.

The American Academy of Pediatrics recommends no added sugar for babies under 2 years of age. This doesn't refer to naturally sweet foods like fruit, but sugar that is *added* to food like flavored yogurt, baked goods, and packaged foods.

Added sugars include cane sugar, beet sugar, high-fructose corn syrup, corn syrup, brown rice syrup, and even so-called natural sweeteners like maple syrup, honey, and agave.

This can be challenging, as even "healthy" foods, like jarred marinara sauce and whole-grain bread, usually contain added sweetener. Our advice is to limit sugar when possible but also don't sweat it when there is a gram or two in something that baby eats infrequently.

> PBJ BOTTOM LINE: Children under the age of 2 don't need added sugar, and eating it regularly can set the stage for sweet preference later in life. The occasional bite of cake on their birthday or lick of ice cream isn't going to kill them, but don't get into the habit of offering sweetened foods. Added sugars are hard to avoid in processed foods, including bread, pasta sauce, etc. Try to pick products with the lowest amount possible, less than 3 grams per serving.

Q: Can my baby have salt?

A: We hate bland food as much as the next person, but under 1 year of age, babies' kidneys have not fully developed and aren't equipped to efficiently filter out large amounts of sodium. A high sodium intake in childhood may lead to high blood pressure in adulthood and increase a child's risk of obesity. It may also alter the body's metabolism of fat, resulting in more fat storage.

In addition to the potential harms to health, eating salty food in early childhood may predispose babies to prefer the taste later in life. Taste bud programming and preferences are established early, and we want to set our kids up for success by getting them used to the taste of whole, minimally processed food.

The US doesn't have an official upper limit for sodium intake for babies under 1 year of age, but other countries do. The UK recommends less than 400 mg of sodium per day for 6-to-12-month-olds and less than 800 mg for 1-to-3-year-olds. The US guidelines are less strict for toddlers, recommending less than 1500 mg of sodium per day for 1-to-3-year-olds, which is a little more than ½ teaspoon.

You don't need to get your measuring spoons and calculator, though. We recommend keeping it simple and avoiding salt for babies under 12 months and using it sparingly for toddlers. This isn't too hard when eating a whole-foods, plant-based diet, which is naturally lower in sodium.

When we cook for the family, we remove the baby's portion before adding salt to the rest of the family's meal. We also purchase no-salt-added or low-sodium tomato sauce and low-sodium canned beans.

 PBJ BOTTOM LINE: Babies' kidneys are not equipped to handle salt. Avoid salt as much as possible for babies less than 12 months and limit it to less than 800 mg per day (approximately ¼ teaspoon) for toddlers 1–3 years of age.

Q: Can my baby have gluten?

A: With the rise in popularity of gluten-free diets and the (unsubstantiated) claims that cutting out gluten helps treat childhood conditions like autism and attention deficit hyperactivity disorder (ADHD), many parents wonder if a gluten-free diet would benefit their baby.

Unless your child has celiac disease, an allergy to gluten diagnosed by a small bowel biopsy, the answer is no. Research does not support the use of a gluten-free diet for any other childhood medical condition. In fact, early introduction to gluten, between 6 and 12 months, may lower the risk of developing celiac disease.

If you or a family member has celiac disease, your child is at a higher risk of developing the condition themselves. You'll want to discuss introducing gluten with your pediatrician.

Not only is a gluten-free diet unnecessary for children without celiac disease, it is typically less nutritious. Grains contain important nutrients for babies like protein (gluten), iron, selenium, and magnesium. Grain-free alternatives often contain nutrient-poor filler ingredients and many are made with rice flour.

 PBJ BOTTOM LINE: Unless your child has celiac disease, a gluten-free diet is not a good idea. Gluten is found in one of the most nutrient-dense foods on earth, grains, which provide much-needed protein, fiber, iron, and zinc for growing bodies.

Q: Is soy safe for kids?

A: Ah, soy. On the list of foods that incite irrational fear, gluten is second only to the poor soybean. Soy has been unfairly demonized for decades following some very old and very poorly done studies in mice. More recent research has revealed that soy is not only *not* harmful, it is likely beneficial for chronic disease prevention including hormone-dependent cancers like breast and prostate cancer. And it seems that the earlier kids start eating soy the better. One study showed that women with a high soy intake had a reduced risk of breast cancer, but those who started consuming soy in early childhood had even greater risk reduction.

Numerous long-term studies have shown that soy is safe for infants and children. Claims that soy consumption results in feminization of boys or reproductive changes in young girls are not rooted in science. Adults who consumed soy formula as children have no differences in endocrine or reproductive functioning compared to those who were fed breast milk or cow's milk formula.

 PBJ BOTTOM LINE: Soy is perfectly safe for babies and an excellent source of plant-based protein as well as other beneficial nutrients like fat, fiber, iron, choline, and phytochemicals. We recommend including 2-3 servings of soy foods per day.

Q: I've heard about arsenic in baby food. Should I be concerned?

A: It's true that recent research has found that many rice products, specifically those intended for babies, contain high amounts of the carcinogenic element arsenic. This is because rice plants take up and concentrate arsenic from soil more than other cereal grains. It doesn't matter if the rice you eat is grown organically or conventionally; all rice plants have the same preference for extracting arsenic from soil. While the FDA regulates the amount of arsenic in our water supply, it does not limit or monitor arsenic in food. Brown rice has more arsenic, as it accumulates in the bran layer of the grain, which is removed to make white rice. Additionally, rice from Texas, Arkansas, and Louisiana has been shown to have higher levels, while rice from California tends to be lower. In order to minimize exposure, we recommend avoiding rice-based products for children, limiting whole rice consumption to 1–2 times a week, and varying your grains. Cooking rice like you cook pasta (using about 6 cups of water for each cup of rice and pouring off the extra water) can cut the arsenic content in half.

 PBJ BOTTOM LINE: Arsenic has been found in potentially harmful levels in many rice products, including those intended for infants and children. We recommend limiting rice intake.

3

First Sips
(0–6 Months)

Whether you breast- or bottle-feed, from day one, you have the ability to foster positive, lifelong dietary habits by adopting evidence-based feeding practices and nourishing yourself properly and selecting the best nourishment available for your little one.

A baby's nutrient needs during the first 6 months of life are higher than at any other time of life to support their rapid growth, both physically and mentally. A baby's brain forms 700 connections per second, operating at twice the activity level of an adult. In just a few short months, your immobile, unresponsive infant will transform into a smiling, giggling, wiggling, interactive ball of energy.

As we'd expect, given the plethora of benefits for adults and children, research suggests that plant-based nutrition during early infancy provides a multitude of health benefits.

For one, a plant-based mama's breast milk may be lower in environmental contaminants. High-fat animal products like dairy, meat, and eggs are the main source of persistent, bioaccumulative chemicals. One study reported that the levels of several toxins in the breast milk of plant-based moms was just 1%–2% of that reported in omnivorous women. Why? Well, the higher up on the food chain you are, the more toxins you accumulate. Persistent environmental pollutants are found in soil, and when animals eat plants, the pollutants accumulate in their tissues. When you eat animals, you consume larger amounts of those pollutants than you would if you only consumed whatever's in the soil. This is why it's better to eat small fish than large, predatory fish, which have higher levels of the neurotoxin mercury in their tissues. Infants are at the very top of the food chain since they derive all their food from human milk and are therefore at the highest risk of exposure to environmental toxins.

Breast milk from plant-based mamas may also be beneficial for babies by setting the stage for more adventurous eating. Our taste preferences are shaped well before

PBJ Quick Bite

Babies double their birth weight by 6 months and triple it by a year!

our first bite, and studies have shown that flavor compounds are present in both amniotic fluid and breast milk. One study showed that infants whose mothers regularly consumed carrot juice during the third trimester of pregnancy and during the first two months of breastfeeding showed fewer negative facial expressions when fed carrot-flavored cereal, compared to infants whose mothers drank plain water. A plant-based diet means that mom not only eats fewer animal products, she also (not surprisingly) eats more fruits and vegetables. An increased intake of these nutrient-rich foods by breastfeeding moms is likely to result in greater acceptance of them by babies.

PBJ Quick Bite

A plant-based mama's breast milk has been shown to be much lower in environmental toxins than omnivorous moms.

In this chapter, we'll dive into the specific nutritional considerations for breastfeeding and bottle-feeding and discuss common questions and concerns. We encourage moms that are having difficulties beyond the scope of this book to see a qualified IBLCE lactation consultant and/or a pediatric Registered Dietitian Nutritionist (RDN).

Feeding Baby Basics

In an ideal scenario, moments after your baby is born, they will be placed on your chest and they'll wiggle their way up to your waiting breast to gently sip their first drops of liquid gold. In reality, this often doesn't happen. Sometimes babies must be separated from mom immediately after birth for medical reasons. Sometimes babies don't latch right away. If this is your reality, try not to stress, Mama. The more relaxed you are in your approach to feeding, the better for both you and your baby.

PBJ Quick Bite

Babies start forming taste preferences in the womb through exposure to flavors in amniotic fluid from mom's diet.

For many new parents, the early days are filled with questions and concerns. *How do I know if my baby is getting enough milk? Is he pooping enough? Is he pooping too much? Should I give him a pacifier or will it jeopardize breastfeeding? Why is he spitting up like a scene out of* The Exorcist?

The litany of obsessive thoughts in the wee hours of the morning is exhausting. We're here to put those concerns to rest with some basic guidelines for infant feeding. You will likely still have those thoughts, which is totally normal for new parents and type A personalities (hello, fellow dietitians), but try to remind yourself that there is a wide range of normal behaviors and bodily fluids. If your baby is peeing, pooping, and growing, they are likely doing fine.

Feeding on Demand

The number one guideline is to feed on demand. This means responding to your baby's hunger cues as quickly as possible and as often as they signal. The exception to this rule is during the first 2 weeks of life (and possibly longer depending on your child). During this time, feed your newborn every 2 to 3 hours, even if they don't ask for it, until they've gained their birth weight back. This adds up to about 8 to 12 feedings per 24 hours.

AVERAGE INTAKE		
First week	**1–6 months**	**6–12 months**
1–2 oz per feeding, 8–12 feedings per day (~12–16 oz/day)	3–4 oz per feeding, 6–8 feedings per day (~24 oz/day)	6–8 oz per feeding, 4–5 feedings per day (~30–32 oz/day)

After they've returned to their birth weight, you can begin to feed according to their cues. This means letting your baby decide when and how much they want to eat—an important cornerstone of proper nutrition that will evolve as your baby grows older. If your child does not wake up hungry at night, you do not need to wake them up to feed. Much to most bedraggled parents' dismay, though, that's rarely the case. One study found that the average 3-month-old infant wakes up about 3 times each night. By about 4 months, most infants do not need middle-of-the-night feeds due to an increased intake during the day.

Responding to your baby's hunger signals as quickly as possible is important for so many reasons. Crying is often a late sign of hunger, and ignoring or delaying feeding, as suggested in some popular parenting books, has the potential to damage the infant-caregiver relationship, disrupt an infant's innate hunger-fullness regulation, and even harm them cognitively. One study showed that infants who were fed according to a schedule at 4 weeks old versus on-demand scored 4 points lower on IQ tests at age 8.

Feeding on demand accounts for the variable nature of a baby's energy needs. Even if you fall into a natural routine, there may be days when they need a little more or a little less, or may need to feed more frequently. Go with the flow. Growth spurts, weather changes, and developmental milestones can all affect feeding patterns. Babies tend to have growth spurts at 2 to 3 weeks, 6 weeks, and 3 months of age. If you're letting your baby lead the way, you cannot overfeed them. Babies have an innate ability to self-regulate their intake.

PBJ Quick Bite
Follow baby's lead and feed on demand. Every feed will be different—sometimes they need more, sometimes less. If you're letting your baby self-regulate, you cannot overfeed.

Keep in mind that breastfeeding infants will often drink smaller amounts and more frequently than formula-fed infants due to the quicker digestion of breast milk. Breast milk also varies in nutritional composition throughout the day, which results in more irregular feeding patterns.

Feeding on demand can be trickier when it comes to formula feeding. Parents and well-intentioned caregivers are often compelled to coax babies into taking one more sip or to finish the bottle, especially if they're worried about a baby's weight. We urge you not to do this and to educate anyone else in your child's care to avoid doing so as well. Forcing babies to finish a bottle disrupts their hunger and fullness self-regulation. When feeding from a bottle, watch your baby closely and monitor for signs of satiety. Hold the bottle at a slight tilt above horizontal, as opposed to a vertical angle, so that they can pace themselves instead of being forced to deal with a waterfall of oncoming milk. We recommend watching a video on paced bottle-feeding for guidance. If your baby gets fidgety or distracted, they are likely done. If your baby finishes a bottle and is still smacking their lips, they may still be hungry. Follow their lead.

Generally, feedings should take about 20 minutes (10–15 minutes per side if breastfeeding) but will vary depending on your baby's feeding style and strength. If feedings are taking a lot longer, your baby could have a poor latch

PBJ Quick Bite
Feedings take about 20 minutes on average (10–15 minutes per side if breastfeeding) but vary from baby to baby.

or be falling asleep at the breast. We recommend talking to your pediatrician or a lactation consultant.

EARLY SIGNS OF HUNGER
· Whimpering or lip-smacking
· Scrunching up arms or legs
· Increased alertness
· Putting hands toward mouth
· Making sucking motions and mouthing
· "Rooting" or nuzzling against your breast

Monitoring Intake

The number one question breastfeeding moms have is: How do I know if my baby is getting enough food? It sounds almost too simple to be true, but the answer is: if they're growing! If your baby is putting on weight and sticking to their growth curve, they're getting enough food. Whether your baby is in the 5th or 95th percentile for weight or height, if they're following that curve, it is healthy and normal. Problems arise when babies jump growth curves in short periods of time. If this occurs, your pediatrician will work with you to determine the cause.

AVERAGE WEIGHT GAIN					
	Days 1–4	Days 5–14	First 3 months	3–6 months	7–12 months
Appropriate Gain	Weight loss	~1 oz/day	~6–7 oz/week	~3.5–5 oz/week	~2.5–5 oz/week
Rule of Thumb	Loss of up to 10% body weight	Return to birth weight	Growth spurts every few weeks	Double birth weight	Triple birth weight

Most parents don't have a baby scale at home. Luckily, there's another more visual (and aromatic) cue—output. That's right, we're talking about poop. In the beginning, you'll want to monitor your baby's wet and dirty diapers for signs of proper intake. Don't worry—after a few weeks, once you've established a breastfeeding routine and your doctor's visits are going smoothly, you can forget all about this.

ADEQUATE OUTPUT*			
Days 1–2	**Days 3–4**	**Days 5–7**	**First month**
A few wet diapers	4–8 wet diapers	6+ wet diapers, pale colorless	6+ wet diapers
1–2 dark, tarry stools (meconium)	At least 2 stools, greenish/yellow	At least 3 stools, yellow, loose, small curds	At least 3 stools (often with each feeding) yellow, loose

Formula-fed babies will often have fewer dirty diapers.

After the first week of life, infants should have about 6–8 wet diapers per day. Wet diapers usually contain about 3 tablespoons, or 45 ml. This amount may be slightly less if your baby is urinating more frequently. If you are unsure of the amount, try pouring water into a clean diaper to compare and get used to the weight.

Dirty diapers are much more variable. Pooping several times a day or every few days can both be considered normal, provided the stools are soft and there is no blood. Baby poop also varies widely in color. Anything green, yellow, or brown is normal. If poop looks white, black, or reddish after the first few days of life, consult your physician.

We recommend using an app in the early days to track wet/dirty diapers and re-mind yourself of feedings every 2–3 hours.

Breastfeeding

We're evidence-based dietitians, as you've heard us reiterate many times. But before that, we're moms. Science aside, we know that not everyone will have the ability or means to breastfeed and that we're all just doing the best we can to care for our babes. We're going to provide an unbiased summary of the research on the subject, but we want you to know first and foremost that it is our belief that "fed is best."

While there are undeniable benefits to breastfeeding, which we'll review, they're not as cut-and-dried as some people would have you believe. If you can breastfeed, we recommend that you do. If you cannot, please know that you still can (and will) raise a happy, healthy, thriving child with the safe, effective formula options that are available.

Properties of Breast Milk

Breast milk is amazing. It is a dynamic, individual, and species-specific fluid that provides both nourishment and protection against harmful pathogens to infants whose bodies and brains are still developing. In addition to the nutritional components, breast milk is rich in antimicrobial, anti-inflammatory, and immunomodulatory molecules that help to develop an infant's digestive tract, promote the formation of a healthy microbiome, and stimulate their immune system.

PBJ Quick Bite

Breast milk provides not only nourishment but also bioactive compounds that support babies' immune system and protect them from disease and infections.

The composition of milk is highly variable from woman to woman. Differences may be due to maternal diet and health status, length of pregnancy, genetics, or the stage of lactation. For example, the protein content of milk is higher during the first few months of life, then levels out around the seventh month, while fat content steadily increases. The composition of milk even changes within the span of a single breastfeeding session, with fat content increasing toward the end of a feed. You may have heard this fat-rich portion of milk called "hindmilk."

Colostrum, also called "liquid gold," is the milk produced during the first few days of life. It is rich in antibodies, white blood cells, growth factors, and other immunological factors intended to protect baby from illness and infections. Colostrum is gradually replaced by "transitional milk," which progresses to mature milk by about the fourth week of life.

BENEFITS OF BREASTFEEDING

- Reduced risk of breast and ovarian cancer and diabetes (mom)
- Reduced risk of ear, nose, and throat infections
- Reduced risk of obesity
- Reduced risk of diabetes
- Reduced risk of childhood cancers
- Reduced risk of SIDs
- Potential cognitive benefits

Research continues to show incredible health benefits for both mothers and babies who breastfeed.

Moms who breastfeed are less likely to suffer from breast or ovarian cancer later in life. One study showed that breastfeeding for more than 12 months resulted in a 26% reduced risk of breast cancer and a 37% reduced risk of ovarian cancer. Women who breastfed also had a 32% reduced risk of type 2 diabetes. Furthermore, breastfeeding helps moms return to a healthy weight postpartum, as it expends calories.

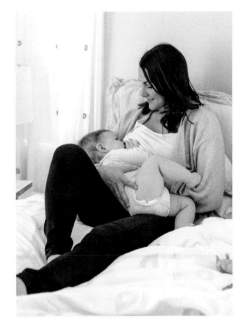

One of the largest and most demonstrated benefits of breastfeeding is the protection against infections. One study of 6-year-olds in the United States found that those who had been exclusively breastfed for 6 months or longer, or at least partially breastfed for 9 months or longer, had significantly reduced rates of ear, throat, and nasal infections in the previous year.

Breastfeeding has also been shown to reduce the risk of childhood obesity. Experts believe this may be related to hormones involved in fat metabolism and appetite regulation. Breastfed infants have higher levels of the satiety hormone leptin, while formula-fed infants have higher levels of the hunger hormone ghrelin. Another factor is exposure to a variety of flavors from breast milk, which could result in greater food acceptance and more adventurous eating. Finally, breastfed infants have shown to have better self-regulation of milk intake than bottle-fed infants, which could bear on future eating behaviors.

Breastfeeding may also reduce the risk of diabetes later in life. One review showed that breastfed infants had a 39% risk reduction compared to formula-fed infants and had lower levels of insulin, a marker of metabolic health. Not only that—research has suggested that breastfeeding results in higher IQ scores in children; however, these findings may be complicated by socioeconomic factors and parental education and intelligence.

Other studies have shown that breastfeeding may reduce the risk of childhood cancers like acute lymphoblastic leukemia, acute myeloblastic leukemia, and Hodgkin's lymphoma, possibly by reducing the risk of early viral infection. One study estimated that 14% to 19% of childhood leukemia cases could be prevented by *any* amount of breastfeeding, partial or exclusive, for 6 months or more.

Finally, breastfeeding reduces the risk of sudden infant death syndrome (SIDS). There are several proposed reasons for this. One is that breastfed infants are more easily aroused from sleep, an important survival mechanism. Another is that breast milk provides essential compounds required for immunity and central nervous system development, which could be lacking in formula. However, it isn't all or nothing. One meta-analysis showed that at least two months of *any* breastfeeding cut SIDS risk in half even when combined with formula. Keep in mind, though, that there are other factors that have been tied to SIDS risk or protection, including maternal smoking during pregnancy, sleep position, bed-sharing, prematurity, room-sharing, and the use of a pacifier.

How Long Should I Breastfeed?

The World Health Organization (WHO) recommends continued breastfeeding along with complementary foods up to 2 years of age or beyond. The American Academy of Pediatrics, however, recommends exclusive breastfeeding for the first 6 months of life and continued feeding until 1 year, though this advice is largely dictated by cultural norms and not by research on optimal nutrition.

Throughout history, traditional societies worldwide typically weaned between 2 and 4 years, and in some cultures, breastfeeding continues until age 6. The immunological factors found in breast milk are maintained in high concentrations throughout the second year of breastfeeding, which suggests continued benefits with extended feeding. However, we acknowledge the physical, social, and economic challenges of breastfeeding and encourage moms to continue as long as it feels positive for both you and your child.

PBJ Quick Bite

When it comes to breastfeeding, the majority of benefits are seen in the first 1–2 years of life.

Nutritional Considerations for Breastfeeding Moms

Breastfeeding, while a beautiful process, is also extremely physically taxing. We fondly recall our early postpartum days like survivors in a postapocalyptic world—stumbling around like bleary-eyed, ravenous zombies, running on adrenaline and takeout.

Energy

The number one complaint we hear from breastfeeding moms is "I'm always hungry!" This is 100 percent normal. Not only do new mamas need nourishment to repair their body after birth, but if breastfeeding, they must also continue to produce and provide nourishment for a voracious little being that will double his weight in just six months.

For this reason, nutrient needs increase across the board, beyond what is required during pregnancy. Breastfeeding expends about 500 additional calories per day to support a healthy milk supply. That's about an extra smoothie and peanut butter sandwich a day, so make sure not to let your intake dip below 1800 calories per day. Fewer calories than this, and you likely won't be able to meet the high nutrient demands of lactation, and your milk supply may suffer.

Though the temptation can be strong to quickly return to your pre-baby weight, we encourage new mamas to set aside societal expectations and focus instead on the incredible journey your body has been through. It took you nine months to grow this baby, and it will likely take an equally long time period (or more) for your body to heal. It may never "get back" to where it was before, and that's OK. Your body is a high-powered machine, capable of far more important things than meeting cultural beauty norms. Instead of worrying about what your body looks like, consider: How cool is it that you grew a human and will continue to provide the sustenance they need to thrive? The female body is truly remarkable. With a nutrient-rich, balanced diet, exercise, and time, your body will settle at its healthiest weight. There's no reason to rush it.

We recommend that breastfeeding moms consume 3 meals and 2–3 snacks per day. While intermittent fasting is all the rage, if you are hungry in the middle of the night while you're up tending to your barnacle (Whitney's nickname for baby Caleb), then eat! A balanced snack will ensure you have enough energy to do your job. Some of our favorite, easy, late-night munchies include: a banana and peanut butter, whole wheat toast with chia jam, and hemp energy balls. You can find recipes on our website and in our Predominantly Plant-Based Pregnancy Guide, found on our website at plantbasedjuniors.com.

PBJ Quick Bite

Breastfeeding moms need 500 extra calories a day. Don't let your intake drop below 1800 calories a day or it could jeopardize your milk supply.

Diet and Supplementation

The beauty of breast milk is that it is a perfectly designed food. It fluctuates to meet babies' changing demands yet maintains a stable amount of certain nutrients. However, some nutrients are subject to changes in mom's diet. Let's review which can be met through diet and which need close attention or supplementation.

DHA

Fatty acid composition varies depending on what mom eats. Women who consume diets rich in poly- and monounsaturated fatty acids, found in plant foods such as nuts, seeds, avocados, and olives, have higher amounts of these fats in their breast milk. Meanwhile, those who consume saturated fat–rich diets tend to have higher amounts of these fatty acids in their milk. Obese mothers are also more likely to have higher levels of saturated fat in their milk. One important fatty acid that is susceptible to mom's intake is DHA. As discussed in Chapter 1, the milk from vegan moms is low in DHA, so if you do not consume seafood, you should supplement with 300 mg per day to support your baby's growing brain.

Some research has shown benefits of supplementation with higher amounts of DHA for preterm infants. This is likely because DHA accumulation increases during the third trimester of pregnancy and preemies miss out on this critical window of DHA accrual. In one study, infants born at less than 33 weeks had increased visual acuity at 4 months corrected age when their moms supplemented with 3 grams of DHA per day.

B12

We won't hammer home the dangers of B12 deficiency, as we already touched on those in Chapter 1, but we will remind you that all plant-based moms must supplement with B12 in order to maintain adequate levels. One study showed 20% of vegan, vegetarian, and non-vegetarian women had inadequate levels of B12 in their milk, and this is despite the fact that 85% were taking B12 supplements or multivitamins. This is likely because the amounts in the multivitamins were not high enough to overcome the low absorption rates of supplemental B12. Plant-based breastfeeding moms should supplement with at least 150 mcg per day. If your pre/postnatal multivitamin does not contain this amount, take an additional supplement.

> *PBJ Quick Bite*
> Make sure your pre/postnatal vitamin has at least 150 mcg of B12 or add a supplement.

Choline

Back to the tricky topic of choline. As discussed, choline is a vital nutrient for baby's brain development, highlighted by the fact that large amounts are present in breast milk. Choline is sensitive to dietary intake, meaning the more moms consume, the more will be present in breast milk. But there are wide variations in the amount of choline in breast milk, regardless of diet. One study of breastfeeding women in Canada eating a typical omnivorous diet and women in Cambodia, whose diet was much lower in animal products, showed no significant difference. Another study showed that supplementation of choline with double the RDA resulted in only a 20% increase in breast milk choline concentration. This suggests that dietary choline may not play as large of a role in breast milk choline concentration as some believe and that increased choline synthesis in the liver may be a larger contributor.

PBJ Quick Bite

Soy is one of the richest sources of choline. Aim to eat 2 servings of soy foods (tofu, tempeh, soy milk, edamame) a day.

There's still a lot we have to learn about choline. We recommend breastfeeding moms go one of three routes to meet their dietary needs—(1) Consume 2–3 servings of soy foods per day, which are rich plant-based sources of choline. (2) Include eggs in the diet, one of the richest animal-based sources of choline. (3) Supplement. Many prenatal and postnatal multivitamins contain some choline, but usually not as high as we'd prefer. If you do not eat soy or eggs, supplement with at least 275 mg per day, half of the RDA for breastfeeding women.

Choline is available in the forms choline bitartrate, phosphatidylcholine, and lecithin. Some breastfeeding moms choose to take lecithin anyway, as it has shown potential benefits for treating and preventing clogged ducts and mastitis.

Iodine

Iodine in breast milk is also dependent on mom's intake. However, all prenatal vitamins are required to contain half of the RDA for pregnancy, which is sufficient for breastfeeding as well. You'll also be getting some iodine from plants and iodized salt, if you use it.

Vitamin D

Breast milk is naturally low in vitamin D, regardless of diet. Historically, babies likely got enough sunlight to generate their own vitamin D. We now know the dangers of sun damage and keep our little ones in the shade, therefore experts advise that all breastfed babies supplement with 400 IU per day of vitamin D. Some research has shown that when breastfeeding moms supplement with very high doses (~6400 mg per day), it is enough to raise vitamin D levels in their infants. However, the upper tolerable limit for vitamin D for breastfeeding women is 4000 IU per day. Therefore, we think the most sensible option is to provide your babe with his own daily drop. There are plenty of plant-based liquid drops on the market that you can give right from the tip of your finger, or on the nipple before feeding.

Iron

Early breastfeeding may be the one time when you don't have to worry much about iron. Iron is very low in breast milk and is not affected by mom's intake. Babies store up enough iron in the womb to hold them over for 4–6 months, when they begin solid food or bridge the gap with a short-term iron supplement. As discussed in Chapter 1, from 4 to 6 months (until they can meet needs through diet) the AAP recommends that all breastfed babies receive a daily iron supplement with 1 mg per kg of body weight.

Iron is the only nutrient that you need *less* of while breastfeeding due to the fact that it isn't found in large amounts in breast milk and many moms don't regain their menstrual cycle until they stop or significantly decrease breast-feeding. Therefore, you're not losing iron through milk or blood.

Continue eating iron-rich foods, but don't worry too much about it unless you were iron deficient prior to giving birth or lost large amounts of blood during delivery.

PBJ Quick Bite

Iron in breast milk is highly bioavailable—50%–70% of it is absorbed. However, breast milk only contains 0.3 mg of iron per liter! This is why all exclusively breastfed babies should receive an iron supplement with 1 mg per kg of body weight from 4 to 6 months.

Calcium

Calcium needs remain the same as during and prior to pregnancy. Calcium in breast milk is not reflective of mom's diet and is maintained regardless of what mom eats. That means that if your diet is deficient in calcium, you're going to suffer—not your babe. Calcium is leached from mom's bones to provide it to baby when diet is deficient, which we suppose is both good and bad news! It's important that just like during your pregnancy, you continue to optimize calcium in your diet with calcium-rich foods like fortified plant milk, calcium-set tofu, cruciferous veggies, legumes, and seeds. If you think you aren't able to meet your needs, an additional daily supplement may be a wise choice. Pre/postnatal vitamins do not contain large amounts of calcium, as it interferes with the absorption of minerals like iron and zinc, so if you decide to supplement, make sure to take calcium separately.

Pre/Postnatal Multivitamins

While most nutrient needs can be met with a balanced, varied diet, moms should continue to take a prenatal or postnatal multivitamin to fill any gaps. For plant-based moms specifically, prenatal vitamins will ensure you're meeting your needs for other nutrients of importance, such as vitamin A, on those days that you fall short. Because there are very few supplements on the market specifically intended for the postpartum period, the majority of breastfeeding women simply stay on their prenatal multivitamin.

Hydration

In addition to 24/7 snacking, many breastfeeding moms report insatiable thirst. This is not surprising, as hydration needs jump from 2.7 liters per day pre-pregnancy to 3.8 liters per day while breastfeeding. That's about 16 cups! Luckily, for those who aren't big fans of plain water, this increased need can also be met through food and other beverages. That means that your daily latte (yes, you can drink coffee—see below), kombucha, soup, and a serving of watermelon all count. We recommend keeping a large water bottle with you at all times.

PBJ Quick Bite

The only beverage infants under 6 months need is breast milk or formula.

Infants under 6 months old will receive all the hydration they need from breast milk or formula. There is no need to provide your baby with any other fluids until they begin solids.

Alcohol and Coffee

After teetotaling for almost 10 months, the last thing most new moms want to hear is that they must continue to limit or avoid certain foods and beverages. Good news, this is not the case. Research shows that the moderate consumption of both alcohol and coffee is safe for breastfeeding moms and their infants.

Alcohol

While the harmful effects of alcohol during pregnancy are well established, there's not a ton of research on alcohol consumption while breastfeeding. (One reason is that ethically we can't intentionally expose babies to alcohol-laden breast milk.)

The American Academy of Pediatrics takes a cautious stance and recommends that moms wait 2–3 hours to breastfeed after having 1 standard drink. This is in order to allow time for mom's blood alcohol level and breast milk alcohol content to decrease. But this isn't practical when you're breastfeeding every 2–3 hours.

Contrary to this conservative advice, studies of alcohol metabolism in lactating women and nursing infants indicate that while some alcohol does end up in breast milk, it's a very, very small amount. Alcohol content peaks between 30 minutes to 1 hour after consumption, and studies estimate that only 2%–6% of the maternal dose ends up in baby's bloodstream. Researchers of one literature review concluded that the amount is likely insignificant and "occasional drinking while breast-feeding has not been convincingly shown to adversely affect nursing infants."

One reason you may want to avoid alcohol is if you have a low milk supply. Contrary to popular belief, research does not support the idea that alcohol increases milk supply—no, not even Guinness. In fact, alcohol has been shown to inhibit the milk ejection reflex and result in decreased production in the hours following consumption. One study showed that women who consumed the amount of alcohol in a large glass of wine expressed 9.3% less breast milk in the next 2 hours. This happens in a dose-dependent fashion, meaning the more you drink, the less milk you'll make. They found that infants also drank less milk after mothers had consumed alcohol, likely due to decreased milk production, but that they made up for it in the next 24 hours. If you're dealing with low supply, it's possible that drinking alcohol may further impair your milk production, at least in the 2 hours following consumption.

PBJ Quick Bite

There is no evidence that alcohol (including dark beer) increases milk supply, or that consuming moderate alcohol while breastfeeding is harmful to mom or baby.

Do what feels right to you. We both felt confident that the state of the evidence supports the safety of drinking in moderation (1 standard drink per sitting) while breastfeeding. If you're concerned, wait 2–3 hours after having a drink. Note that there is never a need to "pump and dump." Alcohol passes freely in and out of breast milk and will decrease in concentration as your blood alcohol level decreases.

Coffee

Despite the fact that all major health organizations approve of moderate caffeine consumption during pregnancy and breastfeeding, don't be surprised if you get side-eye from your barista at Starbucks. The myth that pregnant and breastfeeding women need to completely avoid coffee and caffeine seems to somehow, bewilderingly, persist.

The truth is there's not a ton of research on caffeine intake during breastfeeding, but the studies we do have suggest that drinking coffee in moderation is perfectly safe and does not influence infant outcomes. In fact, caffeine is often given directly to pre-term babies in the hospital to help with breathing problems, which results in much larger concentrations than you'd get from drinking a latte-drinking mama's milk. One study estimated that only 1.5 mg of caffeine ends up in a liter of breast milk within an hour of consuming 1 cup of coffee (150 mg caffeine).

And don't blame coffee if your babe isn't sleeping. Two studies of breastfeeding moms' caffeine intake and baby's sleep quality showed no differences in episodes of night waking or duration of sleep. One of these studies also demonstrated that there was no difference in an infant's heart rate following the consumption of milk from their mothers drinking 500 mg caffeine (~5 cups of coffee) per day for 5 days.

In line with the American Academy of Pediatrics, Australian Breastfeeding Association, and European Food Safety Authority, we think 200–300 mg of caffeine per day, approximately the equivalent of 2 cups of coffee or lattes per day, is completely safe for breastfeeding moms and their babes.

Breastfeeding Troubleshooting

What we both found so astonishing about breastfeeding was the fact that something supposedly so innate could be so difficult. Whether due to a low supply, an oversupply, or mechanical issues, it's practically the norm for it to be a challenge. Many external and internal factors also impact a woman's ability to produce milk, including mental health, body image, work constraints, hospital and familial support, mode of delivery, length of gestation, and socioeconomic factors. You are not alone. We've compiled a list of the usual suspects when it comes to breastfeeding issues to help troubleshoot your issues. This is just a broad overview—if you need more help, consult your doctor or a lactation consultant.

PBJ Bottom Line: The following recommendations will ensure plant-based breastfeeding moms are properly nourishing themselves and their babes:

- Eat a little more than usual. Your body burns an additional 500 calories per day.

- Include good sources of unsaturated fats on a daily basis such as avocados, plant oils (e.g., avocado, flax, extra-virgin olive), nuts, and seeds.

- Take a daily pre- or postnatal multivitamin.

- Ensure your multivitamin contains at least 150 mcg/day of B12 or take an additional vitamin B12 supplement.

- Ensure your multivitamin contains at least 150 mcg/day of iodine or take an additional iodine supplement.

- Supplement with at least 300 mg/day of DHA from algae oil.

- Provide your baby with a daily 400 IU vitamin D supplement.

- From 4 to 6 months, provide your baby with a daily iron supplement containing 1 mg/kg/day.

- Consume at least 2 servings of soy foods per day, 1 or 2 eggs, and/or supplement with 275 mg of choline a day to meet choline needs.

- Hydrate! Breastfeeding moms need a lot of water. Keep a stainless steel bottle on you at all times. Add flavor with fresh berries, a lemon wedge, or a few cucumber slices if you get sick of plain water.

- Limit caffeine to 200–300 mg/day (approximately 2 cups of coffee).

- Limit alcohol to ≤1 drink per day. If possible, drink after feeding and wait 2–3 hours until feeding again.

Problems with Low Supply

It's estimated that about 5%–15% of women suffer from delayed or failed lactation. Early recognition and intervention is key. While there are often ways to increase supply, it's a good idea to try to identify why you're experiencing a low supply before you take action.

SIGNS OF INEFFECTIVE BREASTFEEDING
· Infant weight loss >7%
· Continued weight loss after third day of life
· No audible swallowing from the baby
· < 6 wet diapers per day after day 4
· < 3 stools per day after day 4
· Infant is irritable/restless or sleepy
· Minimal/no breast changes by day 5 after delivery
· Persistently/increasingly painful nipples

Ways to Increase Supply

Breastfeeding is about supply and demand. At the risk of making you feel even more like a human milk factory, one of the first strategies to try to increase production is to tell the warehouse manager that you need more product!

Feeding on demand and feeding frequently help establish a robust supply by signaling to your brain that you need more milk. When your baby sucks at the breast, it stimulates the release of the hormone prolactin from the pituitary gland, which triggers the mammary glands to produce milk. The frequency and intensity of an infant's sucking determines the amount of prolactin produced. To maximize production, you should aim to feed every 2–3 hours during the day, and every 3–4 hours at night. This may mean that you wake up to pump even if baby is sleeping longer stretches as they age.

Pumping immediately after feeding is another way to help boost supply, especially in the early days. Pumping maximizes breast stimulation and ensures complete breast emptying. Even if nothing is coming out, stimulating the breast tells the body that milk is in demand.

PBJ Quick Bite

Feeding on demand and feeding frequently are the best ways to boost milk supply.

Galactagogues, aka Foods, Beverages, and Herbs to Boost Supply

Talk to any mom who has had trouble breastfeeding and you're likely to hear a long list of common herbs, foods, and concoctions believed to boost production. Fenugreek, lactation cookies, and dark beer are commonly recommended. Despite positive anecdotal accounts and wide use in other countries and in alternative medicine, research on the benefits of supplements is, unfortunately, lacking.

We know that mamas who are having trouble producing milk want all the help they can get, so our stance on galactagogues is this: As long as a food/herb has shown to be safe during breastfeeding, it can't hurt to give it a try. Keep in mind, however, that the majority of herbs have not been shown to be safe for breastfeeding. Talk to your doctor before incorporating any supplement into your routine.

Fenugreek

The one herb that we feel comfortable recommending is fenugreek. In one study, fenugreek tea was shown to increase milk volume more than a placebo. While the Academy of Breastfeeding Medicine states that there is insufficient evidence to support using fenugreek as a galactagogue, we say that for most people, it can't hurt to try.

Alex's midwife encouraged taking enough fenugreek to make her smell like maple syrup, though we don't advise you to supplement based on smell. The recommended dosage is 1000–1500 mg 3x/day.

Fenugreek should not be used if you have hypothyroidism, diabetes, or an allergy to peanuts or chickpeas, as they are in the same family. Fenugreek should also be avoided during pregnancy, as it has been shown to cause contractions, premature labor, and miscarriage.

Oats

Another frequently recommended milk booster is oats. While these oatmeal-eating mamas would love to tell you that there is a bulk of research out there, there is not a single scientific study showing their benefit. But—absence of evidence isn't evidence of absence. Many mamas we've talked to report increased milk production by adding oats to their diet. One potential reason for this is that oats are a good source of plant-

> **PBJ Bottom Line: Most herbs that are promoted as galactagogues have no scientific evidence of efficacy, and may be harmful to infants. Fenugreek is the only herb with ample research supporting its use. Always consult your pediatrician or ob-gyn before taking a new supplement. Remember that many herbs, including fenugreek, are not safe during pregnancy.**

based iron, and iron deficiency has been linked to poor milk production. Considering that oats are safe and super nutritious, we say give them a try.

Oversupply

If you're a mom suffering from low supply, having "too much milk" may seem like a champagne problem. Trust us, it's not. Oversupply can be incredibly distressing to a new mom and cause a host of problems.

While there is no set amount of milk production that defines an oversupply, some indications that you may be an overproducer include:

- Baby chokes and sputters at the breast
- Baby cries or lets go during feeding due to a forceful ejection reflex
- Baby arches back when feeding
- Baby's stools are green and frothy (possibly due to lactose overload)
- Recurrent plugged ducts
- Recurrent mastitis

What to Do if You Have an Oversupply

We recommend working with a lactation consultant to figure out a proper course of action for managing your oversupply. Trying to decrease your supply can be tricky and is not recommended in the first three months, as it can have the reverse effect and lead to low milk supply. Drinking less fluid in particular is not recommended. Breastfeeding moms need to stay hydrated!

What you can do is take steps to prevent the painful side effects of oversupply.

Preventing and Treating Plugged Ducts

The best way to describe a plugged duct to someone who has never experienced it is to imagine a golf ball lodged inside your boob—yeah, not fun. Whitney got them on a near daily basis while breastfeeding her son and spent many hours in the shower massaging her chest with the back of an electric toothbrush.

Plugged ducts occur when milk is obstructed from moving through the mammary ducts. Frequent causes include infrequent or incomplete emptying of the breast, injury, poor latch, or oversupply. In order to prevent them, moms should avoid going for long periods of time without nursing or pumping, avoid wearing tight or ill-fitting bras, and be evaluated by a lactation consultant for proper latch and breastfeeding position.

Plugged ducts usually resolve within a day or so, but there are a few things that may help relieve them:

- Nurse as frequently as possible on the side with the plug. Some mamas find that breastfeeding in a position that capitalizes on gravity, like kneeling on all fours over their babe (on a soft floor or bed), can work.
- Take a warm bath or shower before feeding.
- Use a warm, wet compress before feeding.
- Massage the area starting behind the plug and working toward the nipple.
- Use a hand massager or electric toothbrush to massage the area.

Supplementing with 1200 mg of soy or sunflower lecithin up to 4 times a day may also be beneficial for prevention by helping breast milk pass more freely through the ducts.

Preventing and Treating Mastitis

Mastitis, aka "the boob flu," is a real pain in the tit. What starts as pain and inflammation in the boob, often due to a clogged duct, can turn into a full-blown infection and potentially a breast abscess that would need to be surgically drained. About 10% of moms will suffer from mastitis, and it often leads to the discontinuation of breastfeeding.

There's no definitive cause of mastitis, but the risk factors are similar to the culprits of clogged ducts. Frequent nursing, complete emptying of the breast, and ensuring proper feeding technique/latch can reduce your risk of coming down with this nasty infection.

Symptoms of mastitis include:

PBJ Quick Bite

Probiotics with *L. fermentum* or *L. salivarius* may help with mastitis.

- Pain in breast
- Swelling and localized red streaks on breast
- Fever of 101°F or higher
- Body aches and/or headache
- Fatigue

Mastitis may clear up on its own, but depending on the severity of the infection, antibiotics may be necessary. Rest, hydration, and massaging the affected area if there is a plugged duct may also help.

Correcting improper feeding techniques or latch issues may prevent the recurrence of mastitis. Additionally, some research shows that certain strains of *Lactobacillus* may prevent and treat recurrent bouts. One study showed that women with mastitis who consumed supplements of either *L. fermentum* or *L. salivarius* for three weeks had more improvement and a lower rate of recurrence compared to women who took antibiotics.

As research in this area is scant and probiotics are strain specific, we do not recommend trying to treat mastitis with probiotics alone. However, we do think they are a safe and potentially beneficial option. Whitney gave them a shot after suffering recurrent bouts of mastitis and believes that they helped her fend off further infections, along with other tactics.

PBJ Quick Bite

Formula doesn't have to be all or nothing. You can supplement your low supply while continuing your breastfeeding relationship if you want to.

Formula Feeding

We know formula isn't many parents' first choice. But as we said before, fed is best. There are so many reasons a mom may not choose to or be able to breastfeed—from low supply to mental and socioeconomic issues, which are unique to each woman. If you're one of the 75% of parents who use formula at some point during the first year—whether out of medical necessity or personal choice—we support you and we want you to feel confident in your decision. Your route of feeding does not dictate your virtue as a mother. Despite the benefits of breastfeeding we've discussed, formula-fed babies grow up to be healthy, thriving children (we were both formula-fed at some point and we think we turned out OK).

We also want you to know that it doesn't have to be all or nothing. You can absolutely combine breastfeeding and supplementing with formula to meet needs due to low production or mom's work schedule.

One of the benefits of formula is that you don't have to worry about whether your baby is getting enough of any essential nutrients. Baby formulas are strictly regulated to contain specific amounts of macronutrients, vitamins, and minerals to mimic breast milk. If you are providing formula on demand, your baby needs no other food or beverages until 6 months of age and no other supplements until they discontinue formula.

Alex's Story

Before I had a baby, I was firmly in the "breast is best" camp. I had read *The Womanly Art of Breastfeeding,* identified lactation groups to join once baby had arrived, and planned on breastfeeding for as long as my baby would let me. My sister breastfed both of her kids well into their second year of life, and I figured that I would likely do the same.

Now that I am a mom, I'm an advocate for *"fed* is best." While we absolutely encourage breastfeeding and are here to help support you in your journey, we also know that it doesn't always come easy. Without a doubt, human milk is superior to formula in many respects, including ways we will probably never fully understand. We can agree on that. However, like so many things in parenthood, not everything happens according to plan, and for many committed, nutrition-conscious moms, that can include breastfeeding.

It wasn't until we were standing in the pediatrician's office on day five, discussing how much weight my baby had lost and how dehydrated he was, that I came face-to-face with reality. I wasn't producing enough milk to meet his needs and I needed to supplement while we tried to increase my supply.

In the breastfeeding community, supplementation is often painted as unnecessary and harmful. However, in the case of chronic low supply, supplementation is absolutely necessary for the health of the baby and can even help preserve supply. It will not lead to the end of your breastfeeding relationship, unless you want it to. Speaking as someone who has dealt with low supply since day one, I can tell you that we were still able to have a beautiful breastfeeding relationship even though he was also on formula since day five.

Whether you choose to breastfeed, formula-feed, or a little of both, remember that love is not measured in ounces and that you are a great mom, whatever nourishment you choose to provide.

Choosing a Formula

For many plant-based parents, the choice of a formula is fairly straightforward. Soy- or pea-protein-based formulas are safe, cruelty-free options. Other parents may decide that although they follow a predominantly or fully plant-based diet and plan to raise their children the same way, they are more comfortable providing a cow's milk–based formula. Certain conditions may also preclude plant-based parents from choosing soy formula. We support whichever route you choose to go. Both options provide reliable nourishment for your babe.

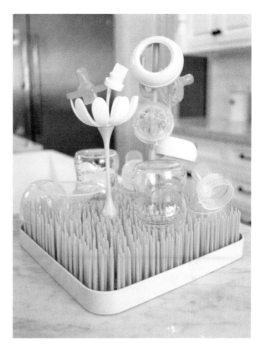

Cow's Milk Formulas

The composition of cow's milk formula for healthy, full-term infants varies by brand and is constantly evolving as we learn more about infants' nutritional needs. Formula typically contains between 19 and 20 calories per ounce, and the US Infant Formula Act sets standards for the minimum and maximum levels of protein, fat, and certain micronutrients such as iron.

Standard formulas contain between 0.4 and 0.5 grams of protein per ounce, which is about 50% more protein than in human breast milk. The protein composition of cow's milk formula also differs from breast milk in that it has a much higher ratio of casein to whey compared to breast milk. Cow's milk contains 80% casein, while breast milk is only 40% casein. It's unclear what this means for human health, but we note it to show that cow's milk is not an identical replacement. Some formulas now add whey protein to try to match the higher whey-to-protein ratio.

The main carbohydrate in both breast milk and cow's milk formula is lactose. Despite the fact that the majority of adults worldwide are lactose intolerant, lactose is the preferred source of energy for infants, and the majority are born with the enzyme required to digest it properly for the first few years of life.

Some formulas contain modified starches or maltodextrin, carbohydrate derivatives that help thicken the liquid. We prefer formulations with as few additives as possible.

Fat makes up about 40%–50% of cow's milk formula and is mainly derived from vegetable oils such as coconut, palm, soy, sunflower, and safflower. These oils are better absorbed than the fat from cow's milk and are mixed to provide an ideal balance of essential fatty acids. Most major brands also add DHA (docosahexaenoic acid) and ARA (arachidonic acid), which provide visual and cognitive benefits for both preterm and term infants.

As formula continues to evolve to more closely resemble human breast milk, companies are also exploring ingredients like human milk oligosaccharides (HMOs), which are believed to be important for infant growth and development. HMOs are indigestible carbohydrates that feed babies' developing microbiome and are abundant in breast milk.

Soy Formulas

Soy formulas have been safely used for infant feeding for over 100 years. They are generally made of soy protein isolate supplemented with the amino acids methionine and taurine and the fatty acid transporter carnitine, as these compounds tend to be lower in soy than in cow's milk and infants are not able to produce their own. As for cow's milk formula, manufacturers add a combination of soy, palm, sunflower, olein, safflower, and coconut oils to achieve a similar amount of fat as breast milk. Plants do not contain lactose, so soy formulas use corn syrup, corn maltodextrin, brown rice syrup, or sugar to provide essential carbohydrates.

Claims that soy formula is harmful to infants are not supported by science. Studies show similar rates of growth, energy intake, and bone mineralization between babies who receive soy and cow's milk formula. In its position paper, the AAP notes, "There is no conclusive evidence from animal, adult human, or infant populations that dietary soy isoflavones may adversely affect human development, reproduction, or endocrine function."

Soy protein has been given to infants for centuries in Asian countries. And while high exposure to soy phytochemicals known as isoflavones has been noted in infants born to Japanese mothers, Asian cultures also tend to have the lowest rates of hormone-dependent cancers.

Likewise, there's no demonstrated increased risk of feminization in boys fed soy formula. One study of adults 20–34 years old who were fed soy formula as babies showed no differences in endocrine and reproductive functioning. It did note a longer duration of menstrual bleeding and more self-reported discomfort in women fed soy formula as children, but researchers cautioned against giving too much weight to this outcome, considering they did not observe differences in total blood flow or in any other of 30 different reproductive indicators measured.

Another concern about soy formula is its aluminum content. For a number of reasons—including natural uptake from the soil—the aluminum content of soy formula is higher than that in cow's milk or breast milk. However, research has found that the amount of aluminum in soy formula falls below established safety limits, and infants drinking cow's milk formula and soy formula have similar blood levels of aluminum. Therefore, while aluminum is not an essential mineral and can be harmful in excessive amounts, we do not think it is a reason to avoid this option for healthy, full-term infants.

An interesting possible benefit of soy formula is its potential to reduce infections. One study tested the antiviral activity of isoflavones in the concentration typically found in soy formula against *Rotavirus*, the most common cause of diarrhea in infants and children, and found that soy isoflavones were able to reduce the viral activity by 66%–74%.

When Soy Formula Is Not Recommended

Soy formula may not be a good choice for infants with congenital hypothyroidism, as the phytates in soy can interfere with the absorption of medication used to treat the condition. This may be overcome with an increased dose of the medication.

Additionally, soy formula is not recommended for preterm infants. Studies show that while bone mineralization is similar in term babies receiving soy formula, preterm infants have a greater risk of osteopenia. This may be in part because preterm infants' kidneys are underdeveloped and they are unable to properly excrete aluminum. Aluminum competes with calcium for absorption and is found in higher amounts in soy formula than in breast or cow's milk, as discussed above.

PBJ BOTTOM LINE: If your baby is premature or has congenital hypothyroidism, cow's milk formula is recommended. If your baby is healthy and full-term, then the decision is personal. Cow's milk and soy milk formula are both safe and promote equal rates of growth. Claims that soy causes endocrine or reproductive problems are unwarranted.

Fluoride

Fluoride is a nonessential mineral found in small amounts throughout the food supply. In many countries, including the US, fluoride has been added to community drinking water since the 1940s, after it was discovered that fluoride consumption reduced rates of tooth decay and dental caries, particularly in children.

Despite criticism of the practice from some groups, the American Academy of Pediatrics, the American Dental Association, and the Centers for Disease Control and Prevention all support fluoridation for the protection of both pre-eruptive and post-eruptive teeth—meaning even before your little one has sprouted chompers, fluoride helps strengthen them.

Common Questions and Challenges

Q: My baby is spitting up a lot. Is this normal? How much is too much?
A: Frequent spitting up after feedings is normal and may be caused by gas, overfeeding, or reflux. Babies' digestive systems are still developing and they don't have the same esophageal control that adults do. Rest assured, the spit-up looks like a lot more than it really is. If your baby doesn't seem distressed and is gaining weight normally, there is no cause for concern. We call these babes "happy spitters." You can reduce the frequency of post-feeding reflux by keeping baby upright for 15 to 30 minutes after feedings.

However, if spitting up occurs extremely frequently or is accompanied by diarrhea, rash, or failure to gain weight, this could be a sign of a food allergy or gastrointestinal issues. Speak to your physician if you are concerned.

> **PBJ Quick Bite**
> Keep baby upright for 15–30 minutes after feedings to reduce spit-up.

Q: Will introducing a pacifier or bottle jeopardize breastfeeding?
A: Contrary to popular belief, infants are pretty smart and don't seem to have a problem differentiating between a cold, plastic apparatus and a human nipple.

Using a pacifier will not jeopardize your chance of a successful breastfeeding relationship. Pacifiers may actually benefit your breastfeeding relationship, as they help infants self-soothe and reduce the chance of baby using *you* as a human pacifier!

(Whitney's son would not take a pacifier, so she learned about this firsthand.) Pacifier use has also been shown to reduce the risk of SIDS.

Similarly, bottle use shouldn't impact breastfeeding, provided that you are still expressing milk when you miss a feeding. Most experts recommend waiting at least two weeks, until your milk production is firmly established, before introducing a bottle.

Q: My baby is very fussy—could it be a food sensitivity or an allergy?
A: It certainly could be, but it's important to differentiate between the two.

Food sensitivities are the result of digestive issues versus an immune system reaction. They are less severe than allergies and do not typically cause rashes or impaired breathing. Because a mom's diet varies widely each day, food sensitivities can be tricky to pinpoint. While there's not a lot of research in this area, some moms report increased infant fussiness following the consumption of spicy foods, cruciferous vegetables, caffeine, or dairy. If you think a sensitivity may be the issue, try cutting out one food at a time for about a week to see if the symptoms improve. Then reintroduce it while monitoring for a return of symptoms.

Food allergies are caused when the immune system identifies and overreacts to proteins in foods. These can be life-threatening, and symptoms in infants may include severe colic, abdominal discomfort, eczema or hives, vomiting, severe diarrhea (often with blood in the stool), or difficulty breathing. If you suspect a food allergy, talk to your pediatrician immediately.

*Q: I'm breastfeeding, and my baby has a cow's milk protein allergy/intolerance—
do I have to eliminate soy too? If so, how do I maintain my protein intake?*
A: Studies show that about 30%–64% of infants with cow's milk protein intolerance—usually demonstrated by frequent vomiting, diarrhea, or bloody stools—also have an intolerance to soy protein. Experts believe that when cow's milk protein damages a baby's gut mucosa, it then allows other proteins like soy to slip through and trigger an immune response.

Breastfeeding moms are frequently asked to remove both dairy and soy from their diet in these cases, which can be challenging for plant-based mamas. We recommend trying an elimination diet first to determine if soy is truly an issue. To do this, cut out all soy and dairy for at least two weeks (be diligent about reading labels during this time for hidden sources of each). Then add soy back into your diet and monitor for a reaction. It may be helpful to work with a dietitian or grab a book on elimination diets.

We like *The 14-Day Elimination Diet Plan: Identify Food Allergies and Sensitivities the No-Stress Way* by dietitian Tara Rochford.

If your child does have an intolerance to soy, you can work around it! There are plenty of other protein-rich, non-soy plant foods to enjoy, including beans, nuts, seeds, and whole grains.

You'll also be glad to know that these intolerances are often age-dependent and most children outgrow them by age 5.

Q: Should I give my baby probiotics?
A: While we don't think routine supplementation is necessary, there are certain cases where probiotics have shown to be beneficial for infants.

Some research has shown that colicky infants have reduced colonization of *Lactobacillus* species in their gut and an increased amount of harmful bacteria like *E. coli*. Several studies have shown that *Lactobacillus reuteri* may benefit these infants by shortening crying times, although these results were mainly demonstrated in breast-fed infants. Research also shows that probiotics may reduce the risk of necrotizing enterocolitis in preterm infants. This is something the hospital will provide if indicated for your child.

If you think a probiotic may benefit your baby, be sure to talk to your pediatrician or dietitian to ensure it is safe. It's important that you not only get the right *species* of bacteria, but also the right *strain*.

4

First Bites
(6-12 Months)

tarting solids is a highly anticipated event for most new parents. We remember eagerly counting down the days until our sons' six-month mark, when we could finally implement the tools and tricks we'd been researching since long before they were born, and putting to use the adorably designed feeding supplies we'd stockpiled and recipes we'd bookmarked.

On the flip side, the simple act of introducing solids can sometimes feel overly complicated. We know from our own experience, and from talking with other parents, that they sometimes feel overwhelmed by the seemingly endless opinions and decisions when it comes to feeding babies. From the "right" style to the "right" first foods, it seems that everyone has a point of view on how to best feed your child. After all, parenting is the easiest thing to have an opinion about, but one of the hardest things to do.

Feeding children should be a time of enjoyment and excitement, not stress. That's one of the reasons we wanted to write this book—to celebrate the fun and exciting role of helping shape our children's palate. While there are a few nutrients that you'll want to ensure to offer, food before one is *somewhat* for fun. It's a time for baby to explore and experiment with food one nibble and slurp at a time. Offering your child the space to get their hands (and face, neck, stomach, hair, feet, high chair, ceiling) dirty is a great first step in raising adventurous eaters.

Let's get one thing straight: There is not a "best" way to introduce solids. We'll discuss both of the two major approaches to infant feeding: traditional purees and baby-led weaning. While we are here to share nutrition science, practical tips, and our own journeys, we want you to feel empowered to choose the route of feeding that feels best for you and baby.

Starting Solids:
Baby-Led Weaning versus a Traditional Approach

Baby-led weaning is essentially the concept of giving babies solid food right from the start, without the use of purees. The term "weaning" can be confusing, as it implies that you're weaning baby off breast milk or formula. That's not the case. Complementary feeding is a more accurate description. You'll still be offering breast milk or formula regularly until your baby's first birthday and possibly beyond. Instead, baby-led weaning refers to gently introducing baby to solid finger foods right from the start, allowing them the opportunity to explore various flavors and textures.

In contrast, a traditional approach to solids starts with spoon-feeding baby purees—smooth, liquefied blends—and gradually increasing the texture and consistency of food until they are eating normal foods around 12 months. Finger foods are often incorporated around 8 months.

Babies develop at different paces. Some are eager to start solids, while others may need more support, and there is no "right" approach. We suggest you let baby take the lead on what they need.

If you explore the baby-led weaning community, you may see various rules about what you should or shouldn't do. Some circles advocate strict baby-led weaning, with no purees at all, even if your baby enjoys them. The argument is that babies will become confused between solids and purees, which may increase their choking risk or delay their feeding abilities. The good news is that there is absolutely no research that says that's true. Like we said, babies are smart; they can differentiate between a pouch, puree, finger food, or spoon-fed food.

Benefits of Baby-Led Weaning

Baby-led weaning may seem like a novel approach, but it's actually a return to how babies were first introduced to solids. Commercial baby-food purees weren't widely available until the 1930s. Prior to this, parents created their own or gave babies the same table food as adults.

There isn't a robust library of research on baby-led weaning, though many feeding experts agree that one of the biggest benefits of self-feeding is a greater understanding of satiety, or how much one needs to eat to feel full. Infants weaned using this approach have been shown to be more satiety-responsive compared to those who are spoon-fed.

As baby is responsible for how much food they eat from day one, there is no pressure for them to take "just one more bite," which can be the case when caregivers coax babies into finishing jars of baby food. Baby-led weaning also gives the opportunity to catch nonverbal cues that baby is full and finished eating.

While childhood obesity is a complex, multifaceted problem, this ability to self-regulate may help prevent it. Several studies have shown that infants fed using a traditional spoon-fed approach were significantly heavier at 18–24 months compared to those fed using a baby-led weaning approach.

At a basic level, it makes sense. We're born to eat, and in infancy the only driving force is true hunger, not external influences. There's no such thing as emotional eating in infancy. If baby isn't hungry, they aren't going to eat. To us, a baby-led weaning approach is a return to what nature intended—trusting babies' innate ability to feed themselves. While more research in this area is certainly needed, we feel that the preliminary results are overwhelmingly positive and encouraging.

Will Baby-Led Weaning Make My Baby Less Picky?

Many parents believe that using baby-led weaning made their child a less picky eater. This is based on the idea that baby-led weaning can expose babies to a wider variety of food, flavors, and textures during the first few months of solid feeding than purees, which some believe leads to a greater acceptance of diverse foods. While this was true anecdotally for Alex's son, the research on this theory isn't conclusive.

While one study showed that baby-led weaning infants were significantly less picky than their spoon-fed peers, others have shown more differences in the types of foods infants prefer versus the range.

In one study, infants who were fed using baby-led weaning showed a preference for carbohydrate-based foods, while infants who were fed using a traditional approach showed a preference toward sweets. In the BLISS (baby-led introduction to solids) study, the largest baby-led weaning study to date, infants who followed baby-led weaning also had greater intake of salt and sugar. This makes sense, as commercial baby food doesn't contain any added sodium or sugar, whereas homemade table food is likely to contain both. Experts recommend limiting sodium and sugar as much as possible before 1 year of age, which is why we recommend that baby-led weaning parents pay special attention to both.

PBJ Bottom Line: Baby-led weaning is an approach to starting solids where babies feed themselves finger food right from the start, skipping purees and spoon-feeding. Research shows this may promote a more positive relationship with food and a reduced incidence of obesity, as it allows baby to self-regulate intake. While some parents report less picky eating with baby-led weaning, there isn't firm research supporting this. Baby-led weaning parents should pay special attention to baby's salt and sugar intake and limit them in family meals.

Baby-Led Weaning 101: When to Start

The decision of when to start solids is ultimately up to you and your pediatrician, but there are a few milestones you'll want to make sure baby has reached before beginning baby-led weaning. First, baby should be close to 6 months old. Both the American Academy of Pediatrics and the World Health Organization recommend waiting until 6 months to begin solids, as babies are more likely to have reached developmental milestones required for feeding.

There is wiggle room, especially if there is a food-allergy risk (more on this later), but for a baby-led weaning approach, they will likely need to be closer to 6 months in order to eat safely.

There are no benefits to starting earlier than 4 months. Research shows that feeding infants solids before that is associated with higher incidences of eczema, obesity, and type 1 diabetes. And in case you're tempted to start early in the hopes that feeding baby solids will help them sleep through the night longer, please know that's a myth.

SIGNS OF READINESS
• Baby is 6 months old.
• Baby can sit up on their own.
• Baby is losing the tongue thrust reflex.
• Baby is excited about food.

In addition to age, baby should be starting to lose the tongue thrust, a natural reflex where the tongue pushes food out of the month. To determine if your little one still has it, try this test: Place a tiny bit of appropriate food thinned with breast milk or formula in baby's mouth with the tip of a baby spoon or your finger. If baby pushes the food right out with their tongue, the thrust is still present.

Baby should also be able to sit up on their own for at least 60 seconds. We want gravity and the esophagus to work in harmony. If baby is slouching forward, that can increase choking risk.

Finally, baby should be excited to eat! Babies are great at letting us know when they are ready for real food. You may start to notice them ogling your plate, attempting to grab food, or moving their mouth in anticipation of feeding while you are eating. These are all signs that baby is raring to go.

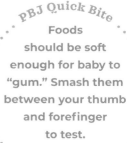

PBJ Quick Bite

Foods should be soft enough for baby to "gum." Smash them between your thumb and forefinger to test.

How to Start

It may seem straightforward—offer baby a piece of food and see what happens. But we both remember Googling "how to start baby-led weaning," so we know most parents can use guidance.

Start by placing age- and texture-appropriate finger food within baby's reach. Have them sit with you and the family at mealtime, and when they are ready, they will grab a bite of food and put it in their mouth. If they seem unsure but interested, you can also place the food directly into their palm. There you go—you've started baby-led weaning!

All food should be soft enough for baby to gum, meaning they can mash it with their gums. If you are able to smoosh the food between your pointer finger and thumb, then it's soft enough.

From roughly 6 to 8 months, your baby will use a palmar grasp to pick up food. This means they'll use their whole hand to create a fist around food and eat whatever sticks out the top. Long strips that are about the width of your pinkie and foods with handles are perfect for this age. The pincer grasp, where baby picks up food using their thumb and pointer finger, doesn't usually develop until 8 to 10 months of age. So at first, baby won't be able to pick up small pieces of food.

Here is a visual example of how common foods should be cut at 6 and 8 months.

BABY-LED WEANING CUTS: 6 MONTHS

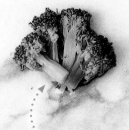

PEACHES

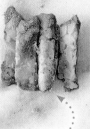

BROCCOLI

TEMPEH

STEAMED CUCUMBER

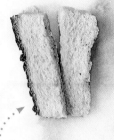

TOAST

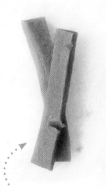

ROASTED SQUASH

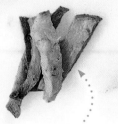

SWEET POTATOES

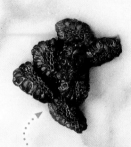

RASPBERRIES

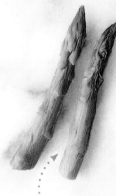

ASPARAGUS

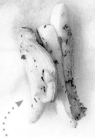

CARROTS

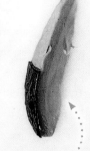

AVOCADO

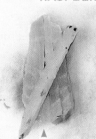

BEETS

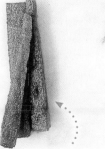

WATERMELON

MANGOES

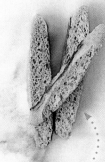

PANCAKES

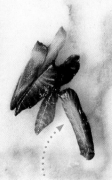

STRAWBERRIES

BABY-LED WEANING CUTS: 8 MONTHS

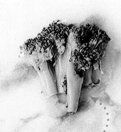 PEACHES

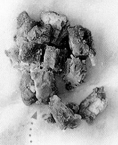 BROCCOLI

TEMPEH

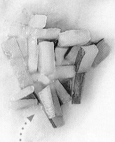 STEAMED CUCUMBER

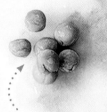 PEAS

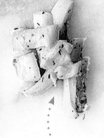 ROASTED SQUASH

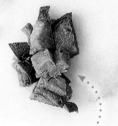 SWEET POTATOES

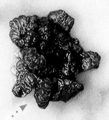 RASPBERRIES

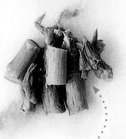 ASPARAGUS

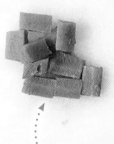 CARROTS

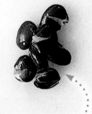 BLACK BEANS

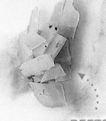 BEETS

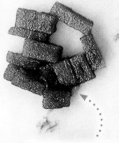 WATERMELON

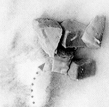 MANGOES

AVOCADO

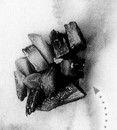 STRAWBERRIES

While you may encounter rare examples on social media of six-month-old babies taking down full plates of food, these are the exception, not the rule. Learning to eat is a slow process. It took Alex's son Vander almost three weeks to understand the concept. She offered him one meal a day to start with, breakfast, then built up from there. For Whitney, it took months before her son would consistently accept meals. Think about it. Breast milk and formula has been an easy source of nourishment up until this point, and eating is a lot of work. If they don't seem interested or get frustrated, stop and offer again at the next mealtime or the next day.

FOOD	PREPARATION	HOW TO COOK	FAVORITE FLAVOR PAIRING
Vegetables			
Asparagus	Halve, depending on size, and remove woody ends. Slice into 3-inch pieces, depending on length.	Steam for 8 minutes; roast at 400°F for 10–15 minutes.	Toss with fresh lemon juice, oil, and chopped tarragon.
Beets	Peel and slice into pinky finger–like shapes.	Steam for 15 minutes; steam roast at 400°F for 25–30 minutes.	Toss with oil and dried dill and/or caraway seeds.
Bell Pepper	Peel and slice into pinky finger–like strips.	Steam for 5 minutes; roast at 400°F for 10–15 minutes.	Toss with oil and garlic powder.
Broccoli	Slice into strips, with at least 1–2 inches of the stalk for baby to hold as a handle.	Steam for 5–7 minutes; roast at 400°F for 20 minutes.	Dip the leafy floret into homemade vegan parmesan cheese or toss with olive oil, ground fennel, ground basil, ground oregano, and ground garlic powder for "pizza trees!"
Brussels Sprouts	Quarter, trimming any tough ends.	Steam for 10–15 minutes; steam roast at 400°F for 20–25 minutes.	Toss with oil and lemon juice or garlic powder.
Butternut Squash	Peel and slice into pinky finger–like shapes.	Steam for 15–20 minutes; steam roast at 400°F for 30 minutes.	Toss with oil and pumpkin pie seasoning.
Cauliflower	Slice into strips, leaving at least 1–2 inches of the stalk for baby to hold as a handle.	Steam for 5–7 minutes; roast at 400°F for 20 minutes.	Toss with oil and curry powder or a salt-free seasoning blend.

FOOD	PREPARATION	HOW TO COOK	FAVORITE FLAVOR PAIRING
Green Beans	Halve, if thick, and remove any pointed ends.	Steam for 5–8 minutes; roast at 400°F for 10–15 minutes.	Toss with oil and lemon juice or garlic powder.
Potatoes	Peel and slice into pinky finger–like shapes.	Steam for 15 minutes; steam roast at 400°F for 25 minutes.	Toss with oil and curry powder.
Sweet Potatoes	Peel and slice into pinky finger–like shapes.	Steam for 15 minutes; steam roast at 400°F for 30 minutes.	Toss with oil and cinnamon.
Zucchini	Slice into pinky finger–like shapes.	Steam for 5 minutes; roast at 400°F for 10–15 minutes.	Toss with oil, ground basil, and garlic powder.
Fruits			
Apple	Peel and slice into strips a little larger than your pinky finger. The apples will shrink during cooking.	Steam for 5 minutes; steam roast at 400°F for 15–20 minutes.	Sprinkle with ground cinnamon and/or ginger.
Avocado	Remove skin and slice into pinky finger–like strips.	N/A	Roll in hemp or chia seeds for easy handling, toss with fresh lemon juice, or mash onto toast strips.
Banana	Peel and slice into pinky finger–like strips or halve, and remove 2 inches of the skin, leaving the rest of the peel on for easier handling.	N/A	Spread with a very thin smear of nut butter, or roll strips into wheat bran, peanut butter powder, or hemp seeds for easier handling.
Berries	Smash berries for pincer grasp. Slice berries into thin strips for palmar grasp.	N/A	Mix into oatmeal or iron-fortified oat cereal. Use a preloaded spoon to allow baby to eat on their own or cool to thicken, then allow baby to scoop the mixture to eat.
Grapes	Diced for pincher grasp or sliced into small strips for palmar grasp. Grapes should never be served whole until ~3–4 years of age.	N/A	Try a grape smoothie! Puree with non-dairy yogurt of choice and a smidge of nut-butter or sesame-seed butter.

FOOD	PREPARATION	HOW TO COOK	FAVORITE FLAVOR PAIRING
Melons	Remove skin and seed. Slice melon into pinky finger–sized slices.	N/A	Roll melon strips into chia, hemp, or flax seeds for easier handling.
Oranges	Peel and remove pith and outer membrane. Slice into sections.	N/A	Simmer with berries for a simple jam to serve with French Toast Fingers on page 222.
Peach, very ripe	Peel and remove pit. Slice fruit flesh into pinky finger–sized slices.	N/A	Try stewed peaches or other stone-fruit as a glaze for tofu and tempeh!
Pear, very ripe	Peel and slice fruit flesh into pinky finger–sized slices.	N/A	Swap pear for apples in your favorite applesauce recipe.
Tomatoes	Peel skin and remove seeds. Slice into pinky finger–sized slices.	N/A	Sprinkle slices with sesame seeds or poppy seeds for added texture and grip.
Grains, Beans, and Other Foods			
Beans	Smash beans for pincher grasp.	See directions in our PB3 Plate Staples handout on page 293.	Use in meatballs or bean-fingers with cooked bean of choice. Puree into hummus and spread onto toast strips or toss with hot pasta for a creamy sauce.
Oatmeal	See our Iron-Optimized Oatmeal recipe on page 57.	Serve thickened oatmeal directly on tray or use preloaded spoon.	Mix in pumpkin or butternut squash puree, ground cinnamon, and ginger.
Pancakes and Waffles	See our BLW Oatmeal Pancakes on page 210 or our Lemon Chia Waffles on page 233.	Slice into finger-width slices.	Serve with thin smear of nut butter and sprinkle with chia seeds and hemp seeds.
Pasta	Penne pasta is perfect for a palmar grasp. Use any shape pasta for pincer grasp!	Cook according to package or slightly longer for easy-to-mash pasta.	Toss pasta with sauce of choice. Consider pureed vegetables (like our Caterpillar Pasta, page 272) or Sunflower Mac 'n' Cheese (page 250).

FOOD	PREPARATION	HOW TO COOK	FAVORITE FLAVOR PAIRING
Quinoa	Use in our Simple Quinoa Breakfast Porridge on page 234 and serve with preloaded spoon.	Cook according to directions in our PB3 Plate Staples on page 295.	For a curried quinoa, add coconut milk, quinoa, tomatoes, and red lentils. Cook until very thick, then serve directly on tray or with preloaded spoon.
Rice	Limit brown rice to 1–2 servings a week to minimize arsenic exposure.	Cook according to directions in our PB3 Plate Staples on page 295.	Use in bean-based meatballs or mix with hummus and roll into balls.
Toast	Soft bread is a choking hazard for young babies. Remove crust, toast bread, then slice into pinky finger–sized slices.	N/A	Spread with a thin smear of nut butters or hummus.
Yogurt	Use tofu or soaked cashews to make your own nondairy yogurt or choose unsweetened storebought options.	N/A	Mix yogurt into iron-fortified oat cereal, use in smoothies and popsicles, or serve on a preloaded spoon.

WHAT IS STEAM ROASTING: Steam roasting vegetables is perfect for all ages, but especially for baby-led weaning. This hybrid cooking method creates tender-on-the-inside and golden-on-the-outside vegetables. Simply cover your baking or roasting pan with foil or a lid for ¾ of the cooking time, then carefully remove cover and continue cooking for the last ¼ of recommended cooking time. By covering the vegetables first, you create a moist environment for steam to cook the vegetables. Removing the cover during the last quarter of cooking allows the vegetables' natural sugars to concentrate and caramelize. While you can also parboil vegetables first before roasting them to get the same results, we prefer this method for easier prep and cleanup. One pan will always trump two pans in our world!

Food Progression

Traditionally, feeding experts have recommended that foods be introduced one at a time, waiting a few days between each new item. These recommendations were created in order to easily identify allergic reactions. However, allergic reactions, unlike food intolerances, are immediate. So waiting one to three days isn't necessary for this purpose; if your baby is allergic to a new food, you will likely see the response right away. Additionally, rapid introduction of a variety of fruits and vegetables has been shown to increase food acceptance and potentially lead to a more adventurous palate.

We see no scientific justification for a single-food, delayed process. Foods with a low allergenic potential can be introduced together and do not need to be spaced out. While it is true that it will be harder to identify intolerances, it is not difficult when babies are only receiving one meal a day with few ingredients.

If you're concerned about a potential allergic reaction, you can certainly introduce the top 8 allergens on their own, which we discuss on page 130.

How Do I Know if They're Eating Enough?

A baby-led weaning approach will mean that baby will likely take in less food than their peers who are being spoon-fed. Self-feeding takes time to master, and we wouldn't expect baby to be an expert from the start. Expect a period of exploration, touching the food, placing the food in the mouth, sucking on the food, and finally chewing and swallowing the food.

Based on the feedback we've received from other moms and clients, it takes an average of 2 to 3 weeks before you'll be able to see food in baby's stool—a great sign that they're taking in solids.

> **PBJ Quick Bite**
>
> It often takes 2 to 3 weeks before you consistently see food in baby's stool.

What About Choking?

"You want me to give my infant *what*?" After months of obsessively policing everything our babe puts in their mouth, we're now supposed to be comfortable with them shoving a large foreign object right in there?

Yup, this was our first concern as well. We vividly remember sitting on our hands the first time we gave our babes solid food, afraid that we were making a terrible decision. Our mommy paranoia was through the roof as we carefully laid a piece of banana (Alex) and a strip of butternut squash (Whitney) on their trays for the first time. *Could our sons really eat on their own?*

Rest assured that research shows there is no difference in the likelihood of choking events between baby-led weaning babies and spoon-fed babies. In fact, one study showed that infants who are fed finger foods the least are at the highest risk of choking.

The most important thing is that you provide appropriate food. Offering your baby a large hunk of raw carrot is an absolute no-no, but giving them a piece of finger-shaped, thoroughly steamed carrot is perfect! There is a wide range of foods that are safe and foods that are not, and we'll get into all the nitty-gritty.

Waiting until the 6-month mark and until baby is able to sit on their own reduces choking risk as well. Choking can occur in infants who have not yet developed the oral motor skills required to safely chew and swallow. If your baby isn't showing signs of readiness at 6 months, it's OK. You can start offering purees and then switch to a baby-led weaning approach once baby is developmentally ready. No matter how we start out, we all end up eating solids at some point.

> Baby-led weaning is not for everyone. Babies with anatomic abnormalities or neurological disorders that put them at a risk of dysphagia should not do baby-led weaning.

Choking versus Gagging

Is it just us or do both of those words sound scary? But gagging and choking are very different.

Gagging is a non-life-threatening occurrence that happens, sometimes multiple times per meal, as a normal part of learning about food. It is usually very noisy and sounds like coughing or sputtering. While an adult's gag reflex is triggered at the back of the tongue, near the esophagus, a baby's gag reflex is triggered closer to the front of the tongue. This means that they will frequently gag in the early feeding days if they take too large a bite to bring the food forward to be chewed more thoroughly. This reflex moves farther backward as baby ages to the normal adult position by about 12 months.

Choking is a life-threatening emergency that occurs when a baby's airway is blocked. Unlike with gagging, choking is mostly silent and baby's hands and skin may turn blue. You may not be able to detect a change in color in babies with dark skin, so looking out for other signs like reaching for the throat or high-pitched, distress sounds is important too.

Choking requires immediate intervention, which is why we recommend that all parents be certified in infant CPR before beginning solids. Gagging does not require intervention, and it is safer to allow your baby to cough up food on their own rather than stepping in, which may lead to choking.

Despite understanding that gagging is to be expected, the first time our sons gagged we just about lost it. It may be normal, but it's not pretty, and we know firsthand how scary it can be. Our advice is to educate yourself on the difference between the two so that when it happens you know how to react. There are plenty of gagging videos online of adorable babies eating solids.

Feeding Baby Safely

1. Never leave baby alone with food. Choking is a silent event. Constant supervision ensures that an adult will be there to respond quickly if needed.

2. Make sure baby is always sitting upright, never leaning backward. We know how tempting it may be to hold baby when they are eating, but sitting upright in a high chair prevents baby from slouching and allows you to watch them the entire time.

3. Allow babies to feed themselves. Babies need to be in control of how quickly they eat and how much food they bite at one time.

4. Test foods to make sure they are the right softness and temperature. Mash a piece of food with your finger and thumb or press the food between your lips. This is about the same pressure as baby's gums and will help you know if baby is able to safely bite the food and to tell if the food is a safe temperature.

5. Offer age- and texture-appropriate foods. Salt and sugar should be limited, and foods that are choking hazards should be avoided.

A Traditional Feeding Approach

We've spent a lot of time talking about the concept of baby-led weaning. For one, it's the approach that we both used with our kids. Alex did mostly baby-led weaning and Whitney used a mixed approach. But we hope we've stressed enough that however you decide to feed your baby is the right way. If you do decide to go with a traditional approach, here is some general information to guide you.

Many pediatricians will give the go-ahead to begin purees around 4 months. Unlike with finger foods, baby is able to mechanically handle pureed food at this age. However, it's still best to still wait until baby has begun to lose the tongue-thrust reflex. If you do choose to start solids earlier than 6 months, single fruits, vegetables, or iron-fortified baby cereal are good options.

When starting purees, the same safety and general guidelines apply. You want to ensure that baby is seated upright in a high chair and that you're always watching them while they eat.

Just as with infant feeding, take your baby's lead. Offer up the spoon and wait until baby opens their mouth to feed them. Never force food into a baby's mouth or pressure or cajole them into eating. Your baby will likely only take 1 to 2 teaspoons during the first meals.

The typical trajectory of spoon-feeding goes like this:

- 6–8 months: pureed fruits, vegetables, and protein/iron-rich foods
- 9–12 months: chopped, ground, or mashed foods and soft finger foods
- 12+ months: age-appropriate family meals

As you can see, it's not all that different from baby-led weaning. The main distinction is that instead of waiting until 8 or 9 months to try finger foods, baby-led weaners enjoy them from the start.

Baby Food Preparation and Safety

If you do choose to feed purees, we recommend making your own as often as possible. Not only is it more economical, it's also more nutritious. Many purees on the market are low in important nutrients like iron and protein, and because they're single ingredients, they expose babies to only one flavor at a time. Making your own allows you to get creative and introduce baby to a rainbow of color and flavor with each bite.

Making homemade baby food doesn't have to be overwhelming. Start with mashing a very ripe avocado or banana for a simple puree that you don't need to heat. From there, almost any fruit or vegetable can be turned into a thin mash or puree.

Just like with solid foods, you'll want to be vigilant about sanitation and ensure that you are cleaning produce before cutting and using clean countertops, cutting boards, and knives. Serve food right away or refrigerate/freeze for later. Most baby food is safe in the fridge for a few days or 1 to 2 months in the freezer. We like the ice-cube-tray technique for freezing baby food in appropriate portions. Most ice cube trays are divided into approximately 1-ounce bites. Simply place the baby food in a clean tray, then freeze. Remove the cubes and put them into a clean, airtight, freezer-safe container. Thaw or defrost as needed, then serve! Once heated, be sure to mix thoroughly and check the temperature before serving to prevent burning baby's mouth.

Since bacteria can be harmful for baby, you'll want to portion out a small amount of food to serve at one time. Any food that had contact with baby's mouth via the spoon or otherwise cannot be saved for later and needs to be discarded. This goes for both homemade and commercially prepared baby food.

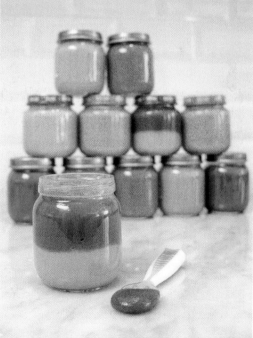

Lastly, we recommend steaming or microwaving with just a little water to retain as many vitamins and minerals as possible. You can also roast veggies with a bit of olive or avocado oil. Compared to other cooking techniques, like boiling, these methods will help retain the most nutrients.

Adding Flavor to Baby's Food

Just as with baby-led weaning, there's no reason that baby can't be introduced to a wide variety of flavors right from the start. Add seasonings to purees anytime during the cooking process to encourage baby to try new flavors and spices. We love combining pureed butternut squash with cinnamon; pureed green beans with Italian seasonings like basil, oregano, and garlic; and pureed carrots with curry powder.

PBJ Quick Bite

Use as little water as possible when steaming fruits and veggies—boiling results in nutrient loss.

You'll still want to omit any salt or added sugar, as babies don't need the additional sweetness and their kidneys are not developed enough to handle added salt. If you are making a meal for the entire family, remove baby's portion before seasoning with salt and then puree.

Nutrition from 6 to 12 Months

Whether you're doing baby-led weaning or a traditional approach, all the same nutritional considerations apply. Baby's main nutritional source is still breast milk and/or formula. Adding food at 6 months of age is intended to complement nutrition, encourage exploration, and develop feeding skills and taste preference.

Breast milk and formula provide the majority of calories, macronutrients, and micronutrients that babies need. For breastfeeding mamas, you'll continue the same supplement regimen you have been following for the first 6 months. Breastfed babies will also continue their vitamin D supplement.

There is one nutrient, however, that we want to discuss in more detail: iron.

Iron

"Start with meat." Pick up most baby feeding books and this is a popular recommendation. Seems like people think that if baby isn't sucking on a hunk of sirloin steak, they're at risk for iron deficiency!

While meat is a good source of iron, it isn't the *only* or the best source when introducing solids. This is one of the reasons the Plant-Based Juniors Instagram account exists. Alex was so frustrated by baby-led weaning books emphasizing the importance of meat that she was determined to prove she could not only do baby-led weaning with her son, but she could do plant-based baby-led weaning.

As discussed in Chapter 1, iron is accumulated in utero, and a baby's stores last until age 4 to 6 months. At around 7 months of age, iron needs jump from 0.27 mg per day to 11 mg per day! Even omnivorous babes are typically unable to meet this high demand without some source of supplemental iron—whether that be from the iron found in formula or from iron-fortified foods. To give you an idea of how much iron we're talking about, your average jar of beef puree contains only 1 mg of iron. I don't know about you, but I don't know many 7-month-olds who can take down 11 jars of baby food in a day.

This is why we recommend including iron-fortified cereal in your baby's diet in addition to iron-rich plant foods—especially for exclusively breastfed babies who are not getting large amounts of iron from formula. Plenty of plant-based foods are excellent sources of iron, including whole grains, legumes, nuts, and seeds. Combining these foods with a source of vitamin C like strawberries, bell peppers, citrus, and potatoes will ensure your baby absorbs them efficiently.

If you started your breastfed baby on an iron supplement at 4 months, you can discontinue it as you start providing these iron-rich foods. Discuss this with your pediatrician if your baby has unique considerations.

The Perfect Pairings

As babe starts the weaning process, make sure to offer energy-dense foods. Baby is growing at an extremely rapid pace, so we want to make sure that each bite is packed not only with nutrients like iron, but also high-calorie, fat-rich foods.

To make things easy, we've created a cheat sheet with ideas for first meals that include iron-rich foods paired alongside high-fat and vitamin C–rich offerings. Our goal here is to simplify feeding and remove the stress that sometimes comes with introducing solids. Mix and match these options and rest assured that babe is getting everything they need.

HIGH IRON	HIGH FAT	VITAMIN C RICH
Red Lentil Pizza Strips (page 216)	Cashew cheese or veggies cooked in olive oil	Lightly steamed broccoli, with handle stem for easy holding
Tofu Marinara Strips (page 218)	Vegan "parmesan" (cashews with nutritional yeast)	Marinara sauce
Lightly fried tempeh strips	Tempeh cooked in olive oil	Very ripe kiwi, cored and sliced
Kidney beans, smashed	Avocado slices, served either plain or rolled in wheat germ or hemp seeds for easier gripping	Strawberries, sliced
Soft toast, sliced into finger shapes	Tahini or nut butter	Raspberries, halved
Tofu frittata cup, sliced into strips or halved	Olives, pitted and quartered	Lightly steamed cauliflower, with handle stem for easy holding
Penne pasta with spinach pesto	Walnuts and olive oil (in pesto)	Lightly steamed bell pepper strips
Iron-fortified cereal pancakes	Pancakes cooked in coconut oil	Ripe cantaloupe, sliced
Chickpea pasta	Broccoli cooked in olive oil	Marinara sauce
Black beans, smashed	Avocado strips rolled in hemp seeds	Tomatoes, thinly sliced
Quinoa-based veggie burger, sliced into finger shapes OR cooked quinoa mixed with hummus and served with a preloaded spoon	Burger cooked in avocado oil	Steam-roasted sweet potato strips

PBJ Bottom Line: Babies will continue to get the majority of their caloric and macro/micronutrient needs from breast milk or formula. Breastfeeding mamas should continue their supplement regimen and breastfed babies should continue to receive a vitamin D supplement. Iron needs are sky-high during this period, so focusing on offering iron-rich foods is important. Pair these with a good source of vitamin C to maximize absorption.

Foods to Avoid

During weaning, we want to expose babies to as many foods, flavors, and textures as possible. But there are certain foods that are not safe for babies, regardless of feeding method.

Foods to avoid between 6 and 12 months:

- Honey before age 1, which may contain *Clostridium botulinum*, bacterial spores that can cause a serious neurotoxic illness called botulism. Make sure to read labels to ensure it is not added to breads or cereals.
- Round foods like veggie sausage, cherry tomatoes, and grapes. These can all block the airway and should be cut into halves or quarters depending on baby's age and skill.
- Food that can break off in large chunks like raw apples and most raw vegetables. Raw vegetables can be introduced around 10 months in shreds or small, bite-size pieces once baby has developed a pincer grasp.
- Foods that form a crumb in the mouth, like French bread or crackers.
- Hard foods like whole nuts, large seeds, and popcorn should be avoided until age 4, as these are major choking hazards.
- Segments of citrus. Oranges, tangerines, and grapefruit should be sliced and membrane removed.
- Large gobs of nut butter, which can get stuck in baby's esophagus. Thin smears of nut butter on toast or swirled into oatmeal are OK.
- Large amounts of cow's milk and plant milk. While it's OK to use milks in small amounts in cooking, we want to avoid giving these as beverages directly until at least 1 year of age. They can displace nutrients in the diet, and drinking cow's milk before 1 year of age may cause damage to the intestinal lining.
- Deli meat and unpasteurized, fresh cheeses. We're guessing you're not planning on serving these foods anyway, but it should be stated that lunch meats and unpasteurized, fresh cheeses shouldn't be offered before 1 year of age as they may contain *Listeria,* a bacteria that can cause a serious illness in babies called listeriosis.

Salt

Under 1 year, baby's kidneys have not fully developed and can't efficiently filter out large amounts of sodium.

We don't add any salt to baby's food under 1 year of age and we severely limit store-bought foods with added sodium. Look for no-salt-added or low-sodium tomato sauce, canned beans, and other packaged foods.

Family-Friendly Feeding Tip!

When cooking for the family, remove baby's portion before adding salt. Have adults and older kids salt their own plates.

Sugar

There's no need for babies to eat added sugar. We want them to develop a taste for natural foods, and consuming sugar at this age may predispose them to a preference for unnaturally sweet food. But we live in the real world and know that even "healthy" foods like jarred marinara sauce and whole-grain bread usually contain some added sweetener. Therefore, we limit it when possible but also don't sweat it when there is a gram or two in something that baby eats infrequently.

Note—"added sugar" does not include naturally sweetened foods like fruit, but sugar that is added to food or isolated from natural sources like flavored yogurts, baked foods, packaged foods, fruit juice, and so on.

The Fruit Obesity Paradox

We often hear parents say they're afraid that if their kids eat too much fruit, they'll gain weight. While fruit does contain large amounts of natural sugar (glucose and fructose), research has shown over and over again that fruit has an *anti*-obesity effect. This is known as the "fruit obesity paradox."

Eating a lot of fruit results in increased feelings of fullness and eating less food overall, likely because it has a lot of fiber and water. Fruit also contains essential micronutrients and phytochemicals, which may provide anti-obesity benefits. Vitamins A, E, and C and zinc, iron, and calcium help with fat metabolism, or the breakdown of ingested fats to use in the body. Therefore, a diet rich in micronutrients, like those found in both fruits *and* vegetables, is helpful.

Hydration

From 6 to 12 months of age, babies don't need a lot of additional fluid, aside from what is provided by breast milk or formula. However, because plant-based babies have a higher fiber intake, you may find that giving a little water helps prevent constipation. Additionally, providing water at meals familiarizes babies with what we hope becomes their primary beverage later in life. We offer baby 1 to 2 ounces of water at mealtimes to assist with digestion and to practice using an open cup.

We know what you're thinking—*Give my six-month-old an open cup, are you crazy?* Bear with us. Yes, your baby will likely drop their cup of water on themselves, repeatedly, but the intention is that they will eventually learn how to use it. Giving infants open cups helps promote mature drinking and develop their oral motor skills. Initially, you'll have to help baby with this.

When you're on the go, obviously, an open cup will not work. We recommend giving baby a straw cup versus a traditional sippy cup with a spout. Straws strengthen muscles in the mouth and face that baby needs to talk and eat, while sippy cups promote immature, infant-like sucking and swallowing and may impact oral development.

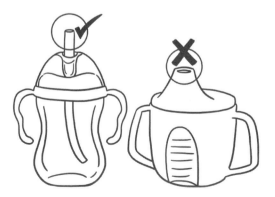

Portion Sizes and Feeding Guidelines

If you're doing baby-led weaning, you'll likely be surprised by how little food baby actually gets into their mouth those first few weeks. A nibble here, a bite there. Similarly, spoon-fed babes often don't immediately take to solids. Luckily, babies don't need that much food, as most of their nutritional needs are still being met by breast milk and/or formula. Again, this is why solid foods at this age are referred to as "complementary." They are designed to complement the uber-nutritious milk that baby will continue to receive until at least their first birthday.

That being said, we know parents like definitive guidance, so we recommend starting with 1 to 2 tablespoons or 2 to 3 strips of food at a time. This gives baby the visual exposure to food, without overwhelming them. It also allows for some food to be discarded, dropped, spit out, or half-eaten. Remember, 6-month-olds will still have the palmar grasp and won't be able to eat every bite that's offered. They will pick up the food in their palm, eat the visible portions, and drop the rest.

PBJ Quick Bite
1 to 2 tablespoons of food/puree or 2 to 3 strips of food at a time is a good starting place.

Meal Timing

Timing is key when it comes to success with new eaters. In the beginning, this means using the "Goldilocks approach": Offer food when baby is not too hungry and not too full. You want them to be hungry enough that they are excited about the meal in front of them, but not too hungry that they become frustrated if they aren't able to satisfy their hunger fast enough. We find that starting a meal about an hour after their last milk feed is a good time.

We recommend starting off with 1 meal per day around 6 months and gradually moving to 2 or 3 meals a day around 9 months. By 1 year, baby will be eating 3 meals and a couple of snacks per day.

Hunger/Fullness Cues

We follow Ellyn Satter's Division of Responsibility in Feeding (something that we go over in depth in Chapter 5), which means that baby is in charge of if they want to eat, and how much. Babies communicate that they're hungry for food in the same way they show they are hungry for milk, though they may use different expressions to indicate that they want more or are finished.

Looking around for more food, smacking lips, looking to you (the food giver) with interest, and/or smacking the tray may all be signs that baby is ready for a second course. Getting distracted, pushing the food around, dropping it on the floor, or becoming increasingly frustrated are all ways that baby may be trying to tell you that she's had enough.

If you aren't sure, you can hold up a piece of food and ask, "More?" before placing it on their tray. You can also place food on their tray and then sign for "more" using American Sign Language (which looks like making a flat O shape with both hands and tapping them together at the fingertips). If baby becomes excited, then they are likely still hungry. If they become irritable, they're likely full.

Sign Language for Toddlers

We both used American Sign Language with our babies to help communicate with them about their hunger/fullness before they were able to voice their desires. While there are many signs that can be helpful, we stuck to the basics: "more," "all done," "eat," and "drink."

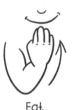

Eat

Drink

All Done

Thank You

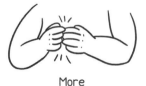

More

Alex introduced these at her son's very first meal, but he didn't easily pick them up. Her pediatrician told her that if he didn't get the signs in the first few weeks, she should let it go. Well, Alex is fairly stubborn, and she continued to use the signs at meals. By 8 months, Vander was signing at every meal and still continues to sign when he's all done.

Don't give up if your babe doesn't get these right away. The more consistently you use these signs, the faster baby will be able to pick them up.

Responsive Feeding

In the beginning, it may be easier to understand when your child is hungry or full. Crying, fussiness, or turning toward the bottle/nipple are all classic signs of hunger, while turning the head away, losing interest, or a slower pace of eating are all signs of fullness. Once solids are introduced, those signals can become trickier to interpret and it's easier to ignore both hunger and fullness cues.

Responsive feeding is learning your baby's individual cues, and responding appropriately. Baby lets you know that they are hungry, and you feed them. When baby shows signs of fullness, you stop. We know this sounds simple, but if you consider how many of us were pushed to join the "clean plate club," or to have one more bite so we could get dessert, or perhaps were underfed in an attempt to control weight, then you can see how easy it is to stray from responsive feeding. Responsive feeding changes as children age with parents providing more structure in order to help support children's natural ability to self-regulate their intake.

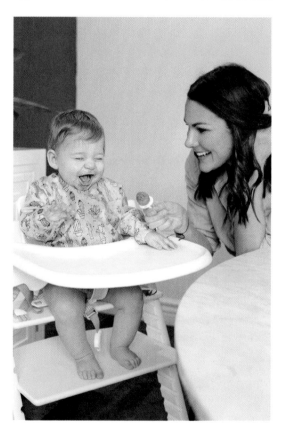

AGE	HUNGER CUES	SATIETY CUES	RESPONSIVE FEEDING ACTION	CHILD LEARNS . . .
0–6 months	Cries, fusses, roots, sucks on hands	Closes mouth, turns head away, slows sipping or sucking, falls asleep	Responds quickly, feeding when hungry and stopping when baby is full	To trust that parent will respond to their needs.
6–12 months	Reaches for food, points to food, uses words or sounds to signal hunger	Shakes head, throws food, spits out food, slows eating	Offers a variety of textures and tastes without pressure or judgment; responds positively to self-feeding attempts	To self-feed; that meals are a pleasant time and a safe space to learn and explore.
1–3 years	Continues to use sounds, movements, and increased vocabulary to signal hunger	Continues to use both actions and vocabulary to signal satiety	Offers consistent, balanced meals and snacks; varies food offerings; responds to child's hunger and satiety cues without judgment or pressure	To trust that food will always be available to them; to try new foods and feeding behaviors.

Food Allergies

Allergies are a major concern for many parents when beginning solids, and rightfully so. Food allergies are on the rise, with some studies showing that they have doubled in the past two decades. Though it has been hard for researchers to get firm estimates, about 10% of the population is affected by food allergies, with the highest numbers in children and people in industrialized countries.

Risk Factors for Food Allergies

Your child may be at an increased risk for developing food allergies if you have a family history of them. Additionally, if your child has one food allergy, then she may also be at an increased risk for developing others. Research also suggests that kids with family members who have a history of sensitive conditions like eczema, asthma, or allergic rhinitis may also be at a higher risk. However, food allergies can develop in children and adults with no family history, so taking measures to prevent them is important for everyone.

Symptoms of a Food Allergy

Allergies affect people uniquely, meaning that one child may have a severe reaction to an allergen while another child is only mildly reactive to it. We discussed the difference between food allergies and food intolerances in the previous chapter, but as a reminder, food allergy symptoms include swelling around the mouth, face, or throat, itchiness, difficulty breathing, and gastrointestinal effects like nausea, vomiting, and diarrhea. In severe cases, food allergies can be life-threatening. Food intolerances are usually isolated to symptoms of digestive distress.

Some children will outgrow food allergies and sensitivities by the time they turn 5 years old, but not all do. Allergies to peanuts, tree nuts, fish, and shellfish often last for life. If you're concerned about your child's risk, it's best to discuss this with your pediatrician. They will also be able to refer you to a specialist, and provide guidance about whether allergy testing is necessary.

Below are the top 8 most common allergenic foods:

- Milk
- Eggs
- Soy
- Shellfish
- Fish
- Peanuts
- Tree nuts
- Wheat

The above 8 foods account for approximately 90% of all food allergies, while the other 10% are other foods, including emerging allergenic foods like sesame seeds and mustard seeds.

Early Introduction for Allergy Prevention

Experts used to recommend delaying the introduction of common food allergens—cow's milk until 1 year, eggs until 2 years, and nuts and fish until 3 years. The belief was that children's immature immune systems weren't able to handle potentially reactive foods.

However, these recommendations have changed based on emerging science. The general consensus today is that waiting to introduce allergenic foods can actually *increase* children's risk of developing allergies. Studies show that introducing children to peanuts and eggs between 4 and 6 months of age may reduce the risk of allergy by about 71% and 44%, respectively.

Based on recent research and the high prevalence of peanut allergy, the AAP now recommends that parents introduce peanuts, specifically, between 4 and 6 months, in an age-appropriate form. The exact timing depends on risk:

- Low-risk babies: Introduce at 6 months. This includes babies who do not have eczema or other allergies.
- Moderate-risk babies: Introduce at 6 months. This includes babies with mild to moderate eczema.
- High-risk babies: Introduce between 4 and 6 months. This includes babies with severe eczema and other food allergies. Exposure should occur in a health-care provider's office versus a home setting. Talk to your doctor about the proper course of action.

How to Introduce Allergens

To introduce potential allergens, experts recommend giving your baby a first taste, then waiting 10 minutes for a reaction, and repeating with a second taste. After that, let your baby finish the serving at a normal speed. Watch for any reactions over a period of around 2 hours, as this is the window of time in which most adverse food reactions will occur. From there, expose your baby to the food at least 3 times per week.

Here are some ways you could introduce common allergy foods to your child:

Peanuts
- A thin layer of unsalted peanut butter on wheat toast, sliced into thin strips for baby-led weaning
- Peanut butter powder mixed into pancake batter or infant cereal

Soy
- Crumbled tofu, scrambled, or blended into a smoothie
- Organic, plain, unsweetened soy milk used in a recipe, soup, or smoothie*

Wheat
- Wheat toast with hummus, sliced into thin strips for baby-led weaning
- Whole wheat noodles, alone or with tomato sauce

Tree Nuts

- Cashew or almond butter, thinned with water and introduced similarly to peanut butter

*Using a small amount of soy milk in recipes is a good option for allergen exposure, but soy milk is not a suitable beverage for children under 1 year.

Allergies and Animal Products

Although there are no standardized guidelines for introducing allergenic foods other than peanuts, it's likely that others should be introduced in the same way, especially if your baby is high-risk for allergies.

Unfortunately, several of the top 8 allergens are animal products—eggs, milk, fish, and shellfish—which creates an ethical dilemma. While we can't make the decision for you, we personally chose to introduce all of the top 8 allergens to our children, with the professional perspective that it may reduce their risk of developing severe allergies later in life. Even if they continue to eat plant-based for the rest of their lives, they may still be exposed to animal-derived food allergens through cross contamination and food processing, and a life-threatening food allergy is something we want to do everything in our power to avoid.

That being said, early introduction to allergens does not guarantee that your child won't develop an allergy, and choosing not to introduce them doesn't mean they will. Additionally, if you do decide to introduce animal-derived allergenic foods to your baby, it doesn't mean that you have to make animal products a part of their diet long-term. Current research suggests that allergen risk is established during the 6-to-12-month period, so that is when you would need to expose them. Biweekly exposure

PBJ Bottom Line: New research has shown that early introduction (between 4 and 6 months) is ideal to reduce the risk of developing an allergy, although how and when depends on a child's individual profile. The strongest research supporting early exposure for allergen risk reduction has been conducted with peanuts, milk, and eggs. However, introducing all of the top 8 allergens may be beneficial.

during this period is likely necessary to provide adequate exposure. We know this can be a scary and confusing topic, so we want to make sure you have all the information you need to make an informed decision that's best for your family. Of course, we also recommend consulting with your pediatrician.

Sample Feeding Schedules

While baby should still be receiving milk on demand from 6 to 12 months, we know it's helpful to have a general idea of how milk and solid feedings might come together.

6 MONTHS

7 a.m. Breastfeed or bottle-feed

8 a.m. **Breakfast**

11 a.m. Breastfeed or bottle-feed

2 p.m. Breastfeed or bottle-feed

5 p.m. Breastfeed or bottle-feed

7 p.m. Breastfeed or bottle-feed

Night wakings: You may also breastfeed/bottle-feed, depending on if baby is sleeping through the night yet.

9 MONTHS

7 a.m. Breastfeed or bottle-feed

8 a.m. **Breakfast**

11 a.m. Breastfeed or bottle-feed

12 a.m. **Lunch**

3 p.m. Breastfeed or bottle-feed

5 p.m. Breastfeed or bottle-feed

6 p.m. **Dinner**

7 p.m. Breastfeed or bottle-feed

1 YEAR

7 a.m. Breast milk or milk/milk alternative

8 a.m. **Breakfast**

10 a.m. **Mid-morning snack**

12 p.m. **Lunch**

3 p.m. **Afternoon snack** + breast milk or milk/milk alternative

6 p.m. **Dinner**

7 p.m. Breast milk or milk/milk alternative

Remember that these are just examples. You'll need to adjust your own routine to fit your child's needs and to work around things like naps and family schedules.

Common Questions and Challenges

While we've tried to cover everything in this chapter, we know there are questions that tend to come up over and over again, especially regarding baby-led weaning. Here are simple answers and solutions to your most common baby-feeding challenges and questions.

Q: My baby is 4 months old. Can I start baby-led weaning now?
A: Breast milk or formula is all your baby needs until around 6 months of age. Though your baby might be interested in food earlier, there are other developmental milestones that they need to meet in order to start baby-led weaning. At 4 months, it's unlikely that baby will be able to sit up on their own or pick up food and bring it to their mouth to eat. All these skills are prerequisites for baby-led weaning.

Q: What's the first food I should give my child?
A: There are no rules about the first foods baby can try (as long as they're not on the Foods to Avoid list found on page 123), but if you're doing baby-led weaning, you'll probably want to start off with something that feels less intimidating for both of you—at least, that's how we felt!

Alex offered banana and avocado slices rolled in wheat germ for easy handling to her son for his first meal, followed by cooked sweet potato sticks. Though she was well versed on gagging versus choking, she was also nervous, so next she gave him pre-loaded spoons with pumpkin, fortified cereal, and yogurt to help her son *and* herself get comfortable with eating.

Whitney spent weeks deliberating over her son's first meal and ultimately settled on butternut squash, which he helped her select at the grocery store. After one bite, he was over it. Desperately wanting a successful first feeding, Whitney ran into the kitchen and promptly cut up an avocado, which Caleb eagerly gobbled up—and mashed all over his hair, high chair, and clothing.

Whatever you choose, try not to get discouraged if your baby isn't into it. Solid food is uncharted territory—it may take them a little time to get comfortable with it.

Q: Should I offer vegetables before fruits?

A: A common myth we hear is that offering fruit before vegetables predisposes baby to sweet preference and makes them less likely to eat their veggies. There is no science to support this idea. In fact, one study showed infants were more likely to accept carrots when they were offered along with fruit.

Q: How often do I offer solids?

A: We recommend beginning with 1 meal per day around 6 months, moving to 3 meals per day around 9 months. By 1 year of age, baby will be eating 3 meals and a few snacks per day.

Q: What if they don't like the food I'm offering?

A: Keep offering it to them. Oftentimes babies seem to dislike a particular food with the first few bites. However, a negative face doesn't always mean they hate it; they may just be getting used to the flavor. It takes time to develop preferences, so keep rotating and offering the food again. Research shows it can take up to 15 exposures before babies will accept a new food. The first few months of eating are among the best times to develop their taste, so make sure you are giving baby a chance to do so. If they still seem to dislike the food after a dozen or so offerings, you can retire it for now.

Q: Can babies have spicy food?

A: Kids want to eat flavorful food, just like adults! Therefore, there is no reason that you can't add various herbs and spices to their meals to develop their palates and introduce them to new offerings. We both introduced a mild curry powder around 7 months and a smidge of chili powder a few months after that.

That being said, most babies do not like spicy food, and you'll likely want to wait until at least 1 year of age before introducing spicy peppers and seasoning blends that contain cayenne or red pepper flakes.

Q: What if they don't want to eat?

A: We subscribe to Ellyn Satter's Division of Responsibility in Feeding at every stage of childhood, from infancy through adolescence (see Chapter 5 for more detail on this). This means that parents are responsible for the what, when, and where of feeding, and the child determines how much and whether or not to eat what you provide. It is up to them to decide if they want to eat the particular food you provide or not.

If they decide to leave a certain food on their plate or not eat at all, that's OK—as frustrating as it might be. You can choose to save the plate for the next meal or offer it again when they seem interested in eating. Follow baby's cues and end the meal if they do not want to eat.

Q: Can I do baby-led weaning and offer purees?

A: Absolutely! There's no research to suggest that offering purees along with finger foods will negate the potential benefits of baby-led weaning.

Q: Can my baby use utensils?

A: Babies won't be able to properly handle utensils until much later, but it's never too early to let them practice.

There are many utensils that were created with infants in mind that are great for serving mashed or pureed foods. We both used the following self-feeding options with our kids and loved the flexibility it provided.

One option is a self-feeding infant spoon, or "pre-spoon." Some have flat, grooved heads that infants can dip into purees or mashes and food will stick to them, as opposed to baby trying to scoop out the food. Others have small, rounded heads that allow for scooping in all directions. You can also preload the spoon and hand it to baby. Giving purees on a preloaded spoon is a great way to offer nutrient-rich foods like bean hummus, fortified cereals, chia pudding, oatmeal, and more. Our favorite self-feeding spoons include the NumNum GOOtensil, the ChooMee FlexiDip starter spoon, and the Olababy Soft-Tip Training Spoon Teether, all of which are made with nontoxic silicone and can be purchased online.

Q: How do I offer runny foods (like soup) during baby-led weaning?

A: Thinner liquids like soups or smoothies can be provided in an open cup once baby masters the skill of drinking.

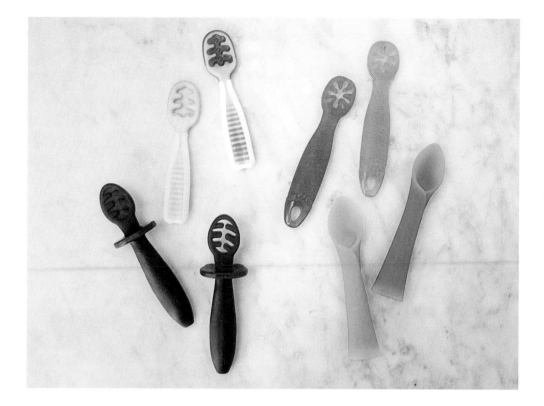

Q: Can babies have grains?

A: With the rise in popularity of grain-free diets, we've heard the erroneous claim that babies under 1 or 2 are unable to properly digest grains. This simply isn't true.

Amylase (the enzyme needed to break down the carbohydrates in grains) is present in both baby's saliva and their small intestine.

Q: What if a baby-led weaning food feels too slimy for my baby to pick up on their own?

A: Slippery foods like bananas or avocado can be rolled in wheat germ, hemp seeds, or bread crumbs to help baby grip the strips.

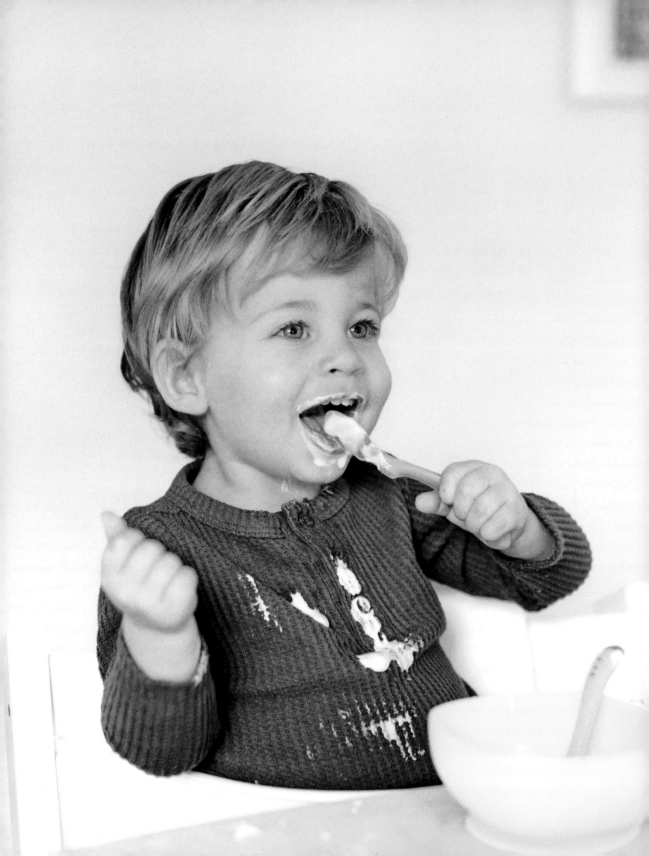

5

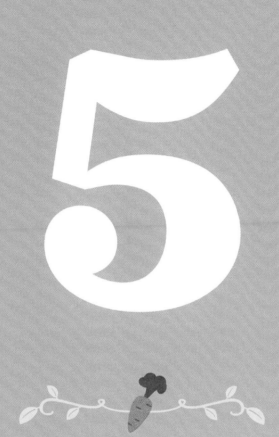

The Independent Eater
(1–3 Years)

Congrats on your baby's first birthday! We think parents deserve some recognition for this accomplishment. Those first 365 days are full of magic, but they are also enormously challenging, so kudos for making it through.

By this time, you are likely more confident in your parenting decisions and ready to tackle toddlerhood. Compared to just a few short months ago, your babe is likely eating at least a few times a day and is much more active. If they haven't done so already, they are likely also letting you know which foods they do—and *don't*—like. That's right, their protests usually get more vocal around this time. The first 6 months or so of solid food introduction is often called "the honeymoon period," a time when baby is much more receptive to new flavors, textures, and options. Things can change dramatically around the first birthday. Growth slows and babe's appetite may wane as well, bringing with it mealtime battles.

But if there's one thing that parenting has taught us, it's that time is fleeting. Just when we think we have the hang of something it changes, and with that comes the gentle reminder that even the hardest phases don't last forever. It's our goal in this chapter to empower you as you navigate periods of selective eating and the new nutrition considerations that come with entering early toddlerhood.

Cow's Milk and Alternatives

The number one question we get from parents, especially as their baby's first birthday looms on the horizon and they are thinking about weaning from breast milk and/or formula is typically: "What do I do about milk?"

Strangely, no other specific food is singled out in dietary recommendations like dairy. It's the only food that is specifically mentioned by the American Academy of Pediatrics (AAP) and mandated by the USDA to qualify for the School Lunch Program.

But contrary to what you may have heard, kids don't need cow's milk to thrive. Whether your child has an intolerance to cow's milk or you've made an ethical decision to raise your child dairy-free, we're here to walk you through all the questions and concerns you may have, talk about the pros and cons of dairy, and explain the best plant-based-milk options.

Milk, Calcium, and Strong Bones

We pride ourselves on being evidence-based dietitians, meaning that we aim to eliminate confirmation bias (selecting only studies that confirm our current viewpoint) and evaluate all the available research—not cherry-pick articles that strengthen our plant-based argument. Therefore, we'd be remiss if we didn't discuss the reasons groups like the AAP recommend cow's milk.

Milk is an easy, concentrated source of calories, protein, fat, calcium, and vitamin D—all important nutrients for growth. Studies consistently show that consuming milk has a positive effect on bone health and bone mineralization in children. Additionally, some studies show that drinking cow's milk is associated with greater height in children. However, these benefits are likely due to the high content of certain nutrients found in milk, like calcium and vitamin D, and not to unique properties of milk itself.

Children need calcium. During periods of growth, like early childhood and puberty, calcium is critical to acquire strong bones, and research shows that the accrual of bone mass in childhood is important for the prevention of osteoporosis later in life. Some studies have shown that children who do not drink cow's milk typically have a smaller stature and lower bone mineral density. However, when we dig a little deeper, we find that the children in these studies had low dietary calcium intake overall, which is likely what caused growth issues, not the avoidance of cow's milk. Those with a high intake of calcium, despite avoiding cow's milk, also had higher bone mineral density. Making sure kids get enough calcium without dairy is not difficult. Studies also show that simply supplementing calcium improves bone density in prepubertal children.

Luckily, fortified nondairy milk, like pea or soy, contains the same amount of calcium as cow's milk. Additionally, calcium is just one of many important factors when it comes to bone health; vitamin D and vitamin K are also critical nutrients. In fact, there is evidence that a lack of vitamin D, not calcium, has a greater effect on later bone density. In a study of 106 Caucasian girls, supplementation with 400 IU of vitamin D per day during the first year of life was associated with higher levels of bone density.

Finally, one of the most important factors for bone mass accretion is weight-bearing exercise, especially in early childhood. The more children use their bones for walking, exploring, running, and jumping, the stronger they become.

We'd also like to mention that research on dairy consumption in adults has shown contradictory results. Despite benefits to bone formation in childhood, many studies have shown that a high consumption of dairy in adulthood does not decrease fracture risk. In fact, some studies have shown an *increased* fracture risk with high dairy intake.

So now, let's talk about why your child doesn't need cow's milk.

IMPORTANT FACTORS FOR STRONG BONES

- Calcium intake
- Vitamin D and vitamin K intake
- Adequate protein intake (not too high, not too low)
- Weight-bearing exercise

A Brief History of Cow's Milk

It's comical to think that we would need to drink cow's milk to get essential nutrients. No other mammal drinks the lacteal secretions of another species! While *Homo sapiens* have been around for 300,000–500,000 years (and the early humans for approximately two million), we only began consuming dairy roughly 10,000 years ago when humans began to domesticate cows as part of a larger shift from hunter-gatherers to an agrarian society.

It began with butter and cheese. Milk consumption didn't start until much later, when proper cold storage allowed for the prevention of spoiling. But the origins of milk don't really matter in our conversation. The important thing is that we didn't evolve to consume milk products because we *had* to for our health. Cow's milk has rather persisted as an important beverage for children as a matter of convenience.

Records indicate that the average length of breastfeeding in traditional societies worldwide varied widely but generally lasted from 2 to 4 years. In ancient Rome, 2 to 3 years was the norm. In ancient Greece, philosophers like Aristotle recommended women feed until the return of menstruation, which can be months or years.

While researchers may debate if there is a biologically natural age to wean, breast milk is incredibly nutrient dense, so it makes sense that babies should receive it as long as possible. Unfortunately, mothers in ancient times encountered many of the same issues we face today, from physical barriers to negative views about breastfeeding in the upper classes. Therefore, animal milk was a popular replacement for breast milk for mothers who could not or chose not to breastfeed and could not afford a wet nurse. In fact, "direct udder nursing" occurred in many hospitals and orphanages in Europe as early as the 1500s!

During the late 1800s and early 1900s, the differences between cow's milk and human breast milk—and the health implications of these differences—were discovered. Cow's milk is very high in protein compared to human milk and causes microscopic tears in an infant's digestive tract leading to blood loss and anemia and an increased risk of type 1 diabetes. When this fact was brought to light, infant formula was developed to use until infants were considered old enough to tolerate cow's milk alone (approximately 1 year). Simultaneously, breastfeeding duration began to shorten during the twentieth century. In colonial America, the average age of breastfeeding was only 12 months. With a large gap between when women chose to wean and how long we were likely biologically meant to wean (2 to 3 years), a recommendation to provide cow's milk to *all* children after weaning fell into place.

The moral of the story is that cow's milk was only ever intended to be a replacement for breast milk as societal obligations moved women away from the anthropological custom of breastfeeding into early childhood. It was never a necessary part of the diet for children or adults, just like human breast milk is not a requirement for older children or adults.

What's Wrong with Cow's Milk?

One of the easiest arguments against the use of cow's milk to replace breast milk is that the two aren't all that similar. Compared to human breast milk, cow's milk has more protein, more carbohydrates, and less fat.

The main carbohydrate in milk is lactose. When we are born, our bodies produce large amounts of lactase, the enzyme that breaks down lactose so that we can properly digest it. About 10,000 years ago, around the time of cattle domestication, a genetic mutation occurred in some populations that allowed people to continue to produce lactase through adulthood. However, this did not occur for roughly 60%–65% of the world's population who are considered "lactose intolerant." After infancy and early childhood, people with lactose intolerance stop producing enough lactase to properly break down lactose, leading to a host of digestive issues, including bloating, gas, and constipation.

Lactose intolerance is the norm; lactase persistence is the exception. It's ironic that public policy worldwide has been shaped to encourage the consumption of dairy when this "evolutionary advantage" is found only in about 30% of the population.

Lactose intolerance is highly prevalent in Asian populations. Yet Asian populations (who typically avoid dairy) have lower rates of heart disease and cancer and an increased lifespan, about 7.8 years longer than the average non-Hispanic white person.

Cow's milk also differs both in the amount and composition of protein, containing roughly three times the total protein of human milk, most of which is from casein, while breast milk contains mostly whey protein.

Some of these casein proteins may increase the time it takes to digest food and have been linked to digestive issues like constipation in children. When a baby has tummy issues, removing dairy is often the first thing pediatricians and dietitians recommend. One study found that 28% of children with chronic constipation experienced relief when cow's milk was removed from their diet.

Milk Consumption and Chronic Disease Risk

The research on milk and chronic disease risk is contradictory and by no means conclusive, but it is worth discussing.

Studies have shown that cow's milk consumption is associated with an increased risk of prostate cancer, and an earlier age of menstruation in adolescent girls, a risk factor for breast cancer, cardiovascular disease, and diabetes. Meanwhile, a high intake of fiber and vegetable protein is associated with a later onset of menstruation. Consumption of more than 3 cups a day has also been associated with childhood obesity, although, counterintuitively, whole milk has a *lower* risk than reduced fat milk.

Milk is one of the biggest dietary drivers of insulin production and a hormone known as insulin-like growth factor (IGF-1), and children who drink a lot of milk have IGF-1 levels that are 20%–30% higher than non–milk drinkers. One study of 8-year-old boys showed that a higher milk intake over the course of 7 days increased their levels of IGF-1, doubled their fasting insulin concentrations, and increased measures of insulin resistance. High IGF-1 levels have also been linked to acne, obesity, type 2 diabetes, Alzheimer's disease, and certain cancers, especially prostate cancer. Not only does cow's milk trigger our own body's production, it contains bovine IGF-1, along with other natural growth factors, intended to help young cows grow quickly. (A baby cow goes from about 85 pounds at birth to 600 pounds when it's weaned about 6 months later. That's a weight gain of 2.5 pounds a day!) Researchers believe that high levels of IGF-1 in childhood may lead to early life programming of the IGF-1 axis that chronically upregulates its production, leading to diseases later in life.

It's unclear how much IGF-1 from cow's milk is absorbed or if it is degraded during digestion, but animal studies have shown that it is absorbed intact upon consumption. IGF-1 is also believed to be one of the reasons dairy consumption is associated with slightly increased height, which creates a bit of a paradox. On the one hand, we want our kids to have optimal growth, but that increased height may come with the baggage of increased disease risk. This remains an area that needs further research.

It's important to keep in mind, however, that we're talking about risk factors and associations. There is no firm evidence that dairy causes disease, and we acknowledge that cow's milk fills an important nutrient gap for some children. It's just not the only option.

Benefits of Plant-Based Milk

Fortified plant-based milk can help little ones meet their daily needs for multiple essential nutrients, including calcium, vitamin D, calories, protein, and fat. While it is possible for your child to get enough calcium through plant-based foods alone, it is unlikely for babies and toddlers. Studies of vegan children show that those who do not consume fortified foods and beverages typically fall far below the RDA. This is due not only to the types of foods that calcium is found in (leafy greens, which tend to be low on the toddler preference totem pole) but also to varying daily appetites and intake.

We strongly encourage parents who avoid cow's milk to provide an appropriate plant-based milk as a replacement, at least during the early years. For the average toddler, enjoying one or two glasses of fortified plant-based milk, like soy or pea, is an easy way to ensure they are meeting their needs. Alex gives Vander a cup first thing in the morning and as a bedtime snack, while Whitney gives Caleb milk with his morning and afternoon snack—sometimes alone, sometimes in a smoothie.

Whichever milk you offer, it's best to keep it to less than 16 ounces a day. More than this and you risk your tot filling up and missing out on other important nutrients like iron that are only found in solid foods.

Which Plant-Based Milk Is Best?

Babies and toddlers have higher nutrient requirements per pound of body weight compared to older kids and adults. This is why we want to make every bite—or sip—count.

There are many plant milks on the market that provide an array of benefits for nutrition, flavor, and cooking, but the only beverages that are appropriate replacements for cow's milk are fortified soy milk and fortified pea milk, which provide the most protein, fat, and calories.

Pea and soy milk are also good sources of the essential amino acid lysine, which can be limited on a plant-based diet, and soy milk is one of the richest plant-based sources of choline.

Again, rice, nut, and oat milks are not appropriate beverages for young children. They are low in protein, fat, and total calories and are nutritionally inferior to soy, pea, and cow's milk. Almond milk, for example, contains roughly a quarter of the calories compared to soy milk. You may have heard about the study that found that 3-year-olds who consumed 3 cups of nondairy milk a day were about 1.5 centimeters shorter than those consuming cow's milk. While critics of plant-based diets used these results to attack plant milk in general, there's a serious flaw with their argument. Namely, the researchers did not differentiate between the type of plant milk or whether they were fortified. Considering nut milks and unfortified milks lack important nutrients, it's no wonder the study showed poor results.

Because toddlers have smaller appetites than older kids, we want to ensure that they aren't filling up on these nutrient-poor milks. A little bit in baked goods or stirred into oatmeal isn't harmful, but they shouldn't be a primary beverage.

PLANT-BASED MILK CHECKLIST

- Soy or pea milk based (approximately 8 grams of protein)
- Fortified with calcium and vitamin D
- Possibly fortified with B12 and DHA as well
- Unsweetened/no added sugar

How to Pick a Plant Milk

The first thing we want to look for is a "fortified" milk, which means that manufacturers have added nutrients like calcium, vitamin D, and sometimes B12 or DHA to the product. They often don't state this on the front of the carton—you need to flip it around and look at the nutrition label. The Daily Value (DV) for calcium and vitamin D should be between 20% and 40%, and you will see words like "calcium carbonate," "tricalcium phosphate," and "vitamin D" in the ingredient list.

Secondly, many plant-based milks have sugar or other sweeteners added. Look for the word "unsweetened" on the bottle. The nutrition facts should also indicate it contains 0% added sugar.

Gums and Stabilizers

Some parents worry about gums, which are additives that stabilize and distribute the added nutrients, in plant-based milks. Current research shows that gums are safe and without gastrointestinal side effects, and we both use fortified milks that contain them. But the truth is that we don't really know the long-term impact, as they haven't been well studied in humans.

If you want to avoid gums, another option is to buy unfortified soy milk and add your own calcium. Pure 100% food-grade calcium carbonate powder can be purchased online or at health food stores and easily added to milk or yogurts. Just make sure to shake the bottle before serving and stir your child's cup frequently to ensure that the powder doesn't accumulate on the bottom, as those stabilizers are what keep the granules suspended. Keep in mind that you will also need to provide a full daily dose of vitamin D, since they are not getting any from fortified milk.

Some plant-based milks use carrageenan, a component of red algae, in order to help thicken and stabilize the fortified milk. There has been controversy on the safety of carrageenan, with some studies showing it may be harmful to the gut and others showing no effect. While the FDA considers carrageenan to be "generally recognized as safe" (GRAS) for use in food products and the amount found in milk falls far below the safe upper limit, many companies are phasing out this additive in response to consumer demand.

PBJ Quick Bite

Choose unsweetened, fortified plant-based milks. Alternatively, you can add food-grade calcium carbonate to unfortified dairy alternatives like yogurt.

Nutrient Considerations in the Second Year

The majority of the nutritional considerations we discussed in Chapters 1, 3, and 4 will continue to hold true as your child enters their second year. You'll still be prioritizing protein, iron, and zinc-rich foods and you'll still want to include fruits and vegetables rich with vitamins A and C with most meals. However, new considerations arise now that the majority of babes will eliminate formula or drastically decrease breast milk and begin to get more of their nutrients from solids.

B12

We apologize if we sound like a broken record, but we cannot stress enough that all vegans, vegetarians, and predominantly plant-based children should receive a B12 supplement from the time they are weaned. Plant foods are not a reliable source of B12, and now that babe is likely off formula completely and either off breast milk or decreasing intake, you'll want to ensure that they are taking their own B12 supplement.

We don't like to assume that fortified foods will provide enough for our children, especially as research shows that despite an intake of B12-containing foods like milk and eggs, vegetarians are still at an increased risk of B12 deficiency. The safest way to ensure your babe gets this vital nutrient is with a supplement.

> **PBJ Bottom Line:** We recommend a daily B12 supplement for all plant-based toddlers who are no longer consuming formula or breast milk (or fewer than 3 feeds per day) containing at least 5 mcg or 1 mcg, 2 times a day.

Iron

After their first birthday, your child's iron needs decrease from 11 mg per day to 7 mg per day, which makes it much easier to meet your toddler's needs through food alone. Continue to offer iron-rich foods regularly along with a source of vitamin C to increase absorption. You may want to continue offering iron-fortified baby cereal throughout the second year if your child does not have a high intake of legumes and/or if they had iron issues in the past.

If it hasn't been done already, your pediatrician will likely check iron levels at your child's 1-year checkup. If your child's iron is low, you'll need to add a supplement to boost his stores.

PBJ Bottom Line: Iron needs decrease at one year, though it remains a nutrient to prioritize. If your child has low iron levels, supplementation is recommended.

Calcium and Vitamin D

As we discussed, ensuring that calcium and vitamin D needs are met on a daily basis is the main reason we prefer offering fortified nondairy soy or pea milk.

We won't sugarcoat it—not including fortified milks makes it much harder to meet calcium recommendations. That's not to say it can't be done, as calcium is abundant in a plant-based diet, but you'll need to ensure your child is offered (and eating!) these foods in high enough quantities, which is challenging if they aren't a fan of beans and broccoli. We like to remind parents of the saying "It's not nutrition unless it's eaten."

We should point out that kids who drink more than 3 cups of milk per day as recommended by the National Dairy Council are at an increased risk for iron deficiency anemia. This is because the calcium in dairy competes with iron for absorption—and wins. Therefore, we prefer to keep our milk offerings to twice a day and serve them separate from our babe's most iron-rich meals: in the morning before breakfast, at snack time with fruit, or before bed, not alongside their iron-rich meals.

Water should still be their main beverage, offered continuously throughout the day. Toddlers' stomachs are small and they don't need much, from solids or liquids, to fill quickly. Allowing babe to drink milk, whether cow's or a plant-based milk, all day long can interfere with nutrient absorption and will likely crowd out other important nutrients.

In the second year, vitamin D needs increase from 400 IU per day to 600 IU per day. For breastfed babes, this means you'll likely continue the supplement you've been providing since birth or find a multivitamin including vitamin D. For formerly formula-fed babes, this is a new consideration.

Similar to calcium, your babe will likely get the majority of her vitamin D through fortified foods like plant milk. But this usually isn't enough. Vitamin D intake from fortified plant milk depends on how often your child drinks milk and which brand you end up choosing. The fortified soy milk that we purchase has 25% RDA of vitamin D per cup, which means our children get 25%–50% of their needs met from this milk alone.

Since vitamin D doesn't naturally occur in plant-based foods (other than specially grown mushrooms, which aren't easy to find), and relying on sun exposure can be tricky depending on the time of year and where you live, cover the rest with a multivitamin or single supplement that includes vitamin D. Make sure you look for a supplement labeled "vegan" or "vegetarian," as some vitamin D3 is sourced from sheepskin, which will be listed as "lanolin" in the ingredients. Vegetarian children can also obtain some vitamin D from eggs, though the amount varies.

PBJ Bottom Line: Consider how much vitamin D and calcium your child is getting from both fortified and naturally occurring food sources. Depending on their diet, you may need to supplement.

Iodine

Similar to B12, once babes are fully or mostly weaned from breast milk or formula, they'll need a dietary source of iodine. Omnivorous toddlers generally get the majority of iodine from cow's milk, but plant milk does not contain iodine. The other major source in the diet is iodized salt, but we try to minimize toddlers' salt intake. The most reliable solution is a supplement. You can buy individual liquid drops or look for a multivitamin that includes it. If you use iodized salt in your toddler's meals (we both use minimal amounts), you may want to provide half of the RDA versus the full amount. Keep in mind that most plants also contain small amounts of iodine.

Remember that the amount of iodine in sea vegetables varies widely and may exceed daily recommendations. For example, one study found that nori (an edible seaweed species) contains about 37 mcg per gram. Your average children's seaweed snack contains about 5 mg of nori, which equals 185 mcg of iodine, more than double the RDA. That's not to say you should never eat nori; we just don't want to give it too much or too often and we want to provide a more reliable source of daily iodine.

PBJ BOTTOM LINE: Toddlers need iodine. A liquid supplement or multivitamin is the most reliable option. We recommend providing half of the RDA (~45 mcg) if you use iodized salt in your child's meals or the full RDA if you don't.

Does My Child Need a Multivitamin?

Intake and food preferences vary widely from toddler to toddler, so it's impossible to say whether every child needs a multivitamin. We also want to be clear that this isn't a plant-based thing—we'd give the same recommendation to an omnivorous child as well.

That being said, providing a multivitamin can be an easier approach to confidently check all the boxes on nutrients that may be harder to find in a plant-based diet, like B12, iodine, vitamin A, and vitamin D, especially for strict vegans. It's true that multivitamins may contain nutrients that your child doesn't need, but they also act as a form of insurance. You will have to consider what makes the most sense for you and your babe.

Though Alex considers Vander to be a great eater who loves his vegetables and iron-rich foods, she has given him a multivitamin since he turned one to help cover any nutrient gaps. It gives her peace of mind that some nutrients don't have to be met through food, especially on days when appetite wanes or Van decides to boycott a meal.

Whitney prefers to individually supplement B12, iodine, vitamin D, and algae oil. The type A dietitian in her doesn't mind mixing up exact amounts of these drops in his water every morning, but this approach doesn't make sense for everyone.

PBJ BOTTOM LINE: Your child's diet and intake will determine their needs. You may find it easier to offer a multivitamin than individual supplements to help cover nutrient gaps that aren't met in the diet.

Picky Eating: What's Normal, What's Not?

As we mentioned, the first year or so of eating solids is the honeymoon period. Many babies are willing to try a wide variety of foods offered, and may even surprise you with which ones become favorites. Alex's son, Vander, happily gobbled up collard greens and sautéed spinach those first few months and couldn't get enough of curried lentils and sauerkraut.

Screech. That's the sound of eating with abandon coming to a halt during the second year. We frequently hear from parents, "My son used to love [insert healthy food] and now he won't even touch it. It's frustrating to see him turn up his nose at vegetables that he used to love." Some kids continue to eat most foods offered and have only short periods of picky eating, but many enter a phase of major selectivity. Or maybe your experience is more like Whitney's, and your babe has avoided all veggies from the beginning. If either sounds familiar, rest assured that it's normal.

For whatever reason, picky eating is sometimes stigmatized, as if you did something wrong. While there are ways to reduce the stress of this period for both of you, selective eating has much more to do with developmental milestones and genetics than it does with parenting. The first thing we like to do is help parents understand why these changes are happening.

PBJ Quick Bite

Picky eating is a totally normal developmental stage. Don't blame yourself!

Slowed Growth

Around age 1, your child's rate of growth will start to gradually decline. Slowed growth means reduced appetite. This begins between 1 and 2 years, and levels off until they reach the next major growth period during puberty. Yes, that means that your 3-year-old may sometimes eat less food than your 1-year-old. Totally normal, and completely OK. For reference, the average caloric needs of a 1-year-old is 900 calories per day, while 2-to-3-year-olds need about 1000 calories per day. (Don't sweat the exact numbers—it's hard to visualize this difference on the plate.)

You also may start to notice that your round baby has started to lean out. Fat stores decrease around this time as baby transitions to a toddler and becomes much more active, coupled with height gains. We bring this up because decreases in appetite typically cause parents to worry that their child isn't getting enough, especially if they are on a plant-based diet. But consistent growth is used to determine proper nutritional status, not appetite. Your pediatrician will continue to plot your child's weight and height on their growth chart and as long as they are following their curve, then there's usually nothing to worry about.

Try not to compare your child's eating to other kids'. Just like adults, children come in all shapes and sizes and have different appetites.

How Parents' Behavior Affects Picky Eating

As with everything in parenting, when it comes to feeding children, we bring our own experiences, feelings about food, and behaviors to the table.

Research professor and author Brené Brown sums it up this way: "We can't give our children what we don't have." Essentially, we cannot foster a healthy relationship with food or teach our children how to honor their hunger and fullness cues if we haven't developed these skills ourselves. Luckily, we can learn from our past experiences and adapt our behavior.

There are four types of parenting styles that are believed to influence feeding: authoritative, authoritarian, indulgent, and uninvolved. In general, authoritative parenting is associated with healthier lifestyles and environments and a reduced risk of childhood obesity, while authoritarian parenting and permissive parenting have both been linked to an increased risk of childhood obesity. Most parents are a mix of these styles, though one tends to dominate. Understanding your current approach will help you modify behaviors and support healthy eating patterns.

Authoritative Feeding Style

We are hesitant to use the word *best* when it comes to parenting, but authoritative feeding is generally associated with more positive outcomes, like increased physical activity and healthy eating. It's also the feeding style that most closely aligns with the Division of Responsibility (more to come on that). Authoritative parents create boundaries around mealtimes and respect their baby's food choices. They honor and respond to children's hunger and fullness cues and allow baby to decide how much and which foods they want to eat. Authoritative parents offer consistent, healthy meals and snacks and treats occasionally.

No pressure, right? As we've mentioned before, we aren't perfect parents and don't always follow this style to a T. It's far too easy to get frustrated when our babes want a cookie for dinner or refuse their broccoli, even though they loved it the day before. But our goal is to align with these principles as much as we can, understanding our responsibilities when it comes to feeding our kids and trusting them to do the rest.

If you weren't raised in a house like this, it probably doesn't feel innate. Alex was raised in a "clean plate" household, where she was forced to sit at the table and finish her dinner before she was allowed to have dessert. Whitney's mom was not so fondly referred to as the "Fruit and Veggie Police," and Whitney recalls the embarrassment she felt when plates of carrots and broccoli were pushed on her friends.

Our moms were just doing the best they could. Many parents believe that forcing certain foods on kids will lead them to be healthy eaters and that restricting junk food will manage their weight. But these demanding behaviors often backfire. It wasn't until well into our adult years that we both learned how to have a healthy relationship with food.

Authoritarian Feeding Style

This is the most common feeding style we see in practice, and the style our parents used. An authoritarian approach gives parents the majority of control. They set the rules around feeding with little regard for a kid's preferences or hunger and fullness cues.

Authoritarian feeding is bossy. It dictates exactly what kids can and should eat and usually involves rewards or punishment for eating certain foods. An authoritarian parent may allow dessert only if and when vegetables are eaten. Or a parent may demand that a child eats a certain amount of food using both pressure and praise.

While rewarding may seem like a positive behavior, it usually backfires. Rewarding kids to eat more or eat specific foods (like vegetables) places junk foods on a pedestal and teaches kids that the only way to really enjoy healthy foods is if there is a reward at the end. Children who are raised in an authoritarian household typically eat fewer fruits and vegetables compared to other feeding styles and are at a higher risk of childhood obesity.

Permissive or Indulgent Feeding Style

This feeding style is known as "yes" parenting—providing few boundaries around food and allowing the child to consume anything they want. Little ones who are raised with a permissive feeding style tend to eat more junk and processed food than their peers.

A permissive style can also be described as an on-demand style: being a short-order cook for meals, allowing kids to graze throughout the day without set meals and snack times, and letting them demand which foods they want (or don't want) to eat.

Neglectful or Uninvolved Feeding Style

The last parental feeding style is an uninvolved or neglectful feeding style. Generally, this means that parents make few demands when it comes to what their children eat, but when kids do ask for food, they aren't supported. We're guessing none of you fall into this category, as you've already taken great strides to support your child's nutrition simply by picking up this book!

The Division of Responsibility in Feeding

One of our favorite tools for building confidence in feeding and raising healthy, joyful eaters is Ellyn Satter's Division of Responsibility in Feeding (sDOR). This model provides parents with a framework to guide children in positive eating habits and sets them up to be lifelong intuitive and mindful eaters.

sDOR is essentially what it sounds like—dividing up feeding responsibilities between the parent and child so that everyone knows their role. Being responsible for your child's nutrition can feel overwhelming, and we find this framework to be incredibly freeing. When you understand your responsibilities as a parent, it makes it easier to accept what you can't control and understand when you must let go and trust your child. No more obsessing over shunned broccoli or beans on the floor. As long as you're fulfilling your responsibilities, your conscience can be clear.

Most picky eating battles are about control. Our babes are learning their preferences and want to affirm them. Dividing control, or responsibility, hopefully makes this stage less painful. As Ellyn says, "When parents do the job with *feeding*, your child will do his with *eating*."

In general, parents are responsible for the what, when, and where of feeding, and babe is responsible for how much and if they want to eat. That means that parents determine the overall menu, where the meal or snack will take place, and what time it will be offered. As we've touched on, this is another reason why having a routine is helpful to everyone. Kids can take comfort in knowing when and where their next meal is coming from, which reduces anxiety or overeating as protection against future hunger. Knowing that you will serve food again also helps us relax and diminishes our desire as parents to push food on our kids when they don't eat a lot at a meal (or at all).

Another opportunity will present itself in a few hours, and kids can choose to eat more then if they'd like.

Once you determine which foods will be offered, it's up to baby to determine if they want to eat it and how much. Yes, that means that they may only want strawberries for breakfast without touching anything else on the plate. You must let go of the reins and allow them to make that decision.

Although you set the menu, this doesn't mean that you should neglect a child's food preferences. The key is to offer both familiar "acceptable" foods along with new foods and avoid catering solely to baby's likes and dislikes. We recommend offering one or two foods you already know your baby likes, along with one new item or even an item they've rejected in the past.

FEEDING RESPONSIBILITIES

Parents'

- Choose and prepare meals and snacks.
- Provide regular meals and snacks.
- Lead by example of how to behave at mealtimes.
- Reduce grazing by not offering additional food and beverages (except for water) in between meal and snack times.
- Be attentive to your child's food preferences, without catering solely to their likes and dislikes.

Children's

- Eat the amount of food that's right for them.
- Grow into the body that is right for them.
- Understand mealtime behavior expectations and learn to behave well.
- Learn to eat the food that the family eats.

Strategies for Promoting Adventurous Eating

Much of what we label "picky eating" is normal developmental behavior. Toddlers are learning to assert their independence and one way to do that is by controlling what they eat. Allowing this phase to turn into a tug-of-war can increase the duration of picky eating behaviors. Instead, playing it cool when new foods are introduced lets our kids know that these are the foods the family eats and we trust their autonomy to partake or not.

While there are many factors that contribute to a child's preferences, the number one recommendation we can make is the benefit of consistent exposure without pressure. Exposure is the number one factor in getting kids to accept new foods. Touching, smelling, seeing, playing, and yes, putting food in their mouth and spitting it out are all ways kids explore foods. That means that you may place the same food on your child's plate a dozen times before they are even willing to touch it, let alone taste it. We know how frustrating it can be, but keep at it. Research shows that continuing to offer a variety of foods during picky eating stages, even if they never actually eat it, increases the likelihood that these foods will be accepted at a later point.

The "without pressure" caveat is a tricky one. The "take a bite" approach can often backfire, as it turns healthy eating into a game of control, rather than trusting children to try to accept food on their own. Pressuring them to try something they don't want to can easily turn into a dinnertime struggle, and we don't know about you, but fighting with toddlers has never ended well for us.

Given our discussion on parenting feeding styles, it may seem obvious that demanding that kids eat their vegetables before they leave the table would be a no-no, but excessive encouragement can also qualify as pressure. Holding a carrot in their face and saying, "Mmm, it's so good. It's so good for you. You'll love it. Mommy loves it!" is considered positive pressure. All foods should be presented with the same appreciation and we should avoid assigning health halos or virtuous labels. The goal is to put vegetables on the plate and allow children the freedom to eat or not, no strings or words of encouragement *or* negativity attached.

Role modeling healthy behaviors seems to have much more of a positive impact than verbally encouraging kids to eat certain foods. Want your babe to enjoy broccoli? Enjoy it yourself!

Finally, letting kids participate in the decision-making process can combat picky eating. Closed-ended questions are important here. For example, "What do you want for breakfast" can lead to a lot of responses that you may not be able to honor. "Cake?!" But "Do you want waffles or oatmeal?" frames a realistic choice of items that you have and are willing to serve.

PBJ Quick Bite

Model the foods you want your toddler to eat by serving the entire family a similar meal.

The same approach works with vegetables. "Do you want broccoli or carrots?" helps kids feel like they have a say in the matter. It's OK if the response is, "None!" In that case, we respond, "I would like broccoli tonight, so we will have that. I will put some on your plate as well and you can choose whether or not you want to try it."

Cooking Techniques to Expand the Plate and Palate

As parents, we know that picky eating phases are hard and often have us questioning whether we are doing things correctly or whether our child is getting the essential nutrients they need. There's no right or wrong way to serve food, but certain techniques and strategies may help.

The first question we ask clients who come in for picky eating is how snacks and mealtimes are structured. Sometimes picky eating is related to hunger and fullness cues being off. If a child isn't excited about eating dinner because they've been snacking all afternoon, it's going to be much harder for them to willingly try a new food. This is another reason that we promote having a meal and snack schedule once your toddler is old enough to wait a few hours in between meals. Limiting grazing, especially before dinner, will boost their appetite when they do sit down at the table and can encourage them to try new foods. We also recommend only water between meals and snacks so they don't fill up on milk or other beverages.

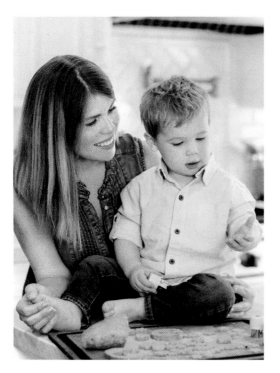

When you do go to introduce a food, there are several approaches you can take to foster acceptance. The first is placing a small, one-bite piece on their plate. This prevents them from being overwhelmed. Remember, exposure is multisensory—for very picky eaters it may take a dozen exposures before they are even willing to touch it. If they do try it, and like it, awesome! You can ask if they'd like more or increase the amount the next time it's offered.

PBJ Quick Bite

Offer one or two foods you already know your child likes along with one new item or even an item he has rejected in the past.

We introduce one new food at a time along with foods that are already accepted. This approach honors our kid's food preferences while also providing an opportunity for exposure. This decreases the chance our kids will leave the table hungry. If we only served them something new, there's a chance that they wouldn't touch any of it, leaving both of us frustrated. Instead, we take the sDOR approach: They are able to eat as much as they want of the foods offered, even if that means they only ate the pasta (*again*) and didn't touch the sautéed spinach (*again*).

Varying the way you offer foods is also helpful. Whitney's son loathes steamed broccoli but gobbles it up when it's finely chopped and mixed into his favorite dairy-free mac and cheese. Alex's son won't touch zucchini or yellow squash if it's sautéed on its own but will happily down it if it's finely chopped in lentil tacos or mixed into an enchilada filling.

Note—we are not promoting hiding vegetables. Making vegetables more palatable or size/texture acceptable for a toddler is not the same as "sneaking" vegetables into a dish and lying about their presence. We don't want to send the message that vegetables are bad and they must be hidden in order for them to taste good. However, purees or finely chopped vegetables are sometimes better accepted than larger chunks, and this is a good way to build on exposure.

PBJ Quick Bite

Offer foods in different shapes, sizes, and textures to increase the likelihood of acceptance.

We've also noticed that cutting fruits and vegetables into fun shapes makes them more likely to be eaten. Alex's son, Vander, refused to eat sweet potatoes for a good six months, until she used small cookie cutters to make star-shaped sweet potatoes. Was it a pain to prep all the stars? Yes. Did it make a difference? You bet. After five or so meals of star sweet potatoes, he started eating regular ol' diced sweet potatoes and asking for seconds.

Lastly, food chaining, an approach that encourages kids to try foods that are similar in taste, texture, color, and/or smell to the food they already enjoy, can also ease the way. For example, if your child loves pizza, she might also like pasta with tomato sauce and dairy-free cheese. From there, you can try to introduce tomato soup and grilled cheese dippers, or add chopped vegetables to their pizza or pasta, and then finally, introduce sliced tomatoes. Or, if your older infant is having trouble moving past purees, you can slowly increase the texture of their foods, gradually making it chunkier until they are able to accept the food in a larger format. Food chaining can take weeks, if not months, but it's a technique that has great success, especially in the pickiest of eaters.

Why Restriction Backfires

Remember how we said that picky eating is often related to control? Imagine how you feel when someone tells you that you can't have something. Is your first inclination acceptance, or do you suddenly want that thing even more? Yeah, we're in the latter camp as well.

As our children start to develop their preferences, you may find them asking for the same items over and over again or choosing to eat only those foods when offered in a meal. Of course, we want our children to have a varied diet, but limiting and restricting their favorites doesn't help. It often backfires, encouraging kids to sneak food when we're not looking or overeat when they are finally allowed off-limit foods.

Our goal is to promote self-regulation—the ability to respond to their own hunger and fullness and learn how certain foods fit into a balanced diet. Kids need to trust that food will be available again, and they also need to trust that they will enjoy eating. Let's

> **PBJ Bottom Line:** Parents are responsible for providing food, but the child is responsible for whether or not they eat it, and how much. Picky eating phases take patience and consistency, but understanding both your and your child's role can help make them less stressful for you both. Repeated exposure without pressure is the best way to handle selective eating. Providing a multivitamin during this time is one way to ease your fears about any nutrient gaps.

prevent any mealtime dread over what's offered and continue to assure our kids that they will have enough to eat. We'll explore this topic in much more detail in Chapter 6.

Common Questions and Challenges

Q: What if my child hates vegetables?

A: If your child refuses to eat vegetables, try not to stress too much. We are all born preferring sweet foods to more bitter ones—a survival mechanism that encouraged us to drink more of our mother's sweeter breast milk and steer clear of sour or bitter things, which are more likely to be poisonous.

Just like with other picky eating behaviors, consistent exposure without pressure is the best way to encourage acceptance. Modeling how you eat vegetables is a great way to spark their curiosity, especially if it's done without coaxing or pushing. Some vegetables are sweeter than others, so peas, carrots, and sweet potatoes are better bets than stronger, more bitter vegetables like asparagus and Brussels sprouts.

No child will love every vegetable. If they adore broccoli and sweet potatoes but shun everything else, consider that a win. Offer broccoli and sweet potatoes often, while continuing to cycle less-accepted vegetables.

Also, keep in mind that fruit contains many of the same vitamins and phytochemicals as veggies. That's why they're grouped together on the PB3 Plate.

Q: What if my child doesn't eat anything at dinner?

A: Despite your best efforts, this will likely occur at some point, or several points. Dinner tends to be the hardest meal for most kids. This is why introducing foods at breakfast or lunch may be easier. Kids are tired later in the day and often have a limited emotional capacity for novelty by dinnertime.

The first thing we recommend is assessing whether their dinner refusal is related to snacking beforehand. If so, try reducing afternoon snacks and limit grazing, or move snack time and dinner further apart.

Here's the truth: It's OK if your babe skips dinner. If they signal that they're done without ever touching a morsel, end the meal. We know what you're thinking: *But what if they go to bed hungry?!* Obviously, don't starve your child. We recommend removing the plate and allowing them to take a break from the pressure of mealtime. Then, after

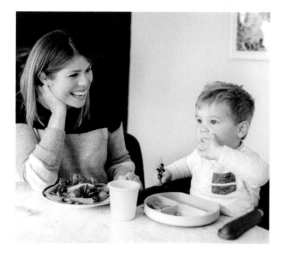

they've had a chance to settle down and understand there is no pressure to eat, you can return to the table and either offer the plate again or another nutrient-dense option for a "bedtime snack," like a peanut butter sandwich. Make sure to let enough time pass between dinner and this evening snack. This shows that you aren't a short-order cook while still recognizing that toddler preferences can be all over the place.

Q: My formerly polite baby has turned into a plate-/food-tossing toddler—what do I do?!

A: We admit this behavior drives us both crazy. The first few times our sons picked up food from the high chair and dropped it on the floor, we smiled and laughed. How cute! When the behavior didn't stop, the cuteness factor quickly wore off and we were left begrudgingly cleaning yogurt off the floor, walls, and ceiling.

First, let's bring it back to development. Food throwing is a normal part of babies' development of fine motor skills and exploration of new foods. Throwing is rarely malicious. Especially as they start to graduate from a palmar to pincer grasp, it may be an unintended consequence of trying to bring food to their mouths.

As babes get older, throwing food is a sport of curiosity. What happens when I throw this fork? Will it come back? What sound will this food make when it hits the floor? Will Mommy laugh or get angry? As infants transition into toddlers, food throwing is usually about getting a reaction and can turn into another power struggle at mealtime.

Understanding where your child falls in these developmental milestones is a good first step to figuring out how to approach food throwing. For both babies and toddlers, remaining calm is a great approach to avoid encouraging the behavior. We recommend picking up the food without returning it to the tray or table and saying something like "I want you to keep the food on your plate." By not giving a reaction and not returning the food, you are letting them know that once the food is thrown, it's done.

Sometimes toddlers throw food to let you know that they don't want it, so you can also set an empty bowl or cup next to their plate. Simply having foods they don't like on their plate may make them feel pressure to eat. Tell your toddler that this receptacle is where they can put food they don't want. This worked wonders for Whitney's son and sometimes he came back to the food later.

Food throwing can also be a sign that baby is done eating or is bored. We recommend calmly removing the tray/plate and your child from the table without making it seem like he is being punished. Again, we want to remove as much emotion from mealtime struggles as possible so we don't encourage battles for control.

Q: I'm worried that my child eats too much or not enough.
A: Alex's son has always been on the larger end of the growth chart. He was almost 9 pounds at birth and has continued to chart in the 80th percentile for most of his short life. He also *loves* food—eagerly requesting breakfast almost as soon as he wakes up in the morning, wanting to try bites of whatever Alex is cooking, and happily enjoying most foods that he's offered. From nannies to day care teachers to friends, his appetite has always been a topic of conversation. "Wow, I wish my child could eat that much." Or "Do you think he needs all that food? That's much more than my child eats."

Some children naturally have larger appetites, some have smaller ones. Kids innately know how much food they need in order to grow appropriately for their body. As long as your child's weight and height are following their growth curve, they are likely eating enough.

If you feel like your child eats "too much," consider their access to food. Children eat more than they need when they are afraid of going hungry. Do you allow for second helpings (or third or fourth!) or do you remove their plate before they are finished eating? Do you limit how often they are able to eat, letting more than three or four hours go by between meals and snacks? Restricting the amount, time, or type of foods and using negative words about how much they eat will all encourage your child to eat *more* than they need, not less. Setting a flexible schedule for meals and snacks and offering balanced meals without restrictions helps provide the structure and consistency that kids need to feel secure about food.

If poor growth is a concern, address this with your pediatrician to rule out any feeding issues that aren't related to nutrition. From there, ensure that you are offering the foods they need to grow: high-fat and higher-calorie foods like avocado, nut butters, oils, grains, beans, and fortified milks.

Our best advice is this: Feed your child as if you weren't concerned about their weight. When making decisions about how much or what to offer your child, ask yourself, *Is this what I would offer if I wasn't worried that they are overweight/underweight?* If you would do something different had the scenario been reversed, that's a sign that you're letting your parental prejudices influence feeding decisions.

Q: My toddler has been constipated lately—are there any foods that can help?
A: Constipation is one of the top issues children struggle with, and many will experience it at some point in their early years. The good news is that by following a plant-based diet you're already adhering to our number one recommendation for fighting it—loading up on fiber!

As discussed, fiber helps support normal digestive functioning by adding bulk to stool and helping it move quickly along the GI tract. Pretty much all fruits, vegetables, beans, seeds, and whole grains are great sources of fiber. A few, however, are exceptionally good at getting the gut in motion. Stone fruits like peaches, plums, cherries, and apricots contain naturally occurring sugar alcohol that acts as a laxative. Very ripe bananas are also helpful because of their fiber and sugar content. Prunes are another helpful fruit. We recommend pureeing them with a little water and offering 1–2 oz with meals as needed.

Speaking of water, hydration is incredibly important to prevent constipation, especially in a high-fiber, plant-based diet. Under 12 months, offer 1–2 oz of water with meals. After 12 months, make sure your tot has unlimited access to water and remind them to drink throughout the day. Busy toddlers often forget!

6

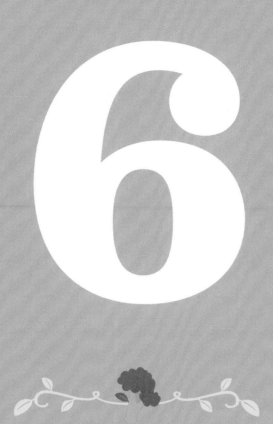

The Plant-Based Toddler and Beyond

We wish we could feed our kids in a bubble. A safe space where artificial colors and unnecessary additives weren't found in their food, where birthday parties served fruit platters instead of cupcake towers and ice cream, and where we didn't have to worry about excessive sugar and salt in *every* little thing.

Unfortunately, even the healthiest kids will eventually be exposed to the world of highly palatable, processed foods—and want in on the action. Alex noticed a big shift in her son's attention and attraction to certain foods around his second birthday. Previously oblivious to what other people were eating, he suddenly started to ask for foods that his preschool classmates ate, like pizza, chips, and candy.

Her first instinct was to ban everything. After all, he was only two. She had hoped she had a few more years of ignorant bliss before he started to realize that the foods served in his house were slightly different from those served at his friends' houses. However, she knew the research—pressuring kids to eat certain foods and withholding others means they will likely eat more, especially sweets, when they are given the chance.

Children need the space to explore foods that we don't always deem "healthy" and the freedom to trust their own bodies without the metaphorical weight of societal norms bearing down on their decisions.

This chapter will address common concerns parents have about raising plant-based toddlers, such as navigating day care, birthday parties, travel, and more. We'll also dive deeper into picky eating challenges and what to do when your parenting partner's diet is different from yours. Finally, we'll leave you with some tips to set your child up for a lifetime of success in the feeding department—from how to establish routines to getting your kids involved in the kitchen.

How to Introduce Sweets and Treats in a Healthy Way

Junk food, forbidden foods, highly palatable foods, whatever term you use, we are likely talking about the same thing—cookies, cake, chips, soda, ice cream, and other snacks and desserts that are high in sugar and salt and low in beneficial nutrients. As discussed in the previous chapters, there's no reason to provide these items to babes under 2, and luckily, they're not on older infants' and young toddlers' radar. However, as your child starts to notice sweets and treats, from the family, school, the grocery store, or friends, handing them a strawberry or shiny toy isn't going to cut it.

So how do you incorporate sweets and treats in a healthy way? First, let's talk about what doesn't work: forced compliance. Forcing kids to eat certain foods (especially in predetermined amounts) before they are able to either get up from the table, have more of another food, or get a separate reward like a toy or dessert, is a bad idea. Turning food into a reward signals to kids that one food is worse than the other and creates additional temptation.

For example, if a child gets dessert only after eating their broccoli, it teaches kids that dessert is a reward and broccoli is a punishment. In order for a child to enjoy their food, they must first choke down a food they dislike. Using food as a reward can also lead to emotional eating. Kids learn that unpleasant situations, like being forced to eat a food they dislike, can be made better with other food. As much as possible, we don't recommend using food as a reward, either for completing certain tasks (like cleaning up their toys) or for eating something else.

Remember our goal is self-regulation. That means that even when we aren't around, our kids will eat moderate amounts of sweets and treats, the same as they do with other foods. Research shows that kids who feel they are restricted from these types of foods eat more of them. One study of preschoolers demonstrated that those who were restricted from palatable food items, like crackers and packaged snack foods, increased their intake of that food when they were finally able to enjoy it. Studies have also shown that food restriction leads to increased weight gain and a greater risk of obesity.

As parents, we want to raise healthy eaters who trust

PBJ Quick Bite
Using sweets as a reward for eating vegetables teaches children that veggies are a punishment and puts treats on a pedestal.

their cravings, hunger, and fullness cues. It's the same thing that we want for ourselves—a healthy relationship with food and our bodies. Withholding or forbidding particular foods tells our kids that we don't trust them to self-regulate, which means they don't learn these important skills that they'll need to navigate a world with lots of tempting food choices.

Structure, Not Restriction

Creating structure is key to developing healthy behaviors around treats. This means setting clear and consistent boundaries about when and where food will be consumed while also considering our children's perspective. Having clear guidelines lets kids know what they can expect from meals and allows them to enjoy food and is also associated with greater behavioral regulation and academic achievement.

RESTRICTIVE FEEDING VERSUS STRUCTURED FEEDING
Restrictive Feeding
• Doesn't allow the consumption of palatable foods
• Doesn't consider the child's perspective
• Doesn't allow for dietary flexibility
• Access is determined by the parent, and the child is unclear when access will become available again
• Takes food away/hides food
• Uses guilt as a deterrent to eating ("I'll be sad if you eat that food." "If you have too much candy, you won't be healthy.")
Structured Feeding
• Allows the child to consume palatable foods with boundaries about when and where they will be consumed
• Considers the child's perspective when creating routines
• Is consistent in the use of routines, but also flexible based on circumstances (allowing for ice cream, cake, *and* candy at a birthday party on occasion)
• Access is determined by the parent, but the child knows when and where foods will be offered again
• Serves appropriate child-sized portions and allows the child to eat as much or as little of what is provided
• Doesn't associate food with guilt or control

Creating Structure for the Plant-Based Toddler

We recommend setting up a routine for how, when, and where these foods will be included in your family's diet. That doesn't mean that snack time will always include chips, chocolate, and cookies. It means that sweets and treats will no longer be placed on a pedestal and will become an unexceptional part of the diet. Know that there is a lot of variability in this approach—so while we will provide a framework for fitting in all foods, it will ultimately come down to what's best for you and your family.

It is up to you as a parent to determine how much and how frequently to offer these foods. We encourage creating general guidelines, such as single servings for dessert on most nights, but also allowing for some flexibility—just as you would with your own diet. We offer dessert to our kids as often as we eat it: a few times a week, without seconds, and we serve it with the same enthusiasm as dinner, so it doesn't turn it into a hyped-up event. As with all meals and snacks, there is no pressure to eat the dessert.

With older children, you can practice this same approach and give them the autonomy to serve themselves so they can regulate their portion. You may still choose to implement the no-seconds boundary while abiding by the Division of Responsibility guideline of allowing your child to consume however much of the portion they plate themselves.

STRUCTURED OFFERING OF SWEETS AND TREATS*

- Pick a few nights a week to offer dessert or a few weekly snacks where treats will be offered and keep it consistent.

- Decide in advance whether seconds are allowed.

- Offer dessert *with* dinner on occasion to remove the perception that dessert is somehow better than the main meal. In this case, you may want to implement the single-portion boundary.

- Set boundaries for situations where treats will be offered in excess such as birthday parties or Halloween. For example, kids can enjoy unlimited candy on Halloween, and then 1 or 2 treats a day or every other day thereafter.

- Occasionally, allow kids unlimited access to sweets and treats to learn self-regulation.

- Create a family ritual—Sundays are vegan ice cream night!

- Make nutrient-dense versions of your favorite desserts in addition to offering traditional sweets and treats.

- Dessert doesn't always mean junk food; fruit can be dessert too.

These are several ideas for how you may choose to incorporate sweets and treats into your child's diet. It's up to you to decide what works best for your family. You do not have to do all or any of them.

Talking to Toddlers About Food and Nutrition

An important part of incorporating sweets and treats in a positive way is refraining from assigning negative labels. So while it may be difficult, we must ignore the urge to explain how terrible sugar is to our toddlers when they're in the middle of enjoying a cookie or a slice of birthday cake. There is a time and a place for discussions about nutrition, but the early toddler years, at the family table, is not it. Conversations about the health benefits of fruits and vegetables can begin as early as your child starts talking, but we'd advise waiting until kids are older (around 4 to 5 years) before broaching the topic of moderation when it comes to less nutritious food. Toddlers are simply too young to understand the concept of food for pleasure versus food for nutrition.

When you do talk about it, nutrition should be discussed away from the table in order to avoid children feeling pressure to eat certain foods or shame about others. We want to avoid framing the conversation as a comparison between "healthy" versus "unhealthy" foods. Try using descriptive versus qualitative words. For example, Whitney's son, Caleb, became much more interested in broccoli when she informed him that it was the same color as his favorite Jedi warrior, Yoda.

HOW TO TALK TO KIDS ABOUT FOOD

Age	Instead of:	Try this:
2–3 years	Eat your broccoli. It's good for you!	Broccoli makes our body and brain strong!
2+ years	Eat your carrots or you won't get dessert.	These are carrots. You don't have to eat them if you don't want to.
2+ years	You can't have another bag of fruit snacks. They're not healthy. Eat this orange instead.	That's all the fruit snacks for today. We'll have more tomorrow. Do you want an orange?
2+ years	You need to watch how much you eat or else you'll gain excess weight.	We listen to our tummy and stop eating when it feels full.
2+ years	You haven't eaten any vegetables today! You need to eat some for dinner.	We eat a variety of foods to help us grow! What kinds of foods haven't we eaten today?
2+ years	Here's a plate of cookies—don't eat too many!	Here's a plate of cookies—enjoy as many as you like.

HOW TO TALK TO KIDS ABOUT FOOD		
2+ years	You can't have pasta again for dinner tonight, that's too many refined carbs.	We eat different foods on different days!
4–5 years	Cookies are bad because they're high in sugar, so we have to limit how many we eat.	Cookies are yummy, but we need to save room for other foods that help our bodies stay healthy and strong. So we don't eat cookies all the time.

Finally, parents can promote positive food behaviors around sweets and treats by demonstrating healthy behaviors themselves. That means ditching diet rules and allowing yourself to consume desserts without shame while also modeling the consumption of more nutrient-rich foods. Enjoy your carrots and your carrot cake with equal enthusiasm and your child will too!

Does Avoiding Meat and Animal Products Qualify as "Restriction?"

With all this talk about restriction, the inevitable question is—"Does preventing kids from eating meat and animal products qualify as restriction?"

We say no. We choose not to eat meat for a variety of reasons. Yes, health is one, but animal welfare and the environmental impact of meat-eating are other reasons. To us, this sets meat apart from other forbidden foods, like cake and cookies, because the reason behind our decision is vastly different.

For many plant-based dieters, avoiding meat and animal products doesn't feel like restriction because unlike treats, these are not foods that one wants to eat but prohibits themselves (or their children) from eating. With junk food, people *want* to eat it but restrict themselves due to fears about the food, which are often weight related. This is how the cycle of avoidance leading to increased desire starts. Most plant-based eaters have no desire to eat meat and animal products and therefore avoiding them doesn't produce a negative eating behavior.

It depends on your family's individual choices about what constitutes food and what does not. Anything that your family does eat—whether regularly or on occasion—should be an option for your child when the food is being served. We both practice a predominantly plant-based approach, and we do consume things like eggs and dairy on occasion. Therefore, while we generally don't serve these items at home, we don't restrict them for our kids when they're offered at a friend's house or a birthday party.

With that said, just because you choose to occasionally serve animal products does not mean you have to always serve them. As discussed in Chapter 5, you are not a short-order cook. Telling your child neutrally that eggs or dairy (or cake) are not on the menu today is not a restriction. Likewise, you don't have to offer treat foods that your family doesn't eat. Neither one of us drinks soda, so we don't have it in the house. When our children are older and begin to ask for soda, we will allow them to order it on occasion when out at restaurants or enjoy it at celebrations, but we aren't bringing it into our homes just for the sake of introducing it to our children.

This is what works for us. We know we may have to reassess this way of thinking as our kids get older and their dietary choices are out of our control. You must decide what works best for your family based on your beliefs.

Whatever your choice, we recommend talking to your children early and often about your family's choices. In these early years, board books geared toward tots can introduce concepts like our love for animals and the importance of protecting our planet. As they get older, you can broach heavier topics like why you choose not to eat animals. There are many online resources to help with these discussions, including great YouTube videos that break down the issues into simple, clear messages that kids can understand. Visiting local animal sanctuaries is another great way to help children make the connection between these issues and the animals at stake. Understanding why your family chooses not to eat animals greatly reduces the chance that your child will ever feel his diet is restricted.

> **PBJ Bottom Line:** Food permission and restriction is a sensitive topic, and research isn't black and white. We recommend providing foods like sweets in a structured fashion with reasonable boundaries, but also allowing for flexibility. Children who are forbidden from eating sweets eat much more when they are given the opportunity to do so.

When it comes to restricting animal foods, the solution isn't so clear. We believe that because our reasons for avoiding or limiting animal foods are different from the main reason many people restrict sweets (weight gain), a different approach is warranted. We choose to restrict meat while allowing for other animal foods on occasion, especially at friends' houses and at celebratory events.

Support for Your Feeding Choices

What's that? Your family isn't as supportive as you'd hoped they'd be about your decision to raise your child fully or predominantly plant-based? We've been there too. We know not everyone is as open to our choices as we'd like them to be—that includes friends, family, and yes, even our pediatricians.

Remember that it's your family, your baby, and your choice. We also think it never hurts to remind concerned parties that the American Academy of Nutrition and Dietetics put out an official statement that well-planned vegan and vegetarian diets are safe for all stages of the life cycle, including pregnancy, infancy, breastfeeding, and beyond. And, of course, the well-planned part is why you picked up this book!

When Your Partner Isn't Plant-Based

How do I raise my child plant-based when my partner isn't on board? We get this question often on our Plant-Based Juniors Instagram page and we'd first like to state that we aren't therapists, so we're not medically qualified to provide advice on how to resolve parenting disputes. There's not a right answer for everyone. But we'll share our point of view and experience from talking to other families.

During the first few years of life, children are learning what, when, and how much to eat largely based on cultural and familial beliefs, attitudes, and practices. This modeling behavior can become a little trickier when children see one parent eating a certain set of foods and another parent enjoying something entirely different.

If raising your child with specific parameters is important to you, it's always a good idea to discuss this with your partner right from the get-go. It may help to sit down with a qualified professional to navigate the decisions you'll need to make—will baby be allowed to eat some meat and animal products? Which ones, and when? Will these foods be served at home? Will the parent who eats animal foods eat them in front of baby?

One option may be that the partner who chooses to consume animal products agrees to eat them outside of the home and enjoy plant-based meals when eating with the family. Another option may be that certain foods like eggs and cheese are allowed in the home, but meat and poultry will only be consumed outside of the home.

If one partner is adamant about eating certain foods, like meat, at the family table, and you intend to keep your child meat-free, this will create a challenge. As we discussed before, kids learn eating habits by modeling. They want to eat what their parents eat. Denying them food that other family members are eating may feel like restriction and lead to an increased desire to consume these foods.

As with all aspects of parenting, you and your partner likely won't see eye to eye on every issue. The best advice we can give is to have these conversations away from the dinner table, when tensions and emotions about food are less charged. You'll have greater success if you are willing to compromise, give space when needed, and not personally attack or criticize. Try to offer the same respect that you'd want someone to give to you about your eating choices, even if you don't agree.

PBJ Quick Bite
Have conversations about food choice away from the family table to keep mealtime positive.

Dealing with Day Care

Navigating day care with a plant-based child can feel overwhelming. Alex will never forget the day she picked up her son from day care and the teacher pulled her aside to let her know that she gave Vander a chicken nugget that was brought in for another child's birthday.

After sobbing for what felt like an eternity, she reiterated her belief system to the teacher and spent the next few days researching new day cares. Once she calmed down, she decided to figure out a more reasonable solution. While Vander was just two years old, she knew that he was aware of the fact that he was the only kid in school who ate different foods from his classmates.

Ultimately, she decided to offer plant-based versions of the same menu items that were offered at his school. Alex made dairy-free mac and cheese on Mondays, tofu nuggets on Wednesday, and calzone strips on Friday. Was it easy to make all these meals every week? No. Did it allow Van to easily fit in with his peers? Absolutely.

We polled our Plant-Based Juniors community and here are a few more solutions that have worked for other families:

1. Find a school/day care that doesn't offer set meals. If you want to be able to pack your child's lunch every day, make sure you pick a school that doesn't have set, communal menus. Some schools participate in the Child and Adult Care Food

Program, where dairy is mandated, and it may be trickier to bring your own food, so be sure to ask.

2. Make your own plant-based alternatives. Like Alex, you can request the school's lunch menu in advance to plan out lunches and snacks that mimic what the other children are being offered.

3. Explore vegetarian and vegan schools. While you'll likely only find them in the most progressive parts of the country, schools that offer only vegetarian or vegan meals do exist.

4. A different approach at school. Many of our families reported that they allow their kids to eat whatever is offered at day care, while continuing to offer plant-based meals at home.

Whatever decision you settle on, it's been our experience that for the most part, staff and teachers are gracious and accommodating when it comes to diet preferences. After the fateful chicken nugget incident, Alex volunteered to bring in tofu nuggets for all the kids one day and often provides recipes for different foods she has packed for Vander that the other kids have been interested in.

Dealing with Birthday Parties

Birthday parties are synonymous with treats galore—cookies, cupcakes, cake, and ice cream in addition to the typical pizza or hot dogs that are often served alongside. In general, we're more relaxed on special occasions but know not everyone feels the same way. Here are the strategies that have worked for us and our friends.

PBJ Quick Bite

Offer to bring a dish to parties and family gatherings when you know plant-based options won't be served.

Alex reaches out to the parents and asks about the food situation ahead of time so she can be prepared to bring alternatives. That way Vander doesn't leave the party feeling hungry or left out. If hot dogs are on the menu, she brings her own veggie dog. Since she isn't asking for any special favors from the host, she's never had a problem with bringing in her own food, and Vander's never been the wiser.

Whitney usually offers to bring a dish to share with the group. At one event where pepperoni pizza was served for dinner, she brought a batch of our Easy Quesadillas (page 282) and they were a big hit. Caleb didn't bat an eye at the community pie.

If you'd prefer your kiddos have vegan treats, you'll want to try a similar approach with items like cookies, cake, and ice cream. As we are predominantly plant-based, we allow our children to enjoy treats containing eggs or dairy at parties while enjoying a meat-free main option.

When it comes time for your child's birthday party, this is your opportunity to show off how amazing plant-based food can be. For Caleb's first birthday, Whitney made a vegan smash cake that he demolished and devoured. It has since become a popular recipe on our website! For Vander's second birthday, Alex had a "Dragons Love Tacos" theme and made a taco bar with lentil tacos, tofu sofritas, rice, black beans, dairy-free cheese sauce, tortillas, and various toppings for the adults. No one missed the meat or the dairy.

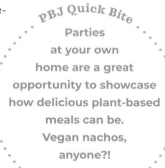

PBJ Quick Bite

Parties at your own home are a great opportunity to showcase how delicious plant-based meals can be. Vegan nachos, anyone?!

The Plant-Based Toddler On the Go

For plant-based toddlers, it can be a little trickier to ensure that appropriate food will be available when hunger strikes (which seems like every other hour with a 2-year-old), but it's not hard with a little planning. This section includes our tips for providing nutritious meals and snacks and sticking to a "rigidly flexible" feeding schedule whether you're out on a daily adventure or an extended family vacation.

Toddler Snacks

There's a reason we dedicated almost an entire recipe chapter to just toddler snacks. Most toddlers are great snackers—preferring to graze all day long instead of sitting down at the table for an actual meal. While snacks are a healthy (and necessary) part of a toddler's diet, it's also easy for snacking to get out of hand. If you notice that your child isn't hungry for meals, or doesn't eat much at meals, consider first how much they are snacking beforehand. Kids who are allowed to graze between meals will likely fill up before sitting down at the table, which can make any struggles you're already having worse.

To remedy this, we recommend sticking to a structured but negotiable schedule of meals and snacks so that kids start to build a routine around hunger and fullness and the trust they will have the opportunity to eat again. Depending on their appetite, this may look like a midmorning and midafternoon snack with the possibility for another snack option before bed.

PBJ Quick Bite

If your child isn't eating much at dinner, think about your snack schedule. On-the-go grazing may be the culprit.

Snacks shouldn't be nutrient-void treats. We've noticed that many products marketed as a "snack," especially to kids, tend to be filled with refined starch, sugar, salt, and sometimes artificial colorings and flavors. Instead, we like to think of snack food as the same food we'd serve at mealtime: fresh fruit and vegetables, whole grains, nut butters, beans/legumes, and healthy fats. Aim to include at least two of the main PB3 categories to ensure a balanced snack that will fill your child up until their next meal. Fresh options might not always be possible when we're on the go, so we also rely on healthy packaged snacks when we are traveling or away from the kitchen. We always have a few stocked up in our purses and diaper bags for those times when we are out and don't have time to stop somewhere and grab a bite.

OUR FAVORITE ON-THE-GO SNACKS FOR KIDS

- Fresh blueberries, bananas, apples, oranges
- Freeze-dried fruit and vegetables
- Chewy Granola Bars (page 244)
- Blueberry Oat Balls (page 257)
- Dried bean and pea bites
- Unsweetened apple sauce
- No-sugar-added fruit and nut bars
- Guacamole and hummus mini-packs with crackers or sliced vegetables
- Baked sweet potato or beet chips

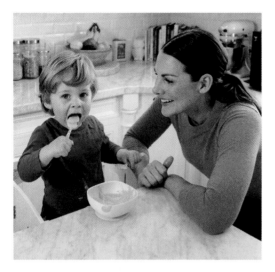

Finally, we know how tempting it is to shove a snack in a screaming toddler's face, but food shouldn't be used as emotional Band-Aids. We've all been there, dealing with a complete meltdown at Target while we pull out every snack in our purse in hopes that they will quiet down. While food can be a fantastic distraction, especially with fussy toddlers, try to resist. We don't want to teach our kids that boredom or sadness are good reasons to eat if they aren't actually hungry. We also don't recommend getting into the habit of offering snacks in the car, unless they need it. Toddler brains are conditioned to form habits quickly, and we don't want them to associate car seats with snacking.

Eating at Restaurants

Unless you're dining at a vegetarian or vegan restaurant, you'll find that most traditional kids' menus leave a lot to be desired nutritionally and usually lack plant-based options. Hot dogs, pizza, grilled cheese, spaghetti and meatballs, and chicken tenders are the usual suspects. Kids' menus cater to highly palatable salty and fatty foods, which, except on special occasions or in accordance with our sweets and treats routine, aren't items we want our kids to fill up on.

We recommend scanning the sides portion of the menu, as that's where you'll typically find vegetables, grains, and sometimes beans. We often make a meal for our kids out of some type of grain or pasta, a vegetable or two, and beans (or tofu if we're lucky). It's completely OK if your restaurant meal doesn't match the PB3 Plate—we don't sweat over individual meals. Proper nutrition is based on long-term dietary patterns.

Depending on what you are eating, you may decide instead to have your babe eat some of your meal. This is

PBJ Quick Bite

Try not to stress when restaurant meals don't resemble the PB3 Plate—good nutrition is a reflection of your child's overall dietary pattern, not a single meal.

especially helpful if portion sizes are large and you aren't sure how much your toddler is actually going to eat. Two large adult portions can easily feed a family of three.

Family Travel

When we travel overnight with our kids, we pack a few extra snacks and foods for easy meals to make in the hotel. Not only does this help keep costs down, it also ensures that we are offering routine, nutrient-rich options at least some of the day. Alex travels with a jar of peanut butter for easy sandwiches and Whitney brings her own rolled oats, chia seeds, and flaxseed. Paired with hot water and a banana, she's easily able to make a yummy bowl of oatmeal for Caleb.

If we're staying somewhere for an extended period of time, we prefer to get a rental with a kitchen. This option allows us to make some of our own meals or enjoy carryout in our rented place.

Our best piece of advice for toddler travel, though, is to enjoy it! We both travel often, and while it can be stressful and challenging coordinating schedules and demands, it's such a blessing to be able to introduce our babes to new environments and cultures. We think any of the added hassles—stroller malfunctions, airport meltdowns, unidentifiable substances from train seats ending up in mouths—are far outweighed by the lifelong memories we make as a family.

> **PBJ Quick Bite**
> Make a game plan for meals and snacks prior to traveling to help vacations go more smoothly. Pack snacks, find kid- and plant-friendly restaurant options, and consider a rental with a kitchen.

The Family Table

We're firm believers in the power of family meals. Eating with your baby right from the start, rather than watching them eat and then serving the rest of the family's dinner later, is important for teaching positive eating habits. Remember, children learn by modeling. Eating with the family teaches them proper feeding behaviors and encourages more exploration with food. Seeing mom enjoy carrots increases the likelihood that baby will try and enjoy them as well.

Studies show that eating together as a family has numerous nutritional benefits.

Family meals have been associated with a higher intake of fruits, vegetables, and essential nutrients and a lower intake of soda, fried foods, and saturated fat.

Children who eat more meals with their family also tend to have healthier body weights. One study of 4-year-old children found that those who ate dinner as a family more than 5 nights a week had a 23%–25% reduced risk of obesity. Another study of kindergartners found that fewer family meals increased the risk of children being overweight by the third grade.

We know that eating every meal together isn't practical for many families, but the more often you can sit down and share a meal, the better. The good news is that the power of family meals doesn't apply only to dinner—these benefits have been demonstrated at other meals as well. One study showed that Latino children who ate a family breakfast at least four times a week were much more likely to consume at least five servings of fruits and vegetables a week than those who did not.

While a family dinner most nights may not be possible, try prioritizing family breakfast or even creating a routine around meals on the weekend. Even having just

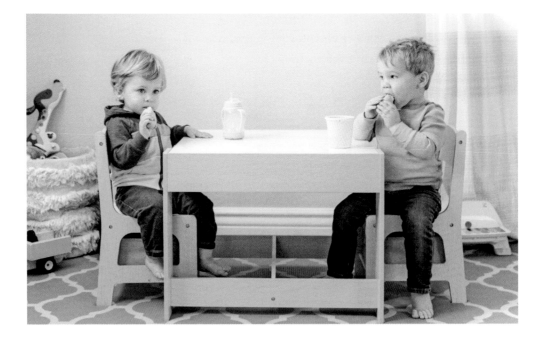

one person eat with baby makes a big difference. That could be you, your partner, or another sibling. If you have another caregiver providing meals for your child, ask that they eat with baby when possible.

Mindful Eating

As we've discussed, babies are born with an innate ability to regulate their intake using hunger and fullness cues. This skill is something we lose with age as societal rules and pressure begin to dictate our food choices and negative eating behaviors hinder our ability to trust our bodies. As a parent, you have the opportunity to help your baby preserve their natural ability to self-regulate by modeling positive mealtime behavior.

One of the most important skills you can teach your child is mindful eating. This means paying attention to our meals in a nonjudgmental way and giving our food the respect it deserves. It means rather than rushing through meals, we slow down and actually taste our food. A novel concept, right?!

Taking the time to savor food allows for better recognition of hunger and fullness cues and reduces the drive to overeat.

Here are a few mindful eating practices you can implement and model for your child:

- Remove distractions like cell phones and televisions.
- Eat food slowly, putting your utensils down between bites.
- Eat seated, at a table.
- Plate your food, rather than eating from a package.

Toddler Table Manners

Let's be honest, toddlers don't have the best table manners. From throwing food to banging utensils on the table to intentionally spitting water all over themselves and other family members, they derive a lot of joy from being the opposite of polite. And while we may shudder at this kind of behavior when we're out in public, we also find ourselves struggling to maintain a poker face when we're cracking up inside. Who doesn't find a baby with a bowl of spaghetti on his head just a little hilarious? This behavior is entirely normal and age appropriate, but at the same time, it's never too early to start teaching proper table manners.

Here are a few of our tips for common mealtime faux pas:

1. Throwing food. We talked about this in the previous chapter, but as a reminder, throwing food is usually a sign that your tot is done with his meal. Rather than scolding, we recommend calmly saying, "I see that you're throwing your food. That means that you must be done," then taking the plate away without fanfare and getting your tot cleaned up. If they didn't eat a lot, you may choose to offer a snack a little later. Another option is to place a small plate or bowl next to their plate and let them know they can put any unwanted food there.

2. Banging cups, utensils, etc. The first time a toddler slams his cup on the table, it's startling, and a little amusing. The second, third, fourth incident of repeated banging—not so funny. We recommend demonstrating to your tot how to gently, properly place their items on the table. You can also designate proper spots for the items, and whenever they place them in the right spot, you praise them for their skill. If your tot continues to slam, take the item away until the next mealtime.

3. Spitting food or beverages. Similar to the slamming, modeling proper drinking and eating behavior is a good first step. Instead of saying, "Don't spit your water," try, "I want you to keep your water in their mouth, like this." If they keep spitting, take away the food or beverage. While we want mealtimes to be enjoyable, this kind of behavior signals that your tot is not hungry and is probably ready to leave the table.

Getting Kids Involved in the Kitchen

It's never too early to get kids involved in the kitchen. Letting children participate in the food-making process empowers them to take an active role in their nutrition. Toddlers are constantly seeking more autonomy and authority, and letting them help with meals is one way to give this to them.

If the thought of cooking with babies and toddlers conjures up images of shattered bowls, perfectly good ingredients lost to the floor or family pet, or dangerously close brushes with stove top burns, let us reassure you, we're not suggesting you hand baby a knife and let them take over as sous chef. There are plenty of safe, (relatively) mess-free ways to make baby a part of meal preparation.

As early as infancy, your babe can join you in the kitchen. From baby-wearing while you're making heat-free meals (avoid this to prevent burns when using the stove or oven) to letting baby lounge in view of the action in a bouncer chair (we love the ones from Babybjörn), they can get in on the action from day one.

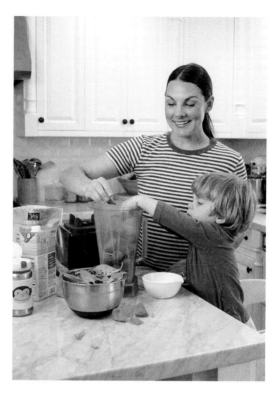

In toddlerhood, baby can begin to help with food prep. Assign activities that require little skill, like pressing the handle on the salad spinner or topping oatmeal with berries. Smoothie making is a great activity to let your little one practice his motor skills and exercise his freedom of choice. Whitney lines up a selection of frozen fruits on the counter and has Caleb select which he wants in his smoothie. Then she lets him scoop the ingredients into the blender, practicing his counting skills as he goes, and press the start button (fully supervised, of course).

Learning Towers are essentially stools that are walled in on all four sides and bring your child up to your level—physically and figuratively. Being able to work alongside you at the kitchen gives toddlers great pride and makes them feel like they are an important part of the process. We love the Kitchen Helper from GuideCraft, but if you're handy with wood, you can make one yourself. There are plenty of tutorials online. Just make sure yours has nonslip legs so it stays in place and a nonslip mat for your child to stand on.

As your child gets older, they will be able to begin using actual, age-appropriate cutlery. Training knives that are made of wood or plastic with blunted tips and non-slip grips teach kids how to cut softer foods without the risk of injury. Assign your child tasks like cutting banana slices or tomatoes and placing them on the family's plates.

Common Questions and Challenges

Q: My child never seems to be hungry at dinnertime. He rarely eats and prefers to play and make a mess of whatever I serve him. Any tips?

A: Toddlers aren't known for long attention spans, and forcing them to sit at the table when they aren't hungry can quickly turn into a power struggle. If you notice that your babe is more interested in playing then eating, check timing of meals. In many cases, not being hungry at dinner typically means that kids ate too much at snack time or had it too late in the day. Because frequent or irregular snacking is often a culprit, we recommend limiting anything other than water between snack and mealtimes. Items like milk or juice can fill up small stomachs and make your child less likely to eat at the following meal.

Q: My son's grandparents don't seem to take our dietary choices seriously and keep giving him animal products. What do I do?

A: Not everyone will understand or agree with your decision to raise a plant-based child, and this can be especially difficult when that person is a relative or regular caregiver. It's important that you clearly communicate your choice and your boundaries to anyone caring for your child. Especially with older generations, plant-based diets may not be something they "get." Framing your position around what's best for your child may help. Try something like this: "I know you may not understand why or agree with our feeding choices, but this is how we have decided to feed _____ and we need you to respect that decision. Research shows that if we don't allow _____ to have these foods at home, but he eats them when he's with you, it will likely cause him internal conflict and confusion and set him up for negative eating behaviors in the future." Establishing the importance of continuity for your child's health and linking it to evidence will hopefully encourage other caregivers to honor your decision.

Q: Are artificial colors harmful?

A: With the introduction of sweets, treats, and snacks geared toward kids comes the exposure to other less savory components of the packaged world, namely artificial colorings.

Despite the fact that the FDA and food companies maintain that artificial dyes are safe, many studies have linked their consumption in children to attention deficit hyperactivity disorder and have shown that removing them from the diet may help reduce symptoms. In the UK, products containing the artificial colors sunset yellow (Yellow 6b), quinoline yellow (banned in the US), carmoisine (banned in the US), allura red (Red 40b), tartrazine (Yellow 5b), or ponceau 4R (banned in the US) must be labeled with the warning "May have an adverse effect on activity and attention in children."

We say, play it safe. There may not be an international consensus on artificial food coloring, but why risk it? Check your labels to make sure products don't contain artificial colors.

There are so many natural options for coloring food. If you're making food at home, try these powders and spices to add vibrant color: beet powder (bright red/pink), paprika (red/yellow), turmeric (yellow/orange), and annatto (red/orange). Whole foods work great too—try adding pureed blueberries, raspberries, sweet potato, purple potatoes, red cabbage, and spinach to dishes to create beautiful natural hues. Crushed freeze-dried berries also make for easy DIY powders to add to frostings for a naturally colored birthday cake.

Q: Is there any credence to the claim that plant-based diets increase the likelihood of developing an eating disorder?
A: Research does not support the theory that plant-based diets cause eating disorders. While more people with eating disorders seem to follow plant-based diets than in the general population, this is likely a situation of reverse causation, meaning that plant-based diets don't lead to eating disorders, but instead people with eating disorders choose plant-based diets because it allows them to restrict certain foods. The motivation behind following a plant-based diet may also be important. One study found that people who chose to eat a plant-based diet because of aesthetics were more likely to have an eating disorder, while those who chose this eating pattern for ethical reasons (like animal welfare or the environment) had no greater risk.

You can avoid potential issues by talking to your children about the reasons for your family's dietary choices and never associating them with weight or appearance. Additionally, monitoring your child's eating habits, modeling healthy behaviors, and sticking to our guidelines for pressure-free feeding as they age and gain more autonomy in their dietary choices will help pave the road toward a lifelong positive relationship with food.

Q: At what age is it important for kids to start exercising?

A: Physical activity is important at all ages! As soon as they start to walk, tots will naturally become very active—eventually running, jumping, kicking, and dancing their way through the day. Physical activity guidelines for 2-to-3-year-olds are as follows:

- at least 30 minutes of structured (adult-led) physical activity
- at least 60 minutes of unstructured (active free play) physical activity
- not be inactive for more than 1 hour at a time except when sleeping

This doesn't mean you should get your toddler a gym membership, but it does mean that you should provide ample opportunities for movement. Structured activities may include family dance parties, neighborhood walks, outdoor games, or toddler sports classes like soccer, ballet, or swimming. Unstructured activities include any time your little one is moving about without your guidance—digging in the sandbox, climbing a jungle gym, chasing the dog, etc.

Conclusion

Our primary goal with this book is to empower parents in their plant-based feeding journey. We know we've packed a *lot* of information into these pages, and we hope we've answered all the questions and concerns you may have. Our intention is that *The Plant-Based Baby and Toddler* becomes your go-to feeding reference and that you'll come back to it again and again for knowledge, support, and inspiration.

In the next section, you'll find 50 recipes covering everything from baby's first solid food to breakfast favorites and family-friendly meals. Additionally, we've compiled a few handouts for easy reference, like our supplement guide, DIY staple recipes, baby-led weaning cooking chart, and more.

We want you to know that we're here for you in every step of your feeding journey. We know what it's like to wonder, *Am I doing this right?* Parenting can be hard. But having a community of like-minded, supportive fellow parents makes it easier. We hope you'll join us on our Instagram page, @plantbasedjuniors, and on our website and blog, plantbasedjuniors.com. We regularly share the latest nutrition information and recipe inspiration, and are a spot for plant-based parents to just generally come together and lift each other up!

Thank you so much for joining us in this journey and we look forward to continuing to support you in the years to come.

Alex and Whitney

Alex Caspero   Whitney English

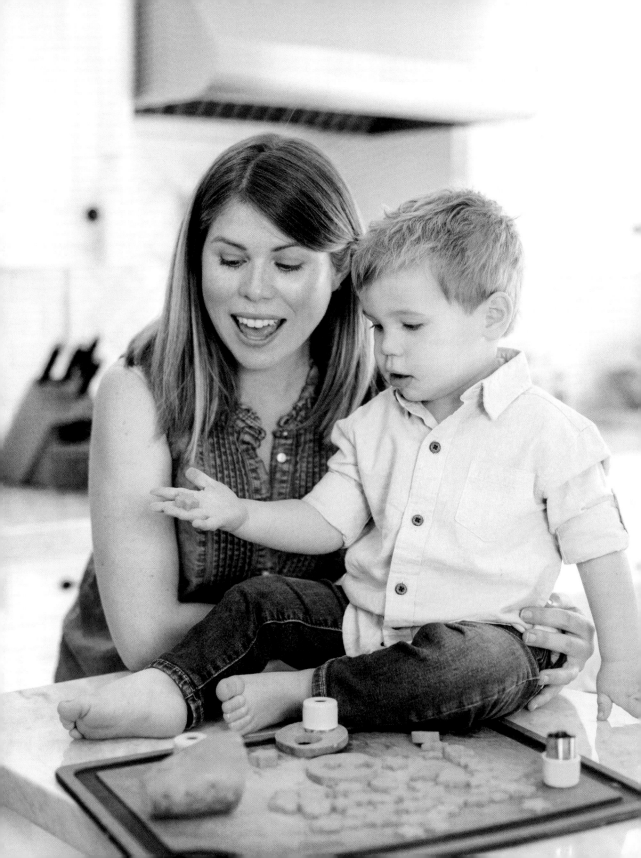

7

Recipes

Recipe Key

These symbols indicate the recipe contains a PB3 Plate nutrient of importance!

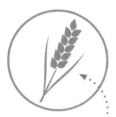

Grains and Starches

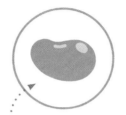

Legumes, Nuts, and Seeds

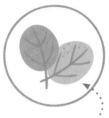

Fruits and Veggies

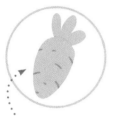

Carotene Queens

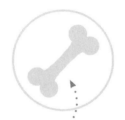

Calcium-Containing Foods

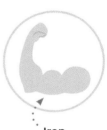

Iron

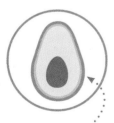

Friendly Fats

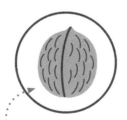

Omega 3–Rich Options

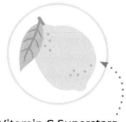

Vitamin C Superstars

Purees and Mashes for Little Mouths

Homemade baby food has many advantages over store-bought. It's cheaper, and you can ensure it contains all the nutrients your baby needs. These purees and mashes focus on iron- and protein-rich plant foods along with fruits, veggies, nuts, seeds, herbs, and spices to expose babies to a wide array of tastes and textures right from the start—which research shows contributes to positive eating behaviors in the future. They are also quick and easy to make—we all know new parents' lives are complicated enough as it is.

   Note: You can add a few tablespoons of water to any of these recipes if your baby needs a thinner consistency. Also, you can adjust how long you process the mixtures to achieve different textures—smoother when you're just starting out, and chunkier as baby progresses.

Notes for safe preparation and serving

- Wash hands and equipment before cooking.
- Thoroughly scrub and peel all fruits and vegetables before cooking.
- Baking, steaming, roasting, or microwaving are the best cooking techniques to prevent nutrient loss.
- Rinse canned beans to remove any sodium and juices.
- Store in airtight containers in the refrigerator or freezer.
- Rewarm before serving, and allow to cool to room temperature. Be sure to stir and taste before serving to ensure proper temperature.
- Individually portion baby food from the main container to serve, and discard any portion that is leftover or has been touched by baby's mouth or spoon.

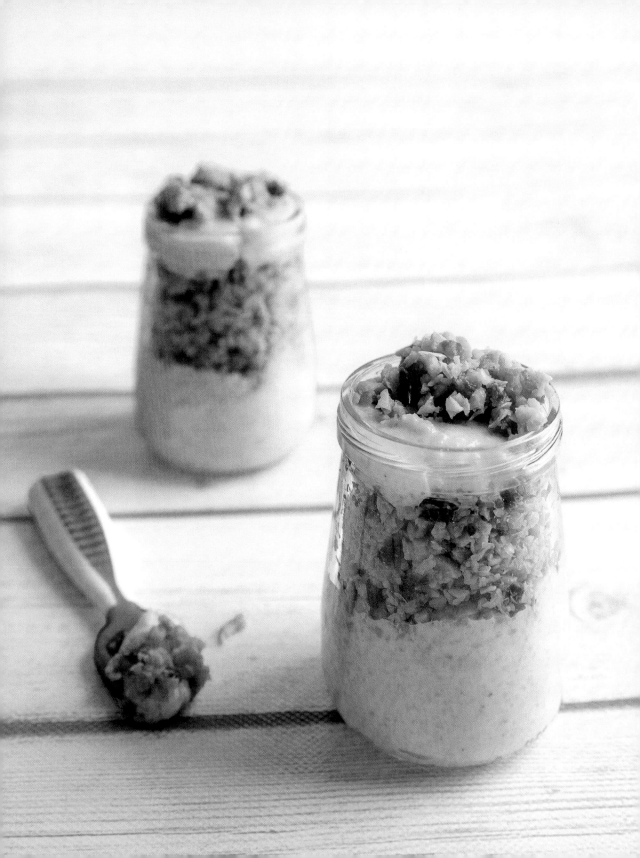

Chicks 'n' Grits

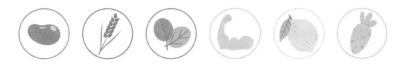

MAKES EIGHT 1-OUNCE PORTIONS

- ½ cup chopped fresh or frozen red bell pepper
- ½ cup cooked polenta*
- ½ cup cooked chickpeas
- 1 teaspoon dried thyme or 1 tablespoon fresh

1 If using fresh bell pepper, toss with ½ teaspoon olive oil. Roast for 20 minutes at 400°F.

2 Place all the ingredients in a food processor, blender, or baby food maker and puree. If needed, add a splash of water to thin.

If using polenta from a tube, add 3 to 4 tablespoons of water to thin out.

Family-Friendly Feeding Tip: Sauté the chickpeas with olive oil and salt. Serve over warm polenta with roasted red peppers and any extra sautéed veggies of choice.

Blueberry Muffin Mix

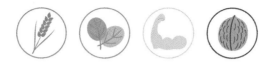

MAKES EIGHT 1-OUNCE SERVINGS

- ½ cup rolled oats
- ½ cup fresh or frozen blueberries*
- ½ cup iron-fortified baby oat cereal
- 1 tablespoon hemp seeds
- 1 teaspoon ground Ceylon cinnamon**

1 In a small pot over medium heat, combine the oats and 1 cup of water. Bring to a simmer and cook until the oats are creamy and soft, about 8 minutes.

2 Place the cooked oats, blueberries, baby cereal, hemp seeds, and cinnamon in a food processor, blender, or baby food maker and puree, or use an immersion hand blender to puree.

If using frozen, add blueberries to the pot with oats so they thaw while cooking.

**We prefer Ceylon cinnamon over traditional cinnamon (also called Cassia or Vietnamese) because traditional cinnamon contains a phytochemical known as coumarin, which has been shown to induce liver damage in large doses.*

Family-Friendly Feeding Tip: Leave out the baby cereal and skip the puree step for older kids and adults. Enjoy topped with blueberries, hemp seeds, and any other favorite toppings.

Cubano Bowl

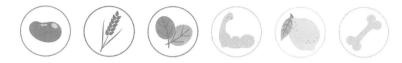

MAKES EIGHT 1-OUNCE SERVINGS

- 1 cup leafy greens of choice (we like collard or kale)
- ½ cup cooked rice
- ½ cup cooked black beans (rinsed if canned)
- 1 large ripe banana
- ¼ teaspoon cumin

1 Place the greens in a steamer basket and steam for about 3 minutes, or until the greens have wilted.

2 Place the steamed greens, rice, beans, banana, and cumin in a food processor, blender, or baby food maker and puree until smooth.

Family-Friendly Feeding Tip: Slice the banana and lightly fry with avocado oil on the stove top until browned. Instead of steaming, sauté the greens with olive oil and cumin. Serve adults' and older children's portions "grain bowl-style," with black beans and rice as a base and greens and banana slices on top. You can also add additional toppings like avocado and tomatoes. Salt and pepper to taste.

Sunshine Bowl

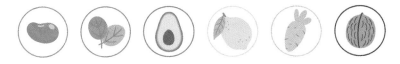

MAKES EIGHT 1-OUNCE SERVINGS

- ¼ cup chopped fresh or frozen carrots
- ½ cup silken tofu, drained
- ¼ cup fresh or thawed frozen strawberries
- ¼ cup fresh or thawed frozen mango chunks
- 1 teaspoon chia seeds

1 Place the carrots in a steamer basket and steam for about 10 minutes, or until soft.

2 Place the steamed carrots, tofu, strawberries, mango, and chia seeds in a food processor, blender, or baby food maker and puree until creamy and smooth.

Family-Friendly Feeding Tip: Enjoy topped with nuts, seeds, and extra fruit as a yogurt alternative!

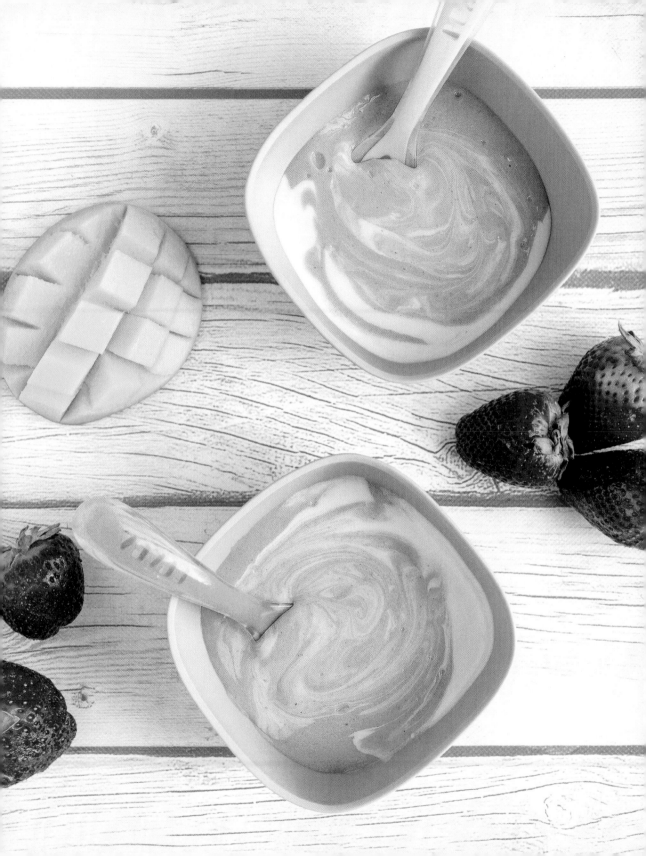

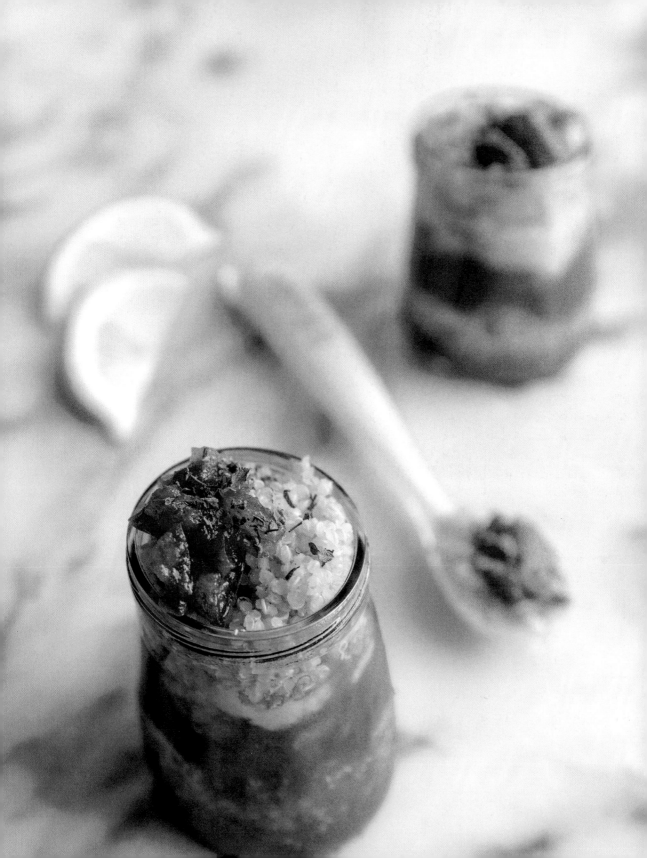

Le Petite Pizza

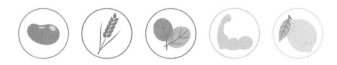

MAKES SIX 1-OUNCE PORTIONS

- ½ cup cooked white beans (rinsed if canned)
- ½ cup cooked quinoa
- ¼ cup tomato sauce (no salt added) or ¼ cup diced fresh tomatoes
- 1 teaspoon lemon juice
- 1 teaspoon dried oregano

1 Place all the ingredients in a food processor or blender and puree until creamy and smooth.

Family-Friendly Feeding Tip: Use as a protein-rich topping for pita pizzas!

Peas Please

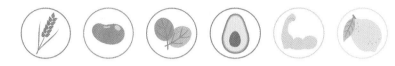

MAKES SIX 1-OUNCE PORTIONS

- ½ cup fresh or thawed frozen green peas
- ½ cup fresh or thawed frozen yellow corn
- 1 medium avocado
- ½ teaspoon garlic powder
- 1 tablespoon lemon juice

1 Place all the ingredients in a food processor, blender, or baby food maker and puree until creamy and smooth.

Family-Friendly Feeding Tip: Serve as a dip with raw veggies or crackers for older kids and adults.

Cheezy Broccoli Cauliflower Mash

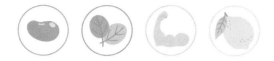

MAKES EIGHT 1-OUNCE PORTIONS

- ½ cup yellow or green split peas*
- ½ cup chopped broccoli
- ½ cup chopped cauliflower
- 1 tablespoon nutritional yeast
- 1 teaspoon lemon juice

1 Sort the peas, discarding any stones, and rinse thoroughly. In a small pot over medium heat, combine the peas and 1 cup of water. Bring to a simmer, cover, and cook for about 25 minutes, or until soft.

2 Place the broccoli and cauliflower in a steamer basket and steam for about 5 minutes, or until soft. You could also steam veggies over the pea pot!

3 Place the peas, broccoli, cauliflower, nutritional yeast, and lemon juice in a food processor, blender, or baby food maker and puree until smooth.

*To save time, substitute with canned white beans.

Family-Friendly Feeding Tip: Thin out the puree with vegetable broth, add a bit of salt, and serve as a soup for the rest of the family.

Beets + Sweets Mash

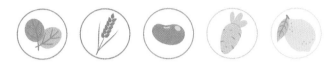

MAKES TEN 1-OUNCE PORTIONS

- 1 small beet
- 1 small sweet potato
- 1 teaspoon olive oil
- 1 small apple, peeled and chopped
- ¼ cup pepitas
- ½ teaspoon ground Ceylon cinnamon

1 Preheat the oven to 400°F.

2 Scrub and rinse the beet and sweet potato. Rub the beet with olive oil, pierce the sweet potato with a fork, and place both vegetables on a baking sheet. Bake for 45 to 60 minutes, or until fork-tender. Allow to cool slightly then remove the skin from both.

3 Place the cooled beet, cooled sweet potato, apple, pepitas, and cinnamon in a food processor, blender, or baby food maker and puree until smooth.

Family-Friendly Feeding Tip: Enjoy as an applesauce alternative or swirled into plant-based yogurt. You can also use this recipe as an opportunity to batch cook cubed roasted sweet potatoes and beets to add to salads or as a dinner side dish.

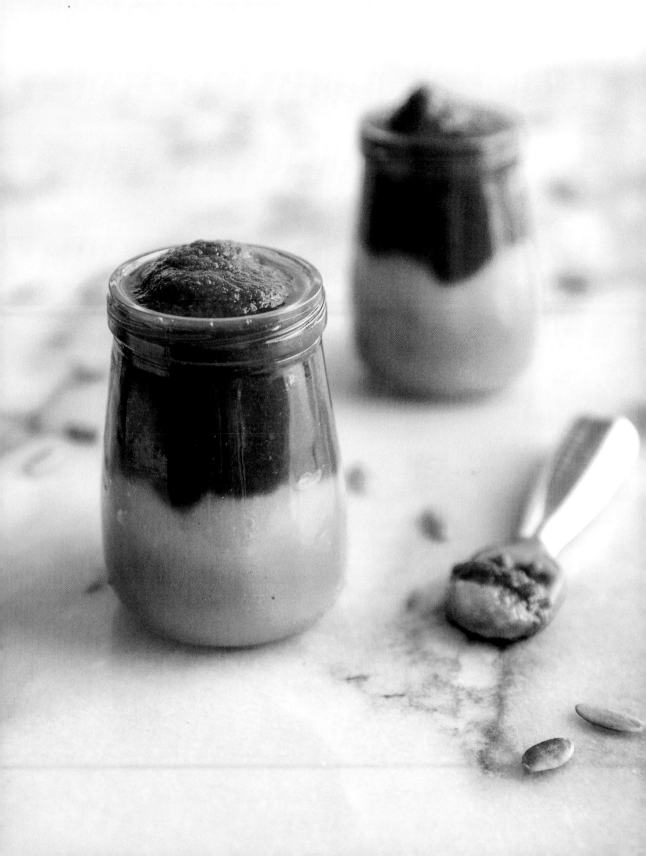

Baby-Led Weaning: Finger Foods for 6+ Months

For parents interested in letting babes feed themselves, our baby-led weaning recipes make it simple for plant-based infants to get all the nutrients they need in an easy-to-grasp form. We focus on key nutrients for the early feeding phase, including iron, fat, and vitamin C. Plus, we show you how to transform these bites into meals everyone can enjoy, because one of the biggest benefits of baby-led weaning is the ability to share food as a family.

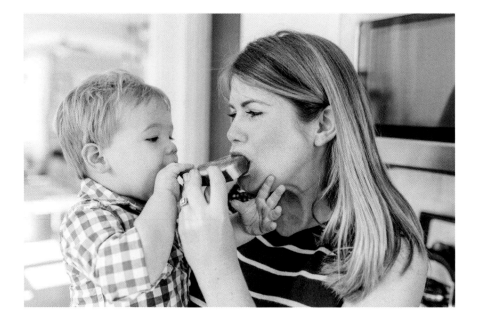

Butternut Squash Fries

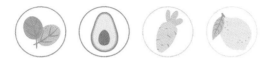

MAKES 2 CUPS OF FRIES

We made these fries at least a few times a week when our babes first started baby-led weaning. These are steam-roasted, which means they soften like steamed vegetables but have the added caramelization from roasting.

The trick is to cover the pan tightly with foil so the veggies create enough moisture to evenly cook. For babies who are just learning to eat, we recommend keeping the foil on throughout the entire cooking process so the squash comes out perfectly tender. Once baby has shown they can handle more texture, remove the foil halfway through to let the outside of the fries crisp while still retaining the soft inside.

You can use this steam-roasting technique for just about any vegetable. Refer to our cooking table on page 297 for more information.

- 1 small butternut squash
- 2 tablespoons olive oil
- ½ teaspoon ground cinnamon

1 Preheat the oven to 400°F.

2 Line a baking sheet with aluminum foil or parchment paper.

3 Peel the squash, halve lengthwise, and scoop out the seeds. Slice into finger-like shapes—about the width of a pinkie. Toss with the oil and cinnamon and place in a single layer on the prepared baking sheet. Cover with another piece of foil and crimp the edges together to form a tight pouch so steam can't escape.

4 Place in the oven and cook for 20 minutes. Then remove the baking sheet and carefully remove the top piece of foil, allowing the steam to escape.

5 Return to the oven and cook for 10 to 15 minutes more, until fork-tender and soft. Let cool before serving.

PBJ's Blender Bean Muffins

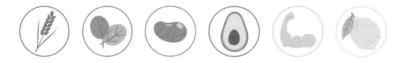

MAKES 12 MINI MUFFINS

These palmar grasp–friendly, convenient muffins are perfect for baby-led weaning. Packed with key nutrients babies need, like iron and protein, these naturally sweetened muffins are a tried-and-true favorite in the PBJ community.

These muffins freeze wonderfully, and we like to cook a big batch of them at a time. When your baby is ready to eat, thaw them in the fridge or on the counter, or defrost in the microwave.

They're also great with a little nut butter on top for toddlers and older children.

- ⅔ cup rolled oats
- One 15-ounce can chickpeas, drained and rinsed
- 1 medium overripe banana
- ¼ cup sunflower seed butter,* or other nut butter of choice
- 1 cup loosely chopped kale
- ½ cup unsweetened soy milk
- ¼ teaspoon ground cinnamon
- 1 teaspoon vanilla extract
- 1 teaspoon baking powder

1 Preheat the oven to 350°F.

2 Grease a metal mini-muffin pan and set aside. Alternatively, use an ungreased silicone mini-muffin pan.

3 Place the oats in a high-powered blender or food processor and process until they reach a flour consistency.

4 Add the chickpeas, banana, sunflower seed butter, kale, soy milk, cinnamon, vanilla, and baking powder and process until smooth.

*We like the brand Once Again because it's both sugar- and salt-free.

5 Fill the cups three-quarters of the way full in the prepared muffin pan and bake for 20 minutes until lightly browned and cooked through.

Tex-Mex Millet Meatballs

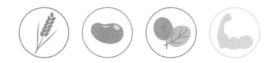

MAKES 20 MEATBALLS

These Tex-Mex meatballs are a great way to introduce millet into baby's diet. This nutrient-dense grain is popular in both African and Eastern European cuisines and is a good source of fiber, iron, B vitamins, and magnesium. You can find millet in well-stocked grocery stores or in the bulk grain section. Or you can substitute equal parts cooked quinoa or cooked bulgur wheat.

Serve for adults and older kids with BBQ dipping sauce. Once baby reaches 12 months, you can add a little salt and chili powder.

To freeze, bake as directed, then let cool. Freeze individually, then store in a large freezer-safe bag or container until ready to use. Microwave or warm in the oven until heated through.

- ½ cup cooked black beans (rinsed if canned)
- ¼ cup seeded, finely chopped tomatoes
- 3 tablespoons tahini
- ¼ cup corn kernels
- ½ teaspoon ground cumin
- 2 tablespoons finely chopped fresh cilantro
- 2 tablespoons oat flour
- ½ cup cooked millet

1 Preheat the oven to 400°F.

2 Lightly grease a baking sheet and set aside.

3 In a medium bowl, place the black beans, tomatoes, tahini, corn, cumin, and cilantro and mash together with a potato masher, fork, or the back of a wooden spoon. The mixture should be fairly sticky and most of the beans mashed, leaving just a little texture.

Add the oat flour and millet and stir. The mixture should easily ball together. If it's too wet, add more oat flour; if it's too dry, add more tahini.

 Scoop 1 tablespoon of the mixture, roll into a ball, and place on the prepared baking sheet. Continue with the rest of the mixture.

6 Cook for 25 minutes, or until golden brown. Let cool before serving.

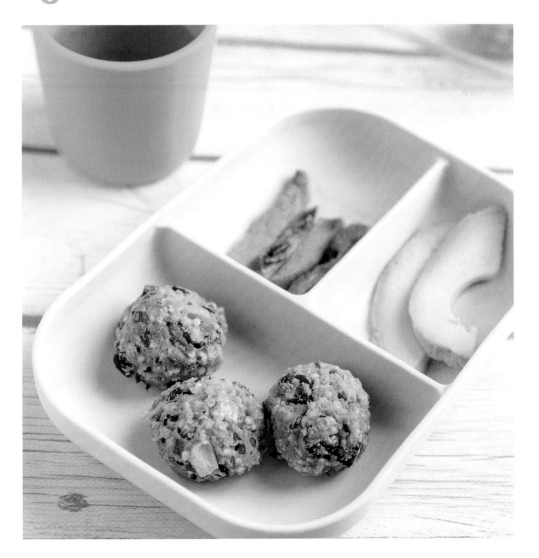

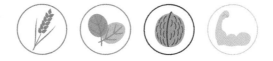

BLW Oatmeal Pancakes

MAKES 8 PANCAKES

These simple pancakes are made in the blender for minimal prep and cleanup. For an extra iron boost, consider subbing in half the rolled oats for iron-fortified baby oat cereal.

- ½ cup rolled oats
- 1 tablespoon ground flaxseed
- 5 tablespoons water or unsweetened soy milk
- ½ teaspoon baking powder
- 1 teaspoon vanilla extract
- ¼ teaspoon ground cinnamon
- 1 large ripe banana
- Coconut oil or nondairy butter, for greasing the pan

1 Place the oats, flaxseed, water, baking powder, vanilla, cinnamon, and banana in a blender and puree until smooth.

2 Grease a large skillet with the coconut oil and place over medium heat.

3 Dollop the batter onto the hot pan, one heaping tablespoon at a time. Cook for 2 to 3 minutes, then flip and cook 1 to 2 minutes more.

4 Let cool before serving. Enjoy as is or with a small smear of nut butter for allergen introduction and additional healthy fats.

Quinoa Prune Bars

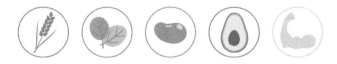

MAKES 12 TO 15 BARS

These baby-friendly granola bars pack in two natural laxatives: ripe bananas and prunes! Coupled with fiber- (and iron-) rich quinoa, these bars are perfect whenever baby's digestion needs a little help.

- 1 cup uncooked white quinoa
- ½ cup prunes
- ¼ cup peanut butter or another nut butter of choice
- 1 ripe medium banana

- ¼ teaspoon vanilla extract
- ¼ teaspoon ground cinnamon
- ¼ teaspoon ground ginger

1 Preheat the oven to 350°F.

2 Line a baking sheet with a Silpat baking mat or parchment paper.

3 Rinse the quinoa. In a large skillet over medium high heat, toss the quinoa with a spatula until it just begins to pop, 3 to 5 minutes. Remove from the heat and let cool slightly.

4 In a small bowl, place the prunes, cover with warm water, and soak for 10 minutes to soften. (This will make them easier to blend.) Drain, then place in a food processor with the peanut butter, banana, vanilla, cinnamon, and ginger. Puree until smooth.

5 Add the quinoa to the food processor and pulse a few times to combine. Spread the mixture onto the prepared baking sheet. Bake for 8 minutes to remove any stickiness. Let cool completely before slicing into finger-width bars.

Sweet Potato Stars

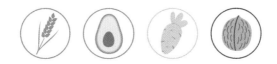

MAKES 10 TO 12 PATTIES

Our sons fell in love with a store-bought version of these patties. We weren't so fond of the sugar content or the ingredient list of said store brand. So we made our own! Just one and a half patties provide all the vitamin A your babe needs in a day along with a hefty dose of protein and plant-based omega-3 fatty acids.

We think of these as a choose-your-own adventure recipe. You can make them sweet or savory, bake them in star shapes, or pan fry for a crispier texture. These make a great portable snack or dinner side dish. They also freeze well if you want to batch cook a bunch at once.

- 1 medium sweet potato
- 2 tablespoons ground flaxseed
- 1 cup oat flour
- 1 tablespoon coconut or avocado oil

1 The sweet potato can be cooked in the microwave, oven, or pressure cooker. Wash and scrub the potato. If microwaving or cooking in the oven, pierce a few times with a fork to let steam escape. Microwave for 6 to 7 minutes or roast for 25 minutes at 425°F, or until soft. If using a pressure cooker, place the potato on the wire rack inside along with 1 cup of water. Seal and cook on high pressure for 16 minutes, then natural release for 10 minutes.

2 Right before the potato is finished cooking, place the flaxseed and 6 tablespoons of water in a large bowl. Let sit until gelled, about 5 minutes.

3 Once the potato is cooked, let cool, then scoop out the tender flesh. You should have about 1 cup of cooked sweet potato. Combine with the flaxseed mixture, oat flour, and any optional flavor add-ins (see below) and stir to combine. If the mixture is too sticky, add more oat flour.

4 To pan fry: Heat the oil in a large skillet over medium heat. Scoop out 1 to 2 tablespoons of the mixture and form into a patty. Wet your hands to make shaping easier. Fry for 2 to 3 minutes per side, taking care as you flip. Repeat with remaining patties.

5 To bake: Preheat the oven to 350°F. Grease a large baking sheet and set aside. If using cookie cutters, lightly flour the cookie cutters and a clean work surface. Turn the mixture out and pat into a rectangle, then cut into desired shapes and place onto the prepared baking sheet. Alternatively, shape 1 to 2 tablespoons of batter into a patty, then pinch five points of the circle to form stars. Wet your hands to make shaping easier. Bake for 23 to 25 minutes, until golden brown, flipping halfway through.

Optional Flavor Add-Ins
Omit salt for babies under 12 months.

Sweet version:
- ½ tablespoon maple syrup
- ½ teaspoon ground cinnamon
- ¼ teaspoon salt

Savory version:
- ½ teaspoon garlic powder
- ¼ teaspoon cumin
- ¼ teaspoon salt

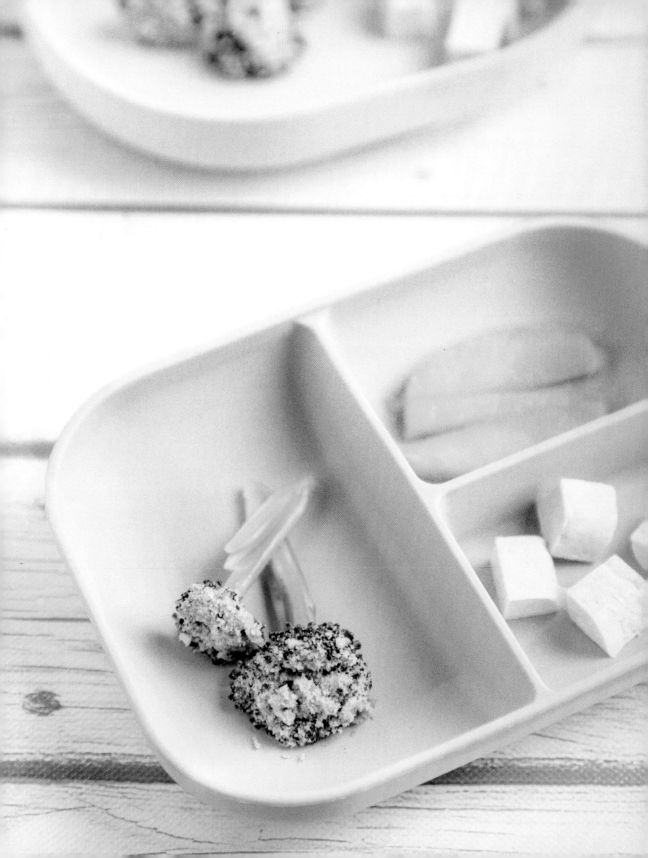

Cheezy Broccoli Trees

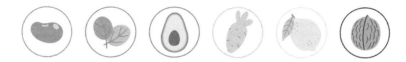

Lightly steamed broccoli florets dipped into homemade vegan Parmesan cheese. Slice the broccoli stalk at least 2 inches long so baby can easily hold it in their palm and gnaw on the cheezy floret end!

- 1 head broccoli
- ¼ cup raw cashews
- 2 tablespoons hemp seeds
- 2 tablespoons nutritional yeast
- 1 teaspoon garlic powder

1 Remove any tough wooden ends from the broccoli and cut into florets, keeping as much of the stalk as possible to make broccoli handles. The broccoli stalk should be about pinkie width in size.

2 Bring a large pot of water fitted with a steamer basket to a boil. Place the broccoli in the basket, cover, and steam until tender, 5 to 7 minutes.

3 While the broccoli is steaming, place the cashews, hemp seeds, nutritional yeast, and garlic powder in a food processor or blender and pulse until the mixture is very fine and thoroughly mixed.

4 In a shallow bowl, place the cheezy mixture. Dip the warm "tree" end of the broccoli into the topping. Repeat with the rest of the broccoli and serve.

Red Lentil Pizza Strips

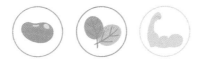

MAKES 1 PIZZA

Pizza! Pizza! To make this iron-rich pizza crust, we use red lentils to create a crispy crust that's ideal for piling on the low-sodium toppings like marinara sauce and homemade Parmesan cheese.

For adults and older kids, add ¼ teaspoon salt to the Parmesan mixture and top with sautéed vegetables of choice.

- ¾ cup red lentils, soaked for at least 3 hours
- 1 small garlic clove
- ½ teaspoon baking powder
- 1 tablespoon olive oil
- ¼ cup raw cashews
- 2 tablespoons nutritional yeast
- 2 tablespoons hemp seeds
- ½ teaspoon garlic powder
- ½ cup salt-free or low-sodium marinara sauce

1 Preheat the oven to 400°F.

2 Place a 12-inch cast-iron pan (or other oven-safe pan) into the oven to warm while it's preheating.

3 Drain and rinse the lentils. Place in a blender with ½ cup of water, the garlic, and baking powder and blend until smooth.

4 Carefully remove the pan from the oven, pour in the olive oil, and swirl to coat the bottom of the pan so the crust doesn't stick while baking.

5 Pour the batter into the pan and return to the oven. Cook for about 30 minutes, or until the edges are golden brown. Remove from the oven and let cool slightly, then gently remove the crust to a large cutting board and set aside.

6 While the crust is cooking, place the cashews, nutritional yeast, hemp seeds, and garlic powder in a blender or food processor. Pulse until the ingredients are well combined and reach the consistency of grated Parmesan cheese.

7 Spoon the marinara sauce onto the crust and cover with the Parmesan cheese. Slice into finger-width shapes and serve!

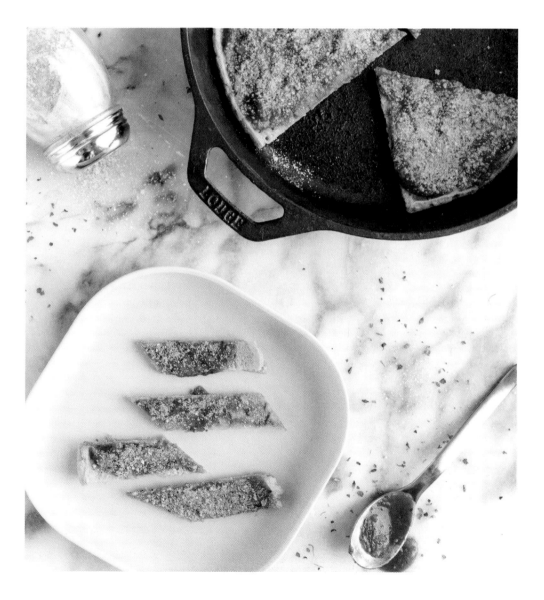

Tofu Marinara

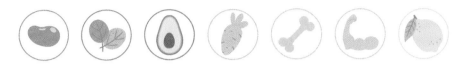

MAKES 12 TO 15 STICKS

This is one of our favorite ways to combine iron and vitamin C. Tofu fingers are first baked in a simple lemon-herb sauce, then topped with marinara sauce and more vegan Parmesan. Omit the parm topping altogether for a speedy meal.

- 6 ounces extra-firm tofu
- 1 tablespoon lemon juice
- 1 teaspoon olive oil
- ½ teaspoon dried basil
- 1½ cups salt-free or low-sodium marinara sauce

- ¼ cup raw cashews
- 2 tablespoons nutritional yeast
- 2 tablespoons hemp seeds
- ½ teaspoon garlic powder

1 Preheat the oven to 400°F.

2 Wrap the tofu in a kitchen towel or paper towel and press a heavy object on top. Let sit for 10 minutes to drain out some of the water.

3 Slice the tofu into finger-width sticks. For older babes, you can cube them.

4 Place the tofu in an oven-safe dish and toss with the lemon juice, olive oil, and basil. Place in the oven and cook for 20 minutes.

5 While the tofu is cooking, place the cashews, nutritional yeast, hemp seeds, and garlic powder in a food processor or blender and process until very fine. Set aside.

6 Remove the tofu from the oven and flip, add just enough marinara sauce to cover, and sprinkle the homemade cheese on top. Return to the oven for 10 minutes more. Then remove from the oven, let cool, and serve.

Smoothies and Breakfast:
Nutritious Foods to Fuel Your Morning

It's easy to get stuck in a rut with breakfast and default to baby cereal. These recipes give you plenty of options to keep mornings exciting.

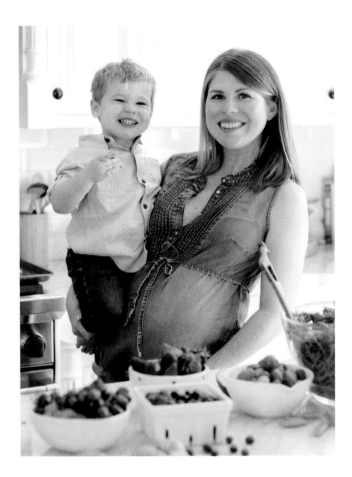

Calcium Creamsicle Smoothie

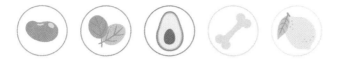

MAKES 2 CUPS

If there's one nutrient we find ourselves struggling to get our kids to eat enough of, it's calcium. That's why we created this Calcium Creamsicle Smoothie with about 400 mg of calcium per serving, depending on which brand of milk and orange juice you use. As a bonus, it tastes like a dreamy creamsicle shake.

- 1 cup calcium-fortified soy milk
- ¼ cup calcium-fortified orange juice
- ½ cup frozen mango chunks
- ½ cup frozen banana
- 1 tablespoon almond butter

1 Place all the ingredients in a blender and puree until creamy and smooth.

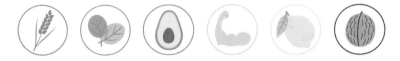

French Toast Fingers with Quick Berry Syrup

MAKES 15 TO 20 FINGERS

We love French toast in the morning but dislike the additional sugary syrup that often accompanies it. These French toast fingers are served with homemade berry syrup, using just frozen berries. You can also serve the fingers by themselves.

Choose thick-sliced, sturdy bread for this recipe, as thinner bread will crumble when sliced into fingers. Alternatively, you can use whole bread slices.

- 1 cup canned coconut milk (regular or light)
- 1 tablespoon ground flaxseed
- 1 teaspoon vanilla extract
- 1 teaspoon ground cinnamon
- 5 thick slices of day-old bread, cut into wide strips
- Coconut oil or nondairy butter, for the pan
- Quick Berry Syrup (recipe follows)

1 In a large, shallow bowl, whisk together the coconut milk, flaxseed, vanilla, and cinnamon. Let sit for 5 minutes while you slice the bread.

2 In a large pan, heat the oil over medium heat.

3 Dip a strip of bread into the coconut mixture, then place in the hot skillet. Repeat with more strips, taking care not to crowd the pan.

4 Cook for 1 to 2 minutes per side, until golden brown.

5 Remove the French toast strips from the pan, and repeat with remaining bread slices.

6 Serve immediately as is or with Quick Berry Syrup for dipping!

Quick Berry Syrup

MAKES 1 CUP SYRUP

It's syrup without the sugar! We like serving this in a little cup for baby to dip the French toast finger into.

- 2 cups frozen berries, slightly thawed
- ½ teaspoon ground cinnamon
- ½ teaspoon vanilla extract

1   In a small saucepan over medium heat, place ⅓ cup of water, the berries, cinnamon, and vanilla and bring to a boil. Using a wooden spoon, gently smash the large berries.

2   Reduce the heat to medium-low and simmer for about 10 minutes, stirring occasionally, until the syrup has reduced and thickened. The syrup should be thick enough to coat the back of a spoon.

3   Enjoy with French Toast Fingers.

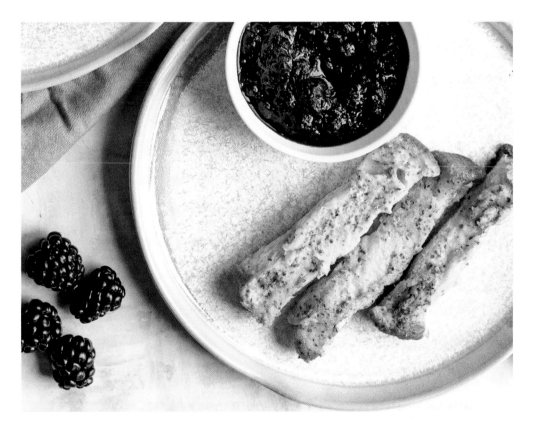

Veggie Omelet Cups

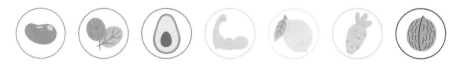

MAKES 9 CUPS

We love a good protein-rich tofu scramble in the morning and wanted a way to serve it in a baby-friendly way. These omelet cups are the answer: tofu "eggs" baked with finely chopped spinach and red bell pepper for additional vitamin C.

We like using kala namak black salt, which lends a familiar eggy taste. You can find it online or in specialty stores, or use regular salt instead. Omit the salt entirely for babies under 12 months.

We prefer to make these in silicone muffin wrappers for easy removal. Serve warm, at room temperature, or make a batch ahead of time and place in the fridge for easy breakfasts on the go. Try serving these like a veggie McMuffin: on a sprouted English muffin with smashed avocado.

- 14 ounces firm tofu
- 1 tablespoon olive oil
- ½ teaspoon salt or kala namak (black salt)
- ½ teaspoon ground turmeric
- ½ teaspoon garlic powder
- 2 tablespoons chickpea flour
- 1 shallot, diced
- ½ red bell pepper, chopped
- 2 cups baby spinach
- 1 teaspoon dried thyme
- 1 teaspoon dried parsley

1 Preheat the oven to 350°F.

2 Lightly grease a muffin pan and set aside. If using a silicone muffin pan, no need to grease.

3 Place the tofu, 2 teaspoons of the olive oil, the salt, turmeric, and garlic powder in a blender and puree until very smooth. Add the chickpea flour and process for another 15 seconds.

In a medium pan, heat the remaining teaspoon of oil over medium heat. Add the shallot and cook until soft, 2 to 3 minutes. Add the red bell pepper and spinach and cook until the peppers have softened and the spinach has wilted, 2 minutes. Stir in the thyme and parsley until combined, then remove from the heat.

 Add the vegetable mixture to the blender and pulse 2 or 3 times to just combine.

 Pour into the prepared muffin pan, filling each cup about three-quarters of the way full. Place in the oven and cook for 15 to 20 minutes. The tops of the omelet cups should be spongy when touched and the edges lightly browned.

7 Let cool slightly, then remove from the muffin pan and serve.

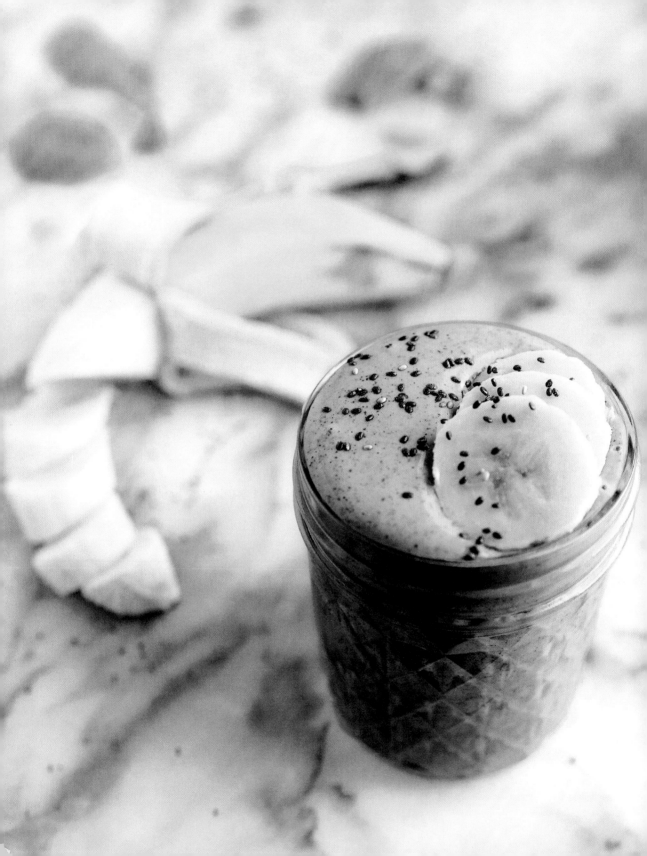

Green Dragon Smoothie

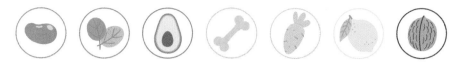

MAKES 2 CUPS

This Green Dragon Smoothie is a yummy way to enjoy the taste of spinach or kale without the accompanying bitterness. Spinach is less potent than kale, so if your kiddos are hesitant about leafy greens we recommend starting with spinach first.

With fortified soy milk, this smoothie is a great source of protein, calcium, and vitamin D.

- 1¼ cup fortified soy milk
- 1 large frozen banana, chopped into large chunks
- 1 tablespoon chia seeds
- 1 to 2 tablespoons nut butter of choice
- ⅛ teaspoon ground cinnamon
- 1 cup loosely packed kale or spinach leaves

1 Place all the ingredients in a blender in the order listed. Puree until very creamy and smooth, adding a little more milk as needed.

Blender Mini Muffins

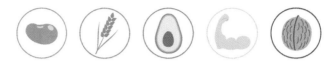

MAKES 24 MINI MUFFINS

These lightly sweetened muffins are ideal for busy mornings on the go. The riper your bananas, the sweeter they will be. You can also omit the maple syrup completely.

For adults, we like these as is, crumbled onto a smoothie bowl, or smeared with a little more peanut butter. We recommend a silicone muffin pan for easy removal if you have one available. As these muffins are fairly dense, we prefer them as mini muffins.

To make your own oat flour, place rolled oats in a blender or food processor and process until fine; store any extra oat flour in the fridge for up to 4 months. While we like the texture that almond meal provides, you can substitute additional oat flour if you don't have it on hand.

- 3 large ripe bananas
- ½ cup peanut butter
- 2 tablespoons chia seeds
- 1 tablespoon maple syrup
- 2 teaspoons baking powder
- ¼ teaspoon baking soda
- ¾ teaspoon ground cinnamon
- 1½ teaspoons apple cider vinegar
- 1 tablespoon cornstarch or arrowroot starch
- ¼ teaspoon salt (optional)
- ½ cup oat flour
- 5 tablespoons almond meal

1 Preheat the oven to 350°F.

2 Lightly grease a 24-cup mini-muffin pan and set aside.

3 Place the bananas, peanut butter, chia seeds, maple syrup, baking powder, baking soda, cinnamon, vinegar, cornstarch, and salt, if using, in a food processor or blender and process until smooth.

Add the oat flour and almond meal and pulse until just combined.

 Scoop the batter into the muffin pan, filling each cup about three-quarters of the way full. We use a tablespoon scoop for easy measuring. Bake for 18 minutes, until slightly golden brown and set.

6 Remove the pan from the oven and let the muffins cool in the pan for 30 minutes. Remove the muffins and place on a cooling rack to finish setting. Store leftovers in the fridge for about 4 days or in the freezer for up to 6 weeks.

Apple Baked Oatmeal

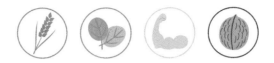

SERVES 4

Alex loves baked oatmeal so much she served it for brunch at her wedding. This is her baby- and family-friendly oatmeal recipe, using finely chopped fresh apples and applesauce as a sweetener instead of any syrup or refined sugar.

Canned pumpkin puree is added for both flavor and vitamin A. You also have the option to add dried fruit, like raisins or dried cranberries, and/or chopped nuts depending on your child's age. For infants, we recommend peeling and grating the apples for easier chewing.

- 1½ cups rolled oats
- 1 teaspoon baking powder
- ½ teaspoon salt
- 1 teaspoon ground cinnamon
- ¼ teaspoon ground nutmeg
- 1 cup unsweetened applesauce
- 1 flax egg (1 tablespoon ground flaxseed mixed with 3 tablespoons water)

- ¼ cup pumpkin puree
- 1¼ cups unsweetened nondairy milk
- 1 teaspoon vanilla extract
- 1 cup peeled, finely diced apple
- ⅓ cup raisins or other dried fruit (optional)

1 Preheat the oven to 350°F.

2 Lightly grease a 9 x 9-inch baking pan and set aside.

3 In a large bowl, whisk together the oats, baking powder, salt, cinnamon, and nutmeg. Set aside.

4 In a small bowl, whisk together the applesauce, flax egg, pumpkin puree, nondairy milk, and vanilla. Add to the oat mixture and stir to combine. Fold in the diced apple and raisins, if using.

5 Pour into the prepared baking pan and bake for 30 to 35 minutes, or until golden brown on top and set.

Note: For adults, we love this served warm in a bowl with nondairy milk, fresh fruit, and a drizzle of nut butter on top.

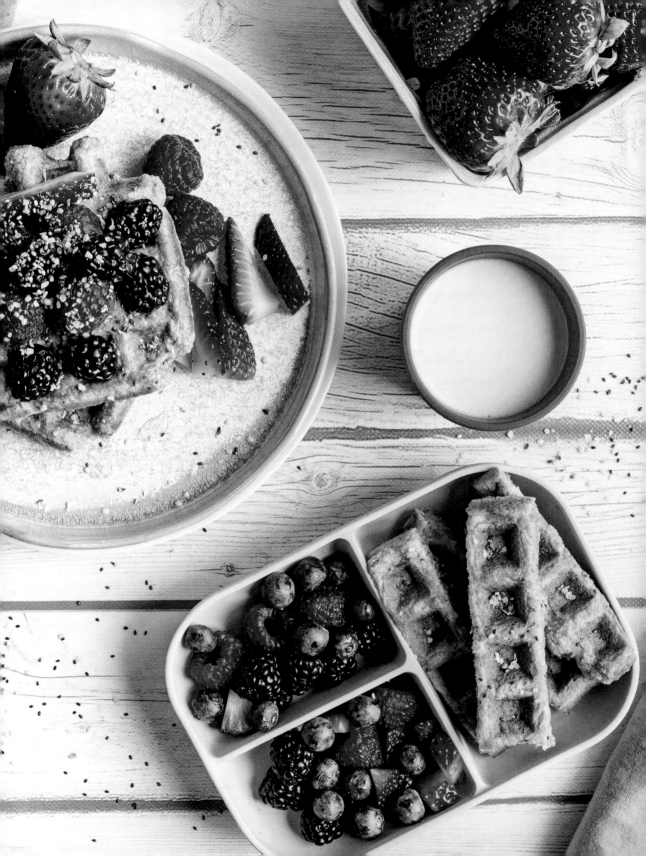

Lemon Chia Waffles

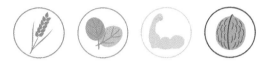

MAKES 8 WAFFLES

Whitney's family has a bit of a waffle obsession, and this zesty version makes an appearance at her table at least a few times a week. They make a double (or triple) batch on Sunday mornings, then freeze the rest for breakfast options.

These are also delicious without the lemon juice and zest and/or with ½ cup of fresh blueberries stirred in at the end. We recommend using a higher setting on your waffle iron to ensure they get a crispy crust and tender middle. They're yummy on their own or served like we do—with a smear of nut butter on top, fresh sliced berries, and a sprinkle of hemp seeds.

- 1 tablespoon chia seeds
- 1½ cups oat flour
- ½ tablespoon baking powder
- ½ teaspoon ground cinnamon
- ¼ teaspoon salt

- 1 medium banana, mashed
- 1 teaspoon fresh lemon juice
- ¼ teaspoon lemon zest
- 1 cup unsweetened nondairy milk
- 1 tablespoon vanilla extract

1 In a medium bowl, combine the chia seeds with 2 tablespoons of warm water. Set aside.

2 In a large bowl, whisk together the oat flour, baking powder, cinnamon, and salt. Set aside.

3 To the chia seed gel bowl, add the banana, lemon juice, lemon zest, nondairy milk, and vanilla and mix together. Add the wet ingredients to the oat flour mixture and mix together until combined.

4 Cook according to your waffle iron's instructions.

Simple Breakfast Quinoa Porridge

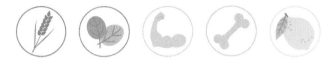

SERVES 2

We love quinoa for its iron, fiber, and protein content. As we often have leftover cooked quinoa in the fridge from meal prep, we created this breakfast porridge as a nice break from oatmeal. Enjoy it plain or with the stir-ins, as listed below.

- 1 cup cooked quinoa
- ¾ cup milk of choice
- ¼ cup fresh fruit of choice
- Optional stir-ins: ground cinnamon, ground nutmeg, toasted nuts and seeds, coconut flakes, nut butter

1 To cook in the microwave: In a microwave-safe bowl, whisk together the quinoa and milk. Microwave for 1 minute, stirring halfway through. To cook on the stove: In a medium saucepan over low heat, place the quinoa and milk and cook, stirring often, until warmed through, 3 to 4 minutes.

2 Stir in the fresh fruit and stir-ins, if using. Serve immediately.

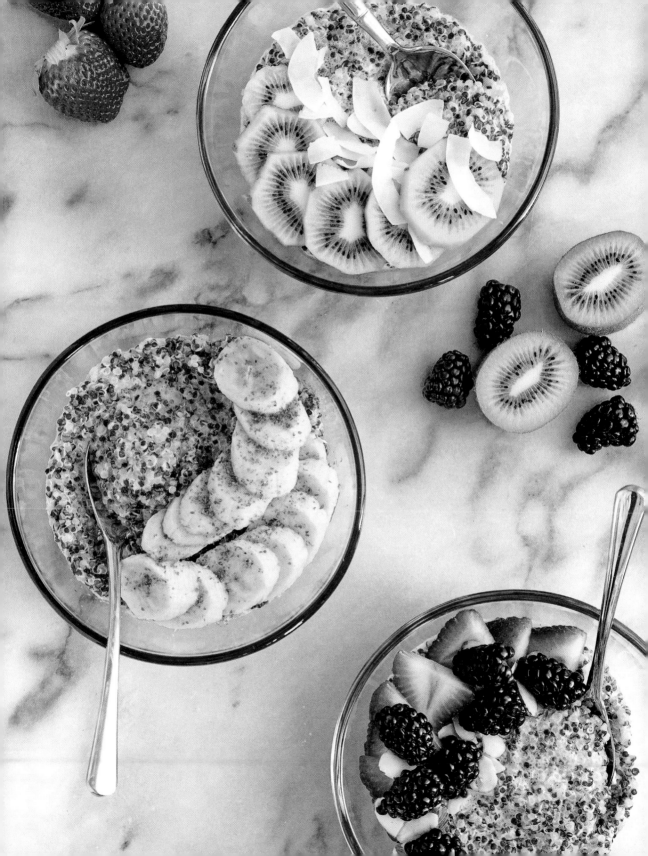

PB&J Smoothie

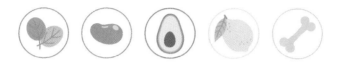

We created this one for moments when it seems like your babe doesn't want to touch any type of fruit or vegetable. Made with fortified soy or pea milk for additional calcium, protein, and vitamin D, plus antioxidant-rich berries and vitamin C-rich cauliflower. You can toss in a handful of greens as well.

- ½ cup frozen blueberries
- ¼ cup frozen raspberries
- ⅓ cup cauliflower florets

- 2 tablespoons almond or peanut butter
- 1 cup unsweetened nondairy milk
- 1 date, pit removed and roughly chopped

1 Place all the ingredients in a blender and puree until creamy and smooth.

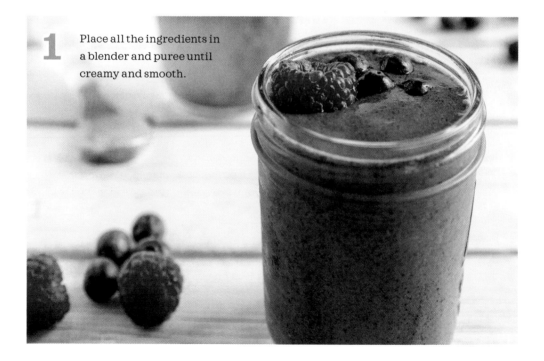

Creamy Bircher Muesli

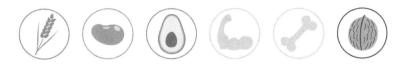

MAKES 2 CUPS

Traditional Bircher muesli uses both whole milk and yogurt, but this creamy version uses soy milk and optional plant-based yogurt. The best part is that it's ready in the morning without any additional prep. Omit the finely chopped sliced almonds/coconut flakes for babies under 12 months.

- 1 cup rolled oats
- 2 teaspoons chia seeds
- 2 tablespoons sliced almonds, finely chopped for younger toddlers
- 2 tablespoons unsweetened coconut flakes, finely chopped for younger toddlers
- 1 date, pitted and finely chopped
- 1 teaspoon ground cinnamon
- 2 cups unsweetened fortified soy milk
- ½ cup plant-based yogurt (optional)

1 In a medium bowl, combine the oats, chia seeds, almonds, coconut, date, cinnamon, and soy milk. Cover and refrigerate overnight.

2 Divide the muesli into bowls and serve with fresh fruit or a drizzle of maple syrup for adults, if desired.

Toddler Snacks and Lunches

Does it feel like your babe eats 24/7? Yup, us too. Providing three meals and two snacks a day can be overwhelming, and it's easy to see why many parents reach for pouches and nutrient-poor packaged foods. These simple, nutritious lunches and small bites can be prepared ahead of time for no-fuss packing and snacking all week long. We also know the struggle parents face when littles head off to day care or preschool and are exposed to chicken nuggets, pepperoni pizza, and corn dogs, and we've come up with plant-friendly versions of common lunch recipes including a nut-free mac 'n' cheese and crispy bean taquitos.

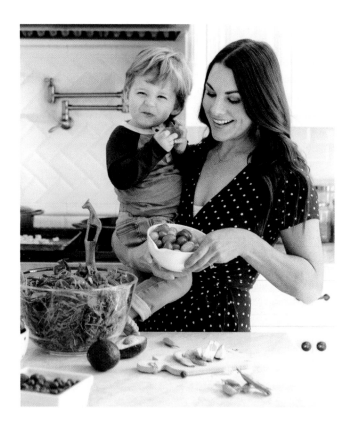

Confetti Guacamole

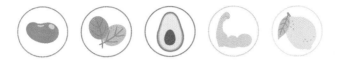

MAKES 3 CUPS

This Confetti Guacamole is a great way to pack in the veggies. We like to add bell peppers, carrots, kale, and tomatoes, but feel free to mix it up. Use a food processor to get the vegetables uniformly chopped in record speed.

- 1 cup frozen peas, cooked then cooled
- 1 large ripe avocado, pitted, peeled, and chopped
- 2 tablespoons lime juice
- 1 cup finely chopped veggies of choice
- ¼ cup finely chopped fresh cilantro
- 1 garlic clove, minced, or 1 teaspoon garlic powder
- ¼ teaspoon salt (optional)
- ¼ teaspoon freshly ground black pepper (optional)

1 Place the peas in a food processor and pulse until smooth.

2 Transfer the peas to a medium bowl along with the avocado, lime juice, veggies, cilantro, garlic, and salt and pepper, if using. Mash with a fork to combine.

3 For baby-led weaners, serve on a preloaded spoon with pita bread or with Bean and Corn Taquitos (page 252) or on its own.

Strawberry Cashew Yogurt

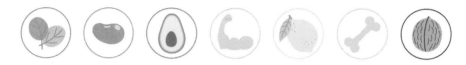

MAKES 3 CUPS

We don't know about you, but we find it difficult to find low-sugar, dairy-free yogurt on the market that also tastes good. So we made our own with a base of silken tofu, raw cashews, and just enough frozen berries for sweetness. We like to add probiotics and food-grade calcium carbonate powder for additional healthy bacteria and calcium, but you can leave them out if you prefer. Almost any probiotic capsule will work, and you can find food-grade calcium powder online. Just ¾ teaspoon in the entire recipe equates to approximately 150 mg of calcium per ½ cup serving. You have the option to add a teaspoon or two of maple syrup for older tots.

- 3 cups frozen strawberries, slightly thawed
- 1 cup raw cashews
- 1 cup silken or soft tofu (about ½ block)
- 2 tablespoons lemon juice
- ¾ teaspoon 100% pure food-grade calcium carbonate (optional)
- ½ probiotic capsule (optional)

   Place the strawberries, cashews, tofu, lemon juice, and calcium powder, if using, in a food processor or blender. If you are using a probiotic capsule, carefully open the capsule and pour half the capsule into the blender. You can always add more, but too much probiotics can lend a chalkier flavor.

2   Blend until very creamy and smooth, scraping down the sides as needed. Depending on the power of your blender, this may take up to 5 minutes. If you are having trouble blending, add in a splash or two of milk of choice.

   Store in an airtight container in the fridge for up to 5 days.

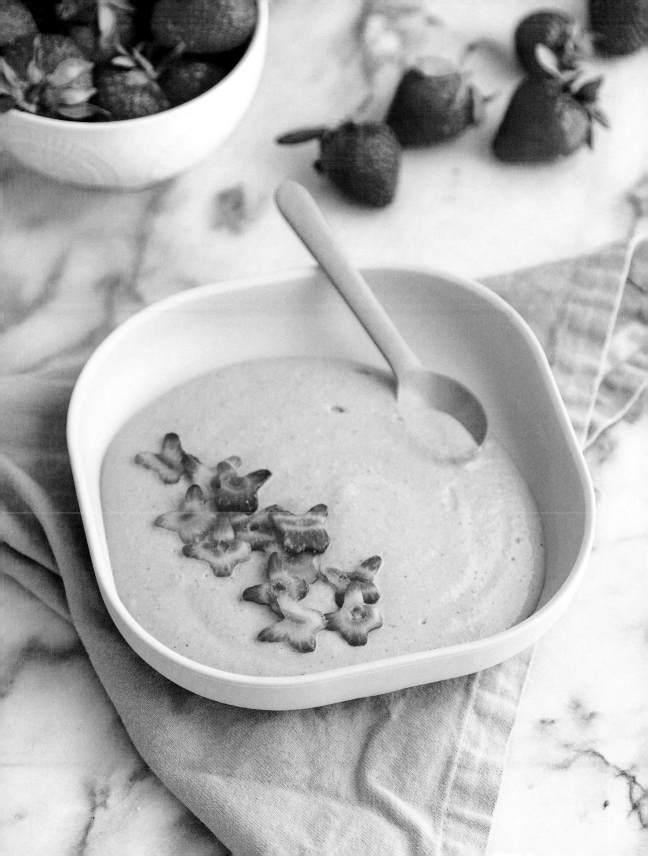

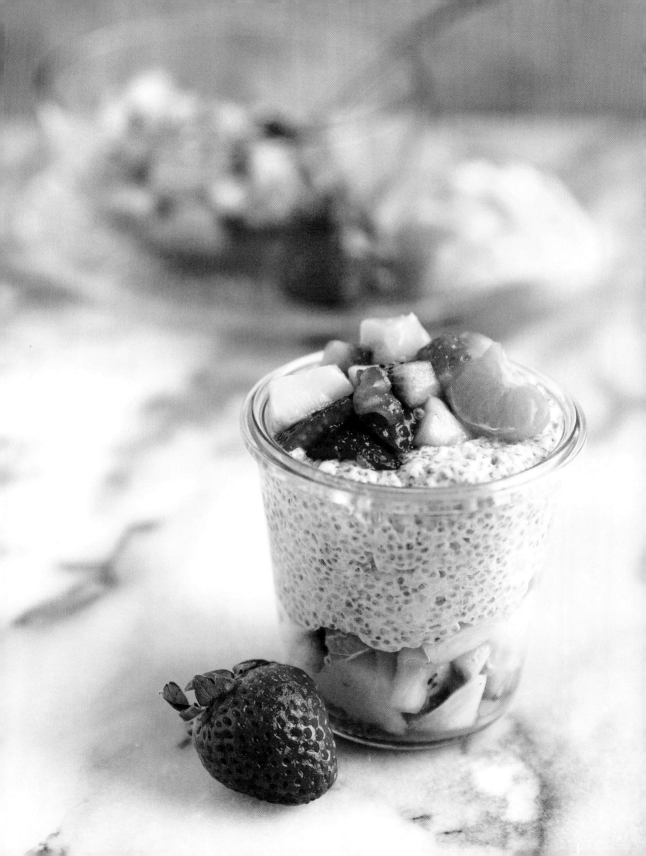

Tropical Chia Pudding

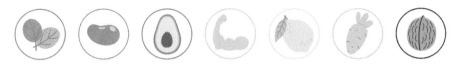

SERVES 4

For younger babes who will eat this with their hands, we recommend bumping up the chia seeds to ⅓ cup for a thick, gelatinous pudding.

- One 14.5-ounce can light coconut milk
- ½ cup mango
- ⅓ cup chia seeds
- 1 cup chopped fruit such as kiwi, orange, mango, or other fruit of choice (optional)

1 Place the coconut milk and mango in a blender and puree until smooth. Pour the mixture into a medium bowl or large mason jar.

2 Stir in the chia seeds and refrigerate for 20 minutes.

3 Remove, mix again, and refrigerate for at least 3 hours or overnight to gel.

4 Serve as is or place in a bowl and top with chopped fruit of choice.

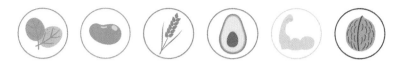

Chewy Granola Bars

MAKES 12 TO 16 BARS

This recipe is a cross between banana bread and granola bars. Sweetened only with fruit, these dense bars are perfect for hungry toddlers, and we love them with nut butter and chia jam. Compared to most no-bake bars, these are sturdy and OK to enjoy at room temperature, which means they are both portable and freezable.

- 1½ cups mashed overripe banana (from about 3 bananas)
- ⅓ cup almond butter
- 1 teaspoon vanilla extract
- 2 cups rolled oats
- ¼ cup unsweetened coconut flakes
- ½ cup walnuts
- ½ cup pepitas
- ½ cup sunflower seeds
- ¼ cup hemp seeds
- 1 teaspoon ground cinnamon
- ¼ teaspoon ground ginger
- ¼ teaspoon salt

1 Preheat the oven to 350°F.

2 Lightly grease a 9 × 13-inch oven-safe dish. For easier removal, line with parchment paper and leave an overhang to lift the bars out of the dish.

3 In a large bowl, mash the banana with the almond butter and vanilla until very smooth.

4 Place the oats, coconut, walnuts, pepitas, sunflower seeds, hemp seeds, cinnamon, ginger, and salt in a food processor and pulse until very finely chopped.

5 Add the oat-nut mixture to the banana mixture and stir together. The mixture should be fairly thick.

6   Place the mixture into the prepared baking dish and smooth out the top using a silicone spatula.

7   Bake for 22 to 25 minutes, or until firm in the center.

8   Remove from the oven and let cool in the baking dish for 15 minutes, then carefully remove and let cool completely on a cooling rack. Slice into bars or small squares.

9   Store in an airtight container in the fridge for 1 week or in the freezer for up to 6 weeks.

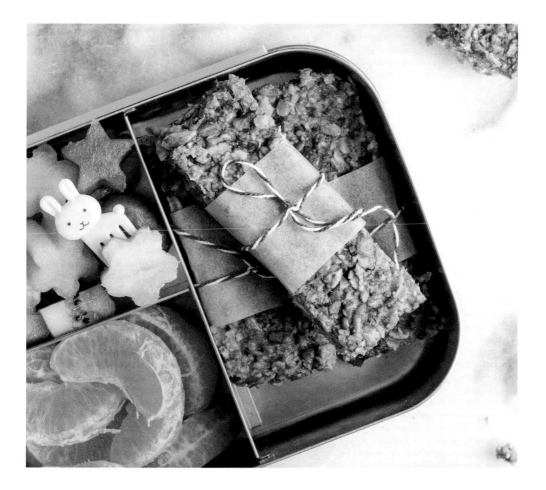

Alphabet Pasta Salad

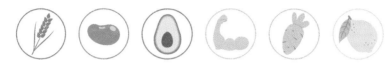

MAKES 3 CUPS

This pasta salad was created with school lunches in mind. We make a batch to add to bento boxes with sliced fruit and a banana muffin or a chewy granola bar. You can sub any type of pasta you have on hand, but you'd be amazed how much quicker tots will gobble up a lunch made with letters!

- 1 cup dried alphabet pasta
- 1 cup frozen corn kernels, thawed
- 1 cup frozen peas, thawed
- 1 tablespoon olive oil
- 1 tablespoon dairy-free mayonnaise
- 1 tablespoon white wine vinegar or lemon juice
- ½ teaspoon salt
- ¼ teaspoon freshly ground black pepper
- 1 tomato, seeded and diced
- ½ cup finely chopped red bell pepper

1 Bring a medium pot of water to a boil. Add the alphabet pasta and cook until al dente according to package directions. Drain and rinse with cold water; set aside.

2 In a small microwave-safe bowl, place the corn, peas, and 1 tablespoon of water and heat for 90 seconds, until warmed through. Drain.

3 In a large bowl, mix together the olive oil, mayonnaise, vinegar, salt, and pepper. Add the cooked and cooled pasta, corn, peas, tomato, and red bell pepper. Toss to gently combine, seasoning to taste as needed.

4 Enjoy as is or store in the fridge for an easy snack or meal. This salad also packs well for day care or school lunches.

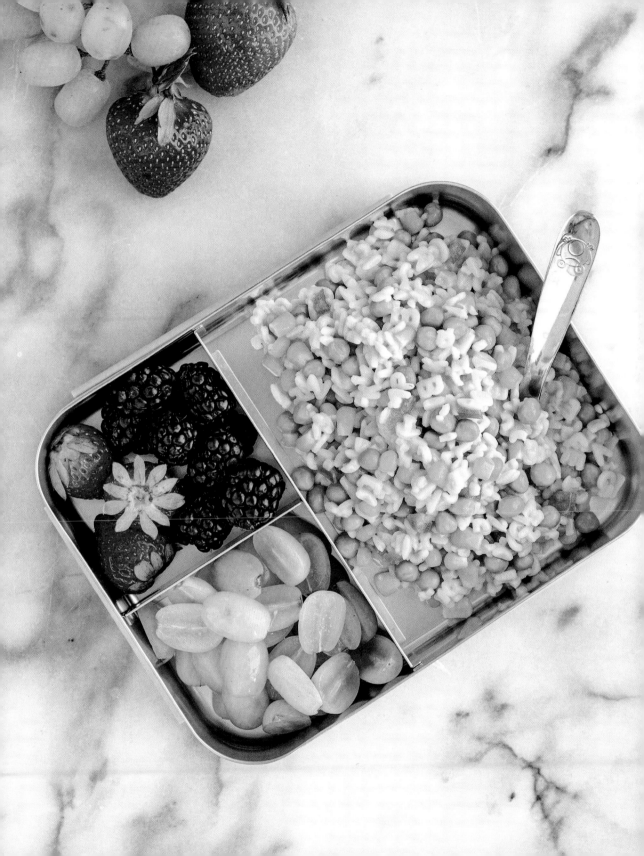

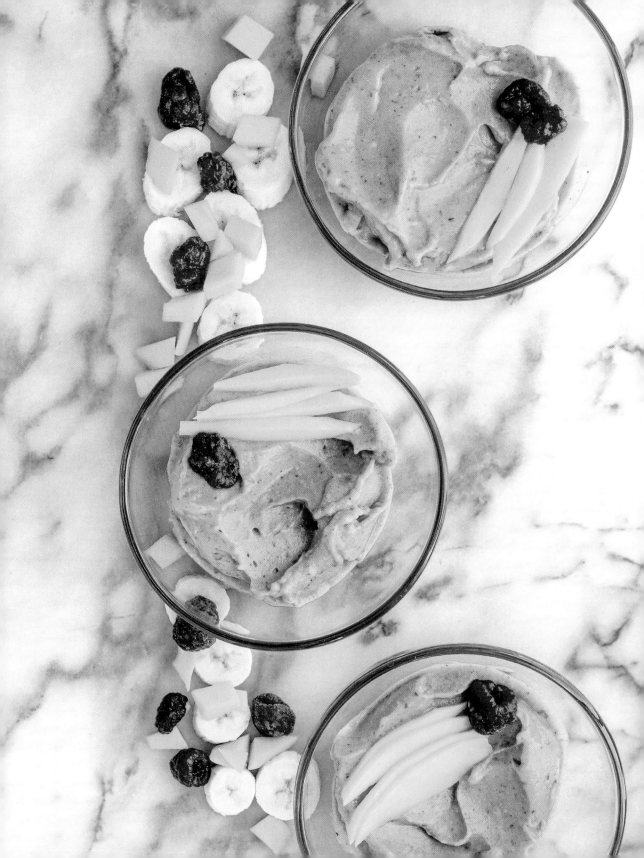

Ice Cream Smoothie Bowl

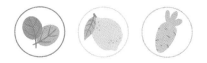

MAKES 2 HEAPING CUPS

Once our kids tasted "real" sorbet and ice cream, it was only a matter of time before they started asking for it at home. This is our fruity version, packed with raspberries, mango, and banana. It's more tart than traditional banana "nice cream," so if you find that your kiddos are sour sensitive, reduce the amount of raspberries and increase the amount of mango or banana.

You can make this in a blender, though you will likely need to stop and scrape down the sides more often. Slightly thawed fruit will also be easier to blend.

- 1 cup frozen raspberries, slightly thawed
- ½ cup frozen mango chunks, slightly thawed
- 1 medium frozen banana

1 Place all the ingredients in a food processor or blender and puree until very smooth and creamy, scraping down the sides as needed. Depending on the power of your appliance, this may take 4 to 5 minutes.

2 Enjoy immediately! Leftovers can be stored in the fridge and enjoyed in a smoothie or poured into popsicle molds and frozen.

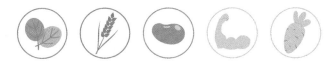

Sunflower Mac 'n' Cheeze

SERVES 4

Would a toddler recipe book be complete without mac 'n' cheese? We didn't think so! Our sons gobble down this dish (or a similar version) on a weekly basis. While we often use cashews as a creamy cheezy base, we made this version nut-free using sunflower seeds so that tots can enjoy it at preschools and day cares with allergy-free policies.

- 1 tablespoon olive oil
- ¼ cup chopped white onion
- ½ cup peeled and roughly chopped carrots
- 1 Yukon Gold potato, peeled and roughly chopped
- 1 garlic clove, minced
- ½ teaspoon salt
- 1½ cups vegetable broth
- ½ cup raw, shelled sunflower seeds

- 8 ounces elbow noodles
- 2 teaspoons cornstarch
- 1 tablespoon lemon juice
- ½ teaspoon ground turmeric
- ¼ teaspoon smoked paprika
- 2 tablespoons nutritional yeast
- 2 teaspoons tomato paste

1 In a large pot, heat the olive oil over medium heat. Add the onion, carrots, and potato and cook, stirring often, for 5 minutes, or until the vegetables have softened slightly.

2 Add the garlic, salt, vegetable broth, and sunflower seeds and bring to a boil. Reduce the heat to low and simmer for 10 minutes, or until the potatoes are soft.

3 While the vegetables are simmering, bring 6 cups of water to a boil in a large pot. Add the elbow noodles and cook until al dente. Drain and set aside.

4 Transfer the vegetable mixture to a blender with the cornstarch, lemon juice, turmeric, paprika, nutritional yeast, and tomato paste. Puree until very creamy and smooth, scraping down the sides as needed.

5 Return the puree to the pot and simmer over low heat until just thickened. Taste and add more salt, pepper, and/or lemon juice as needed. Add the cooked pasta and stir to combine. Serve!

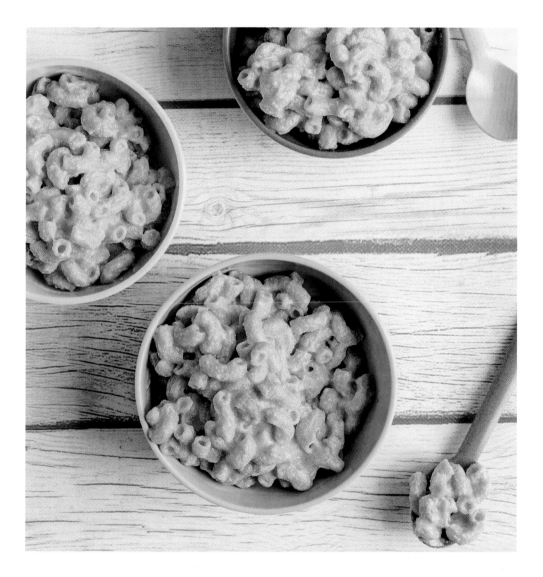

Bean and Corn Taquitos

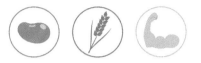

MAKES 10 TO 12 TAQUITOS

These taquitos are a fun way to get your kiddos to enjoy beans: seasoned refried beans tucked into corn tortillas, then baked until crispy, to be precise. Serve as is or with our Confetti Guacamole (page 239). Canned refried beans will vary in terms of added sodium, so it's up to you whether or not you need to add more for flavor.

- 1 cup vegetarian refried beans of choice*
- ¼ cup cooked black beans (rinsed if canned)
- ¼ cup corn kernels
- ½ teaspoon ground cumin
- ½ teaspoon paprika
- ¼ teaspoon chili powder
- 2 tablespoons mild salsa
- Ten to twelve 4-inch corn tortillas

1 Preheat the oven to 425°F.

2 Grease a large baking sheet and set aside.

3 In a medium microwave-safe bowl, mix together the refried and black beans, corn, cumin, paprika, chili powder, and salsa. Microwave for 1 minute, then remove and stir again. You want the mixture to be just warm enough that you can easily spread it onto the tortillas.

4 Right before rolling the taquitos, warm the tortillas so they don't break while rolling or cooking. Place 2 or 3 tortillas at a time in the preheated oven for 1 minute or microwave for 15 seconds.

5 Spread 1 to 2 tablespoons of the bean mixture in the center of a tortilla. Roll up, then place seam side down on the prepared baking sheet. Repeat with the remaining tortillas and beans. Lightly spray the outside of the tortillas with cooking spray, or brush them with more oil.

6 Bake for 15 to 20 minutes, or until the taquitos are golden and crunchy. Remove and let cool slightly, then serve as is, or with more mild salsa or with Confetti Guacamole (page 239).

You can also mash your own beans if you do not have refried beans.

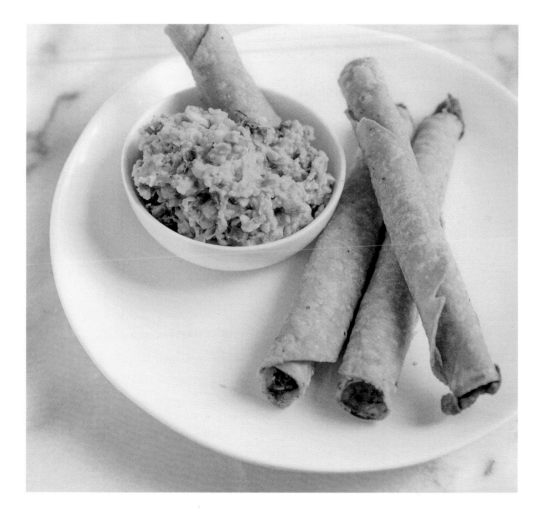

≈ Savory Corn Muffins ≈

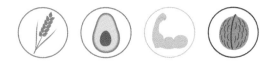

MAKES 12 MUFFINS

Muffins are a champion packable snack for playgroups, day care, and school lunches. These savory corn muffins contain nutritious whole-grain flour, omega-3 fatty acids, corn, bell peppers, and just a hint of spice. Omit the maple syrup for younger tots.

- 1 tablespoon ground flaxseed
- 1 cup cornmeal
- 1 cup whole wheat flour
- ½ teaspoon dried cilantro
- 2 teaspoons baking powder
- 1 teaspoon baking soda
- ½ teaspoon salt
- ½ teaspoon ground cumin
- ¼ teaspoon chili powder
- 1¼ cup soy milk
- 1 teaspoon lemon juice
- ¼ cup avocado oil or other neutral oil
- 1 tablespoon maple syrup (optional)
- ⅓ cup finely chopped red bell pepper
- 1 cup frozen corn kernels, thawed

1 Preheat the oven to 400°F.

2 Lightly grease a muffin pan and set aside.

3 In a small bowl, whisk together the flaxseed and 3 tablespoons of water and set aside.

4 In a large bowl, whisk together the cornmeal, flour, cilantro, baking powder, baking soda, salt, cumin and chili powder.

In a separate bowl, whisk together the soy milk, lemon juice, avocado oil, and maple syrup. Stir in the flaxseed mixture and pour into the cornmeal bowl. Gently stir together until just combined.

 Pour into the prepared muffin pan, filling each cup about three-quarters of the way full.

7 Bake for 20 minutes, or until a toothpick inserted in the center of a muffin comes out clean. Remove from the oven and let cool for 10 minutes before removing from the pan.

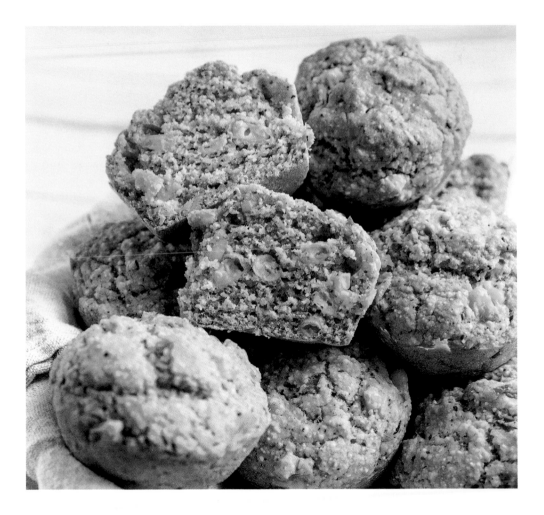

Cherry Chia Popsicles

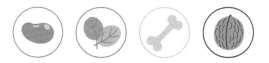

MAKES ABOUT 6 POPSICLES, DEPENDING ON MOLD SIZE

These popsicles are another fun, delicious way to expose your babes to omega-3-rich chia seeds. Feel free to swap in other fruit instead of cherries, and we recommend using nontoxic silicone popsicle molds.

- 1 cup frozen cherries, thawed
- 1 cup fortified soy milk
- 1 pitted date (optional)
- 2 tablespoons chia seeds

1 Place the cherries, soy milk, and date, if using, in a blender and puree until creamy and smooth.

2 Add the chia seeds and pulse 1 or 2 times to just combine. Pour into popsicle molds and place in the freezer for at least 3 hours.

Blueberry Oat Balls

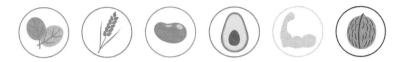

MAKES 20 TO 22 BALLS

Our boys both love oatmeal balls, and these pack in antioxidant-rich blueberries, protein-rich hemp seeds, and a hefty dose of peanut butter. Enjoy thawed from the freezer for an easy, make-ahead snack.

- 1 cup frozen blueberries
- 1 cup rolled oats
- 1 cup raw cashews
- 6 Medjool dates, pitted
- ¼ cup hemp seeds
- ¼ cup peanut butter

1 Line a large baking sheet with parchment paper. Set aside. Place the blueberries, oats, cashews, and dates in a food processor and pulse 8 to 10 times, until the ingredients have broken down.

2 Add the hemp seeds and peanut butter and process until smooth, 30 to 45 seconds.

3 Form into teaspoon-size balls for younger toddlers and tablespoon-size balls for older toddlers and kids.

4 Place the balls on the prepared baking sheet and freeze for 1 hour.

5 Store in the freezer and allow to thaw for a few minutes before serving.

Pumpkin Oat Cookie Drops

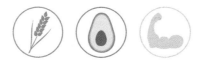

MAKES 16 COOKIES

Alex created these one afternoon after Vander asked for cookies. Naturally sweetened and ready in less than 20 minutes, these are ideal for afternoon snacks or lunch box treats.

If you don't have pumpkin pie spice on hand, substitute ½ teaspoon cinnamon, ⅛ teaspoon ground ginger, and a dash of nutmeg.

- 1 cup rolled oats
- ¾ cup oat flour
- 1 teaspoon baking powder
- ¼ teaspoon salt
- ¾ teaspoon pumpkin pie spice
- 1 large very ripe banana, mashed
- ½ cup pumpkin puree
- 1½ tablespoons almond butter
- 1 teaspoon vanilla extract

1 Preheat the oven to 350°F.

2 Line a large baking sheet with parchment paper and set aside.

3 In a medium bowl, whisk together the oats, oat flour, baking powder, salt, and pumpkin pie spice.

4 In a separate medium bowl, or in a blender, thoroughly mix together the mashed banana, pumpkin puree, almond butter, and vanilla. There should be no visible chunks of banana. Pour the banana-pumpkin mixture into the oat bowl and mix together until just combined.

5 Using a small cookie scoop or spoon, drop the dough 2 inches apart onto the prepared baking sheet. Bake for 12 to 14 minutes, or until slightly golden. Remove from the oven and let cool completely on an oven rack.

Note: For older kids, you can mix in mini chocolate chips, chopped nuts, or dried fruit such as raisins.

Family Dinners

Making separate meals for each member of the family isn't practical for busy parents and is counterintuitive to building positive eating habits. Our dinners are crafted with toddlers' special needs in mind but can be easily adapted to appeal to the whole family. Look for "Family Feeding Tips" with each recipe to explain how to add or subtract ingredients to make them more appetizing for parents and older children or more age appropriate for babies.

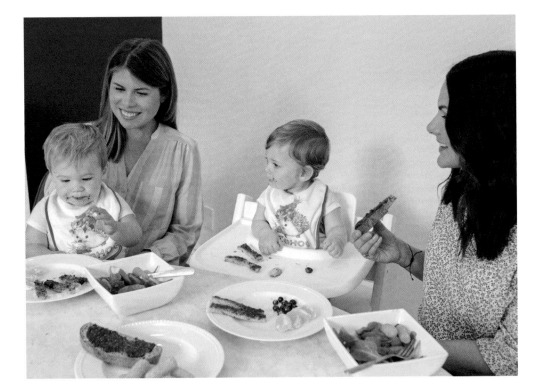

Lentil-A-Roni

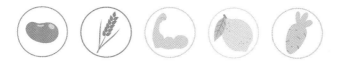

SERVES 4

This is our interpretation of that classic childhood meal Pasta-Roni. It combines our love for a quick and easy pasta dinner with iron- and protein-rich lentils.

How much chili powder you use is up to you. Start with 1 teaspoon and add from there. This recipe also makes for a great chili mac 'n' cheese base; simply add shredded dairy-free cheddar cheese or a homemade Vegan Cheese Sauce (page 291) at the end of cooking. Or swap in bean pasta for an extra legume boost!

- 8 ounces uncooked elbow noodles
- 1 tablespoon olive oil
- ½ cup chopped onion (1 small onion)
- 1 garlic clove, minced
- ½ teaspoon dried thyme
- 1 to 3 teaspoons chili powder, depending on spice preference
- ¼ teaspoon salt
- ⅛ teaspoon black pepper
- 1¼ cups cooked lentils
- 2 cups tomato sauce

1 Cook the pasta according to the package directions. Drain and set aside.

2 While the pasta is cooking, heat the olive oil in a large skillet over medium heat. Add the onion and cook, stirring constantly, for 8 to 9 minutes, or until the onions are very soft. Take care not to burn the onion.

3 Stir in the garlic, thyme, chili powder, salt, pepper, and lentils. Cook for another 2 to 3 minutes, until warmed through, then stir in the tomato sauce and cooked noodles.

4 Cook for 1 to 2 minutes more. Season to taste as needed.

Note: Add dairy-free shredded cheese for a cheesier version.

Pasta Fagioli

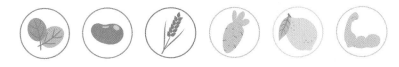

SERVES 4

Our healthier version of SpaghettiOs—pasta and white beans in a simple tomato sauce. We recommend salting the water to cook the pasta, as you will use this to flavor the overall soup. However, if you are making this for babes under 12 months, skip this step and salt the finished dish after removing their portion.

- 1 tablespoon olive oil
- ½ small white or yellow onion, finely diced
- 1 cup finely diced carrots
- 1 cup finely diced celery
- 3 garlic cloves, minced
- One 15-ounce can tomato sauce
- One 15-ounce can cannellini or white navy beans, drained and rinsed
- 1 tablespoon salt
- 1 cup ditalini pasta or other small-shaped pasta
- ½ cup finely chopped fresh parsley

1 In a large saucepan, heat the olive oil over medium heat. Stir in the onion, carrots, and celery and cook, stirring occasionally for 5 to 8 minutes, or until the vegetables have softened slightly.

2 Stir in the garlic and cook for another 30 seconds. Add the tomato sauce and drained beans. Reduce the heat to low, and simmer for 30 minutes while you make the pasta.

3 In a separate medium saucepan, combine the salt with 6 cups of water and bring to a boil. Add the pasta and cook, stirring occasionally, until al dente according to package directions. Drain, reserving 2 cups of the pasta cooking water.

4 Stir the cooked pasta into the bean mixture along with the parsley and ½ cup pasta water. Add more pasta water to reach the desired consistency. We usually end up adding about 1¼ cups pasta water; the dish should be hearty but brothy.

5 Serve as is or topped with vegan parmesan cheese!

15-Minute Black Bean Tacos

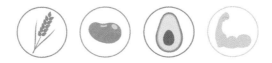

MAKES 4 TACOS

If you're looking for an easy way to encourage your family to eat more beans, these tacos are it. You can substitute equal amounts of cooked lentils, pinto beans, or kidney beans instead of black beans. This recipe can easily be doubled (and tripled) depending on how many you are planning to serve.

As with most of the family-friendly recipes, you'll want to reduce the salt for babies under 12 months. Therefore, we recommend using a homemade, salt-free taco seasoning and no-salt-added beans.

- 1 tablespoon olive oil
- ¼ cup mild pico de gallo
- 1 tablespoon taco seasoning (see Note)
- One 15-ounce can black beans, drained and rinsed
- 2 tablespoons vegetable broth
- 4 tortillas
- Taco toppings of choice

1 In a large skillet, heat the olive oil over medium-high heat. Add the pico de gallo and cook, stirring occasionally, until just softened, about 3 minutes.

2 Stir in the taco seasoning, black beans, and vegetable broth. Cover and reduce the heat to medium low and cook for 3 to 4 minutes, until warmed through. Remove the lid and gently mash the beans, leaving some whole.

3 Serve in warmed tortillas with toppings of choice.

Note: While you can use store-bought taco seasoning, we like to make our own and store it in the pantry for quick meals. We use a mild chili powder that the whole family loves. If you are sensitive to spice, then you'll want to cut down to 2 to 3 tablespoons here. For babes under 12 months, we also recommend cutting down the salt and salting adult portions upon serving.

Homemade Taco Seasoning

- ¼ cup chili powder
- 2 tablespoons ground cumin
- 1 tablespoon paprika
- 1 tablespoon salt
- 1 teaspoon garlic powder
- 1 teaspoon onion powder
- 1 teaspoon oregano
- ½ teaspoon freshly ground black pepper
- 1 tablespoon cornstarch (optional; will help to prevent caking while stored)

1 Mix everything together in a mason jar and cover tightly with a lid. Store in the pantry for up to 6 months.

Sheet Pan BBQ Tofu Bowls

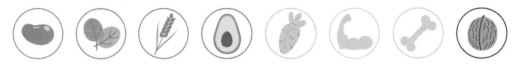

SERVES 6

These bowls can be as simple or fancy as you want. Some nights we opt for just the sweet potato, tofu, and quinoa with a squirt of BBQ sauce on top, and other nights we make a few pans of roasted vegetables and top with creamy avocado sauce (recipe below).

We've included portion sizes to make this a dinner and meal-prep recipe. If you want to serve just for a meal, divide the recipe in half.

Sheet Pan BBQ Tofu:
- Two 14-ounce packages extra-firm tofu, drained, pressed, and cubed
- 2 tablespoons olive oil
- 2 tablespoons cornstarch
- 2 teaspoons smoked paprika
- 2 teaspoons chili powder
- 2 teaspoons onion powder
- 2 teaspoons garlic powder
- 1 teaspoon salt

Sheet Pan Vegetables:
- 1 large sweet potato, peeled and diced
- 4 teaspoons olive oil
- ½ teaspoon salt
- 3 small zucchinis, chopped (about 2 cups)
- 1 cup frozen corn kernels
- Cooked quinoa, rice, or farro, for serving

1 Preheat the oven to 400°F.

2 Grease 2 large baking sheets and 1 medium sheet pan and set aside.

In a large bowl, toss together the tofu, olive oil, cornstarch, paprika, chili powder, onion powder, garlic powder, and salt. Place in a single layer on a prepared baking sheet and set aside.

 In the same bowl (no need to wipe clean), mix together the sweet potatoes, 2 teaspoons of the olive oil, and ¼ teaspoon of the salt. Place in a single layer on the prepared sheet pan and place both the sweet potato tray and tofu tray in the oven. Cook for 25 minutes.

 While the potatoes and tofu are cooking, place the zucchini and corn kernels in the same bowl (again, no need to wipe clean) and toss with the remaining olive oil and salt. Place in a single layer on a prepared baking sheet and set aside.

6 Remove the tofu and sweet potatoes and stir. Return to the oven along with the zucchini pan and cook for another 15 minutes, or until the zucchini is tender.

7 Serve over cooked grains of choice. For a simple sauce, drizzle adult bowls with prepared BBQ sauce, tahini, or Creamy Avocado Sauce (recipe follows).

Creamy Avocado Sauce

1 ripe avocado, juice of 1 lime, 3 tablespoons olive oil, 3 tablespoons shelled pistachios, ¼ cup water, and a handful of fresh cilantro pureed in a blender.

Very Veggie Enchilada Casserole

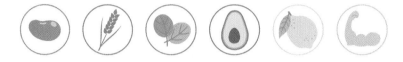

SERVES 6 TO 8

Our simplified version of enchiladas—layers of corn tortillas, enchilada sauce, refried beans, veggies, and a cashew "cheese" sauce. The can of mild green chilies heightens the Tex-Mex flavor of the sauce, but you can leave out completely if your family is sensitive to spice.

- ½ cup + 1 tablespoon raw cashews
- One 4-ounce can mild green chilies
- 2 tablespoons nutritional yeast
- ½ cup water
- 1 tablespoon olive oil
- 3 bell peppers (any color), diced
- ½ red onion, finely diced
- 2 cups frozen corn kernels
- 2 teaspoons chili powder
- 2 teaspoons ground cumin
- ½ teaspoon salt
- Two 15-ounce cans vegetarian refried beans
- 2 cups mild red enchilada sauce
- 18–20 corn tortillas

1 Preheat the oven to 400°F.

2 Place the cashews, chilies, nutritional yeast, and ½ cup of water in a high-powered blender and puree until creamy. Depending on the power of your blender, this may take up to 5 minutes. Set aside.

3 In a large skillet, heat the olive oil over medium heat. Add the peppers and onion and cook for 8 to 10 minutes, or until vegetables are very soft. Add the corn, chili powder, cumin, and salt and cook for another 2 minutes.

4 In a medium bowl, mix together the refried beans and ¼ cup of the enchilada sauce. If the beans are too hard to stir, microwave for about 30 seconds to soften.

5 Assemble. Slice the tortillas into thick strips, about 4 to 6 strips per tortilla, as this will make it easier to layer in the casserole dish. Lightly grease a 9 × 13-inch baking pan, then spread a thin layer of enchilada sauce on the bottom. Layer in order: one-third of the tortilla strips, half of the beans, half of the veggies, half of the enchilada sauce, and half of the cheese sauce. Then layer with half of the remaining tortilla strips and the rest of the beans and veggies. Top with the remaining tortilla strips and cover with the remaining enchilada sauce and cashew sauce.

6 Lightly tent with foil and bake for 20 minutes, until the sauce is bubbling. Remove from the oven and let cool for 5 to 10 minutes before serving. We love this served with guacamole and chopped fresh cilantro.

Lentil Sloppy Joes

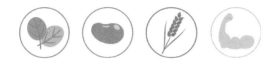

MAKES **8** SANDWICHES

These sloppy joes are high in both iron and plant-based protein, and a great way to introduce mushrooms. The trick is finely chopping the mushrooms and letting them cook down with the onions; their natural sweetness helps boost the flavor of traditional sloppy joes without the use of refined sugars, ketchup, or BBQ sauce. To keep prep time at a minimum, we use our food processor to finely chop the vegetables and we use canned lentils.

For adults, serve with whole-grain sprouted bread or buns, pickles, and BBQ sauce. For toddlers, offer it up as is or in a sandwich cut into smaller pieces. For baby-led weaners, mash the lentil mixture onto whole-grain toast, then slice into strips.

- 1 tablespoon olive oil
- 2 medium sweet onions, finely diced (about 3 cups)
- 10 ounces white mushrooms, finely diced
- 2 cups cooked brown or green lentils
- ¼ teaspoon dried thyme
- ¼ cup all-purpose flour
- 1 cup canned crushed tomatoes

- 1 cup low-sodium vegetable broth
- 1 tablespoon 100% maple syrup
- 1 tablespoon white vinegar
- 1 tablespoon vegan Worcestershire sauce
- ½ teaspoon salt (optional, for adult portions)
- Freshly ground black pepper to taste
- 8 mini buns, for serving

1 In a large skillet, heat the olive oil over medium heat. Add the onion and cook, stirring often, until the onion is very soft, 12 to 15 minutes. If the onions are browning too quickly, add a tablespoon or two of water.

2 Add the mushrooms to the skillet, and cook until they have released their juices and the liquid has evaporated, 6 to 8 minutes. Add the lentils and thyme and cook another minute or two, gently smashing some of the lentils with a spatula or wooden spoon.

3 Sprinkle the flour over the lentil mixture and stir to coat. Add the tomatoes and broth and cook for 5 minutes, stirring often so the mixture doesn't stick to the bottom of the pan.

4 Reduce the heat to low and stir in the maple syrup, vinegar, Worcestershire sauce, salt, if using, and pepper. Simmer, stirring occasionally until the mixture is cooked through and the sauce has thickened, 3 to 5 minutes.

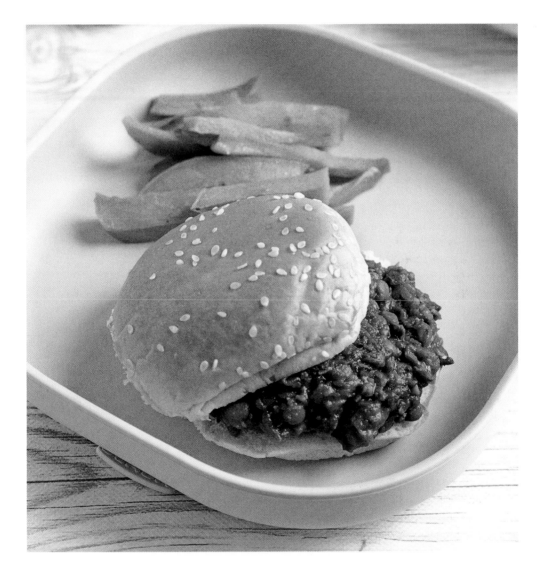

Caterpillar Pasta

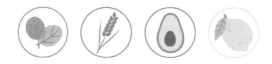

We don't know about you, but after our kids turned 18 months, it became harder and harder for us to find ways for them to enjoy leafy green vegetables like kale. Thankfully, they both gobble up this creamy pasta sauce.

We rotate between regular pasta, whole-grain pasta, and legume-based pasta, so choose whichever one you enjoy most. It is made extra delicious with a little nutritional yeast either in the sauce or sprinkled right on top. For adults, we like a pinch of red pepper flakes on top as well. This recipe easily doubles or triples to batch cook for the week.

- ¼ cup olive oil
- 2 smashed garlic cloves
- 6 ounces torn kale leaves, stems removed (about 2 packed cups)
- 2 tablespoons lemon juice with 1 teaspoon fresh zest
- ½ teaspoon salt
- ½ teaspoon freshly ground black pepper
- 8 ounces pasta of choice, such as linguine, spaghetti, or fettuccine

1 Bring a large pot of 8 cups water to a boil. In a medium bowl, place 2 cups of ice cubes and enough water to cover. Set aside.

2 While the pasta water is heating, add the oil to a small skillet and place over low heat. Add the garlic and cook, stirring constantly so the garlic doesn't brown, for 1 to 2 minutes. Once you begin to smell the garlic, remove from the heat and set aside to cool.

3 Using tongs or a slotted spoon, add the kale to the boiling pasta water for 60 seconds, then promptly remove and place in the prepared ice water bowl.

4 Strain the kale and place in a blender along with the garlic-infused oil, lemon juice and zest, salt, and pepper.

5 Add the pasta to the same boiling water you used for the kale and cook until al dente. Strain, reserving ½ cup of the pasta water.

6 Add ¼ cup of the reserved pasta water to the blender with the kale mixture and puree until creamy and smooth. Add more salt, pepper, and/or lemon to taste. If the mixture is too thick, add a little more pasta water, 1 tablespoon at a time. The sauce should be slightly thin.

7 Return the kale pasta sauce and cooked pasta to the pot and toss well to coat. Serve immediately!

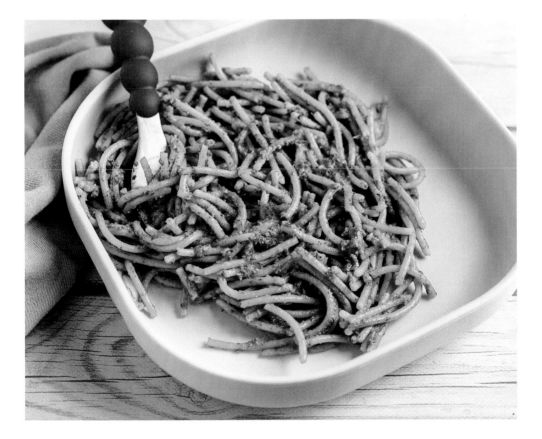

Chickpea Coconut Curry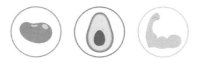

SERVES 4 TO 6

We're both suckers for anything Indian inspired, and this uncomplicated meal fits the bill for being family friendly and easy. If you don't have garam masala, sub in another tablespoon of curry powder.

- 1 tablespoon olive oil
- 1 medium white or yellow onion, finely diced
- 3 garlic cloves, minced
- 1 inch fresh ginger, finely chopped
- 1 tablespoon curry powder
- 1 tablespoon garam masala
- 1 teaspoon chili powder (optional, for older kids/more heat)
- 1 cup tomato puree
- One 14-ounce can light coconut milk
- Two 15-ounce cans chickpeas, drained and rinsed
- Salt to taste
- Cooked whole grains, for serving

1 In a large saucepan, heat the olive oil over medium heat. Add the onion and cook until soft and translucent, about 5 minutes.

2 Stir in the garlic and ginger. Cook for 1 minute. Add the curry powder, garam masala, and chili powder and cook until just fragrant, 30 seconds.

3 Whisk in the tomato puree, coconut milk, and chickpeas and let simmer. Reduce the heat to low and cook for 10 to 15 minutes until slightly thickened, stirring occassionally.

4 Serve with cooked grains of choice.

Tofu Fish Sticks

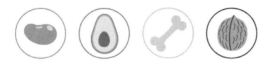

Seaweed powder turns these crispy tofu fingers into "fish sticks." To make homemade seaweed powder, place a handful of dried nori sheets into a coffee or spice grinder and pulse until pulverized, or crush by hand. Alternatively, you can purchase nori powder or kelp granules online or at a natural foods grocery store. We like Braggs and Maine Coast Sea Vegetables. Or you can leave it out completely! These are still great without that "fishy" taste. If you omit the nori powder, you will likely need to add in a little extra salt to the bread crumb mixture.

Given babe's fat needs, we don't stress about the added oil that gives a crispier coating when pan-fried. If you choose to bake these, spray them with cooking spray before placing in the oven. Look for brands that don't use propellants, like Chosen Foods.

The addition of finely ground cornmeal provides wonderful texture, but you can also use all panko bread crumbs, regular bread crumbs, or a mixture of the two. If your lemon pepper has salt, then you may not need additional salt. As this recipe is fairly time intensive compared to the others in this book, we recommend using two blocks of tofu for extra sticks throughout the week.

- Two 14-ounce packages extra-firm tofu, drained and pressed
- ½ cup all-purpose or whole wheat flour
- ½ cup unsweetened soy milk
- 1 tablespoon low-sodium soy sauce
- 1 tablespoon fresh lemon juice, lime juice, or apple cider vinegar
- ¾ cup bread crumbs
- ¼ cup finely ground cornmeal
- ½ teaspoon smoked paprika
- 2 tablespoons nori powder (see header note)
- 2 teaspoons lemon pepper seasoning (see header note)
- ½ teaspoon salt
- Avocado oil or cooking spray

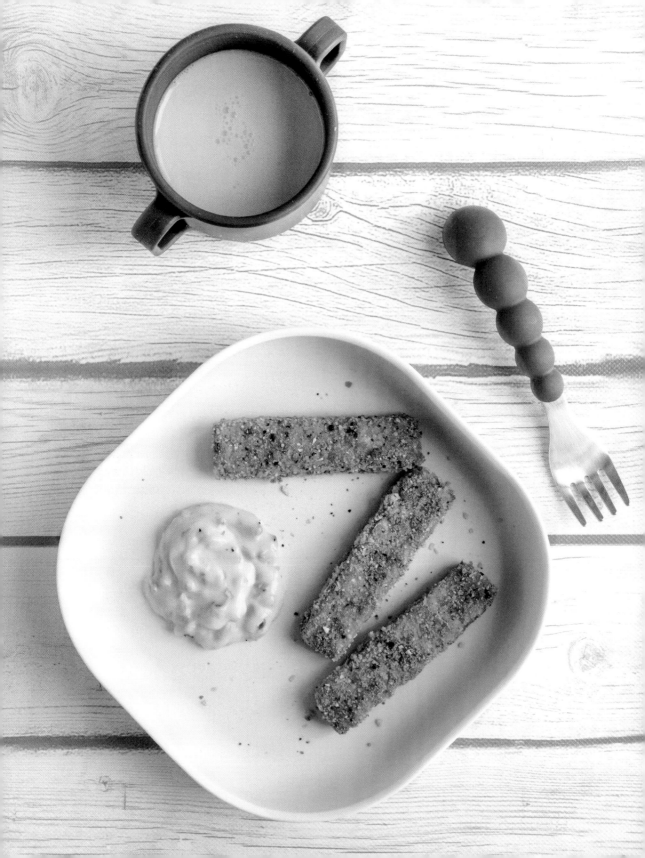

1 To panfry: Line a plate with paper towel and set aside. To bake: preheat the oven to 375°F.

2 Slice the tofu widthwise into 1-inch-thick strips, then lengthwise into 2 strips to create finger shapes

3 Place the flour on a plate. In a shallow dish, whisk together the soy milk, soy sauce, and lemon juice. In another shallow dish, combine the bread crumbs, cornmeal, paprika, nori powder, lemon pepper seasoning, and salt.

4 Now you have your stations! Dip a tofu finger into the flour, then into the soy milk mixture, and finally into the bread crumb dish. Repeat for all the fingers.

5 If panfrying, heat a small layer of oil (we like avocado for higher-heat cooking) in a large skillet and add the tofu fingers. Cook for 2 to 3 minutes per side, until golden brown and crispy. Remove to a paper-towel-lined plate and repeat with the rest of the fingers.

6 If baking, preheat the oven to 375°F. Place the tofu fingers in a single layer on a greased baking sheet. Lightly spray the fingers with cooking spray or drizzle with oil, then bake for 25 minutes. Flip, spray with a little more cooking spray, and bake for 10 minutes more, until crispy and golden brown.

7 Serve as is, with sauce of choice, or in fish tacos (see Notes).

Notes: For a full family meal, we make these as fish tacos for the adults and deconstructed fish tacos for the kids. For a quick and easy slaw, toss together a bag of pre-shredded coleslaw mix with a little vegan mayo, fresh lime juice, salt, and pepper. Serve with crispy tofu sticks and tortillas.

Veggie Calzone Night

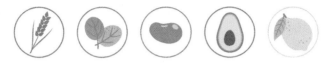

MAKES 4 CALZONES

We have fond memories of Friday pizza nights growing up—complete with a trip to the video store to rent the latest hit. These days, we're serving up calzone night, a fun twist on those dinners. To make this a family-friendly meal, slice the calzones into strips and serve with extra marinara sauce for dipping.

For babes learning to like vegetables, finely chop the veggies and allow kids to pick and choose which ones they want to tuck inside their calzones.

Cashew Mozzarella Cream:
- ¾ cup raw cashews
- 2 teaspoons olive oil
- 1 teaspoon all-purpose flour
- 2 teaspoons nutritional yeast
- ½ teaspoon onion powder
- ½ teaspoon garlic powder
- 1 teaspoon lemon juice
- ½ teaspoon salt
- All-purpose flour, for rolling
- 1¾ pounds pizza dough
- 1 cup prepared pizza sauce
- Favorite vegetable toppings, chopped and cooked as desired (see Notes)
- 1 recipe Cashew Mozzarella Cream (below)

1 Preheat the oven to 450°F.

2 Lightly grease two large baking sheets and set aside.

3 Make the mozzarella cream: Place the cashews, olive oil, flour, nutritional yeast, onion powder, garlic powder, lemon juice, salt, and 1 cup of water in a blender and puree until very creamy and smooth. This may take up to 5 minutes depending on the power of your blender. Transfer to a medium saucepan over medium heat and simmer for 2 to 3 minutes, stirring constantly until just thickened, taking care not to burn. Remove from the heat.

4 Lightly flour a clean work surface. Divide the pizza dough into 4 pieces. Roll out 1 piece of dough into an 8-inch circle about ¼ inch thick. Spoon ¼ cup of the pizza sauce onto the middle of the dough, then top with the mozzarella cream and preferred toppings.

5 Gently fold the dough in half and dampen the edges with water. Pinch the edges together, then crimp the edges all around. Repeat with the remaining dough.

6 Transfer the calzones to the prepared baking sheets. Brush the tops with oil. Using kitchen scissors or a sharp knife, make 2 or 3 slits in the top to create steam vents.

7 Bake for 15 to 20 minutes, or until the tops are golden and the filling is bubbling. Let cool for 5 minutes before slicing into strips for kids.

Notes: While any topping works in these calzones, we like sautéed greens like spinach or kale, sautéed bell peppers, finely chopped broccoli, pineapple, and cooked tempeh bacon crumbles.

> *Quick Tip:* If you don't have pizza dough on hand, or for a super-quick and easy alternative, use these same toppings on pitas. Place the pita on a greased baking sheet and add your favorite toppings. Bake for 10 minutes at 400°F.

One Pot Teriyaki Stir-Fry

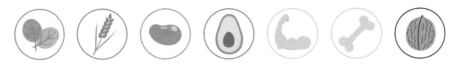

SERVES 4

This is another of our favorite quick meals, using frozen edamame and stir-fry vegetables. It's perfect for busy weeknights and is customizable depending on what vegetables your family likes. You can also sub in baked tofu or tempeh if you don't like edamame.

This recipe uses white basmati or jasmine rice for a faster cook time. Don't worry, though; it still packs in the fiber thanks to the vegetables and edamame.

As always, we recommend omitting the soy sauce for younger babies and adding to adult and older kid portions after plating.

If you have a microplane, use that for fast ginger and garlic prep.

- 1 tablespoon olive or sesame oil
- 3 garlic cloves, minced
- 1 inch fresh ginger, minced
- 1 cup uncooked basmati or jasmine rice
- 12 ounces frozen stir-fry vegetables

- 1 cup frozen edamame
- 2 tablespoons low-sodium soy sauce
- 1 tablespoon maple syrup
- 2 teaspoons toasted sesame oil
- 2 scallions, sliced

1 In a large, deep skillet, heat the oil over medium heat. Add the garlic and ginger and cook until fragrant, about 1 minute. Add the rice and cook for 1 to 2 minutes, or until the rice is toasted.

2 Add the frozen vegetables, edamame, and 2 cups of water. Raise the heat to medium-high and bring to a boil. Cover, reduce the heat to low, and simmer for 10 minutes.

3 In a small bowl, whisk together the soy sauce, maple syrup, sesame oil, and scallions.

4 Fold the sauce into the cooked rice and vegetables and serve.

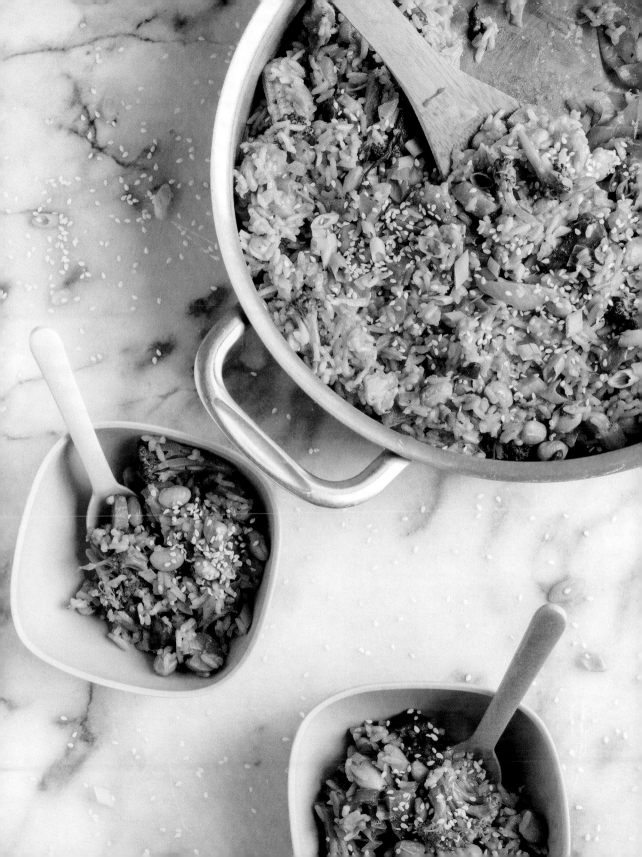

Easy Quesadillas

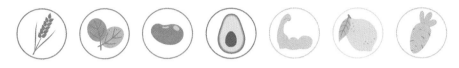

MAKES 4 QUESADILLAS

These effortless quesadillas were inspired by our need to come up with a dinner recipe that we could get on the table in roughly 10 minutes. Throw the cashews in a blender, sauté the vegetables, assemble, and eat.

- ½ cup raw cashews
- 1 cup boiling water
- 2 teaspoons olive oil
- 1 medium red bell pepper, seeded and finely chopped
- 1 cup spinach leaves, roughly chopped

- One 15-ounce can low-sodium vegetarian refried beans of choice*
- 1 medium garlic clove, roughly chopped
- Salt and freshly ground black pepper to taste
- 8 tortillas

1 Place the cashews in a medium bowl. Pour the boiling water over the cashews and let sit while you prep the rest of the ingredients.

2 In a medium pan, heat the oil over medium heat. Add the bell pepper and cook for 5 minutes, or until soft. Add the spinach and cook until wilted, about 2 minutes. Transfer the cooked vegetables to the bowl with the refried beans and stir to combine. Wipe out the pan.

3 Drain the cashews and place in a food processor or blender with ⅓ cup of water, the garlic, and salt. Puree until very creamy and smooth, scraping down the sides as needed. Adjust salt and pepper to taste.

4 Assemble the quesadillas: Spread the cashew cheese on 4 of the tortillas and the bean mixture on the remaining 4. Place 1 of the cashew cheese tortillas on the bean mixture, then heat in the pan over medium heat for 1 to 2 minutes per side, until warmed through and golden brown.

5 Continue with the rest of the quesadillas. Slice into strips or small triangles for older infants and toddlers.

*If you can't find vegetarian refried beans, you can sub any mashed bean of your choice.

> *Quick Tip:* For super-fast quesadillas, you can skip the homemade cheese and use a plain vegan cream cheese or shreds. We prefer the brands with minimal ingredients, like Miyoko's Creamery. These also stick together pretty well without any cheese thanks to the sticky refried beans.

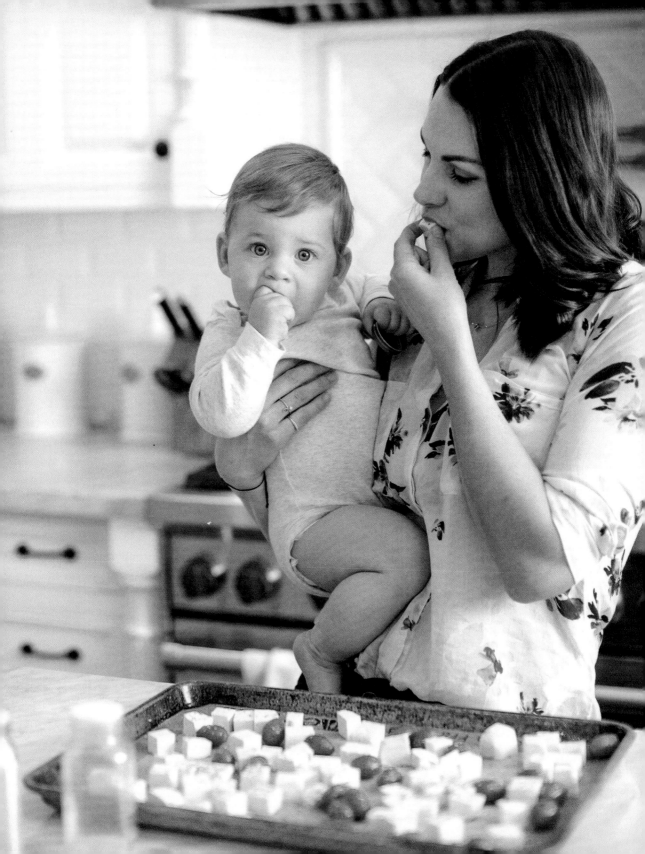

Handouts and Resources

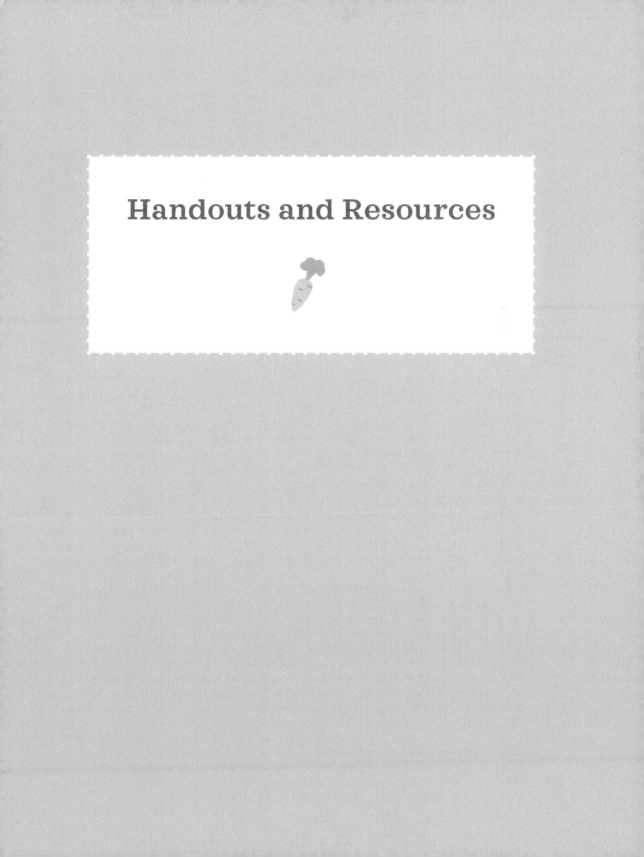

Nutrients of Importance: RDA Quick Guide

Energy:
1-3 years: 1000-1400 calories (depending on age, weight, sex, and activity level)
Breastfeeding: ~500 extra calories per day

Carbohydrates:
0-6 months: 60 g
7-12 months: 90 g
1-3 years: 130 g (45%-65% daily intake)
Breastfeeding: 210 g (45%-65% daily intake)

Protein:
0-6 months: 9 g
7-12 months: 11 g or 1.5 g/kg
1-3 years: 13 g or 1.1 g/kg
Breastfeeding: 71 g or 1.1 g/kg

Total Fat:
0-6 months: 30 grams
7-12 months: 31 grams
1-3 years: 30%-40% daily intake
Breastfeeding: 20%-35% daily intake

DHA:
0-6 months: 20 mg/kg DHA
7-12 months: 15-20 mg/kg DHA + EPA
1-3 years: 15-20 mg/kg DHA + EPA (~170-230 mg for a 25-lb. baby)
Breastfeeding: minimum of 300 mg*

Up to 3 g/day for premature babies

Iron:
0-6 months: 0.27 mg
7-12 months: 11 mg
1-3 years: 7 mg
Breastfeeding: 9 mg

Zinc:
0-6 months: 2 mg
7-12 months: 3 mg
1-3 years: 3 mg
Breastfeeding: 12 mg

Calcium:
0-6 months: 200 mg (AI)
7-12 months: 260 mg (AI)
1-3 years: 700 mg
Breastfeeding: 1000 mg

Iodine:
0-6 months: 110 mcg (AI)
7-12 months: 130 mcg (AI)
1-3 years: 90 mcg
Breastfeeding: 290 mcg

Selenium:
0-6 months: 15 mcg (AI)
7-12 months: 20 mcg (AI)
1-3 years: 20 mcg
Breastfeeding: 70 mcg

B12:
0-6 months: 0.4 mcg
7-12 months: 0.5 mcg
1-3 years: 0.9 mcg*
Breastfeeding: 2.8 mcg*

Supplementation recommendations far exceed the RDA due to bioavailability factors.

Vitamin D:
0-6 months: 400 IU
7-12 months: 400 IU
1-3 years: 600 IU
Breastfeeding: 600 IU

Vitamin A (RAE):
0-6 months: 400 mcg (AI)
7-12 months: 500 (AI)
1-3 years: 300 mcg
Breastfeeding: 1330 mcg

Choline (AI):
0-6 months: 125 mg
7-12 months: 150 mg
1-3 years: 200 mg
Breastfeeding: 550 mg

Create Your Own Supplement Regimen

NUTRIENT	BREASTFEEDING MOMS	0–6 MONTHS	6–12 MONTHS	1–3 YEARS
Vitamin D	Included in pre/postnatal	Breastfed babies: 400 IU/day	Breastfed babies: 400 IU/day	
Iron*	Included in pre/postnatal	Breastfed babies: 1 mg/kg/day from 4 to 6 months	Only if deficient	Only if deficient
B12	At least 150 mcg/day if not high enough in pre/postnatal	N/A	N/A	At least 5 mcg/day
Iodine	Included in pre/postnatal	N/A	N/A	
DHA (algae oil)	300 mg/day	N/A	N/A	

Plant-based babies' and toddlers' supplement needs will vary and change depending on a variety of factors—age, formula or breast milk, amount of fortified milk intake for toddlers, and dietary pattern (vegan vs. vegetarian vs. predominantly plant-based).

We've included a few blanket recommendations but left blank the sections that will depend on your child's unique needs. Use Chapter 1 to determine which supplements your child will need and how much and fill in the blanks so you have an easy reference for the future.

Here are a few questions to consider when filling in the blanks:

1. Vitamin D: Does your child consume cow's milk or fortified plant milk? How much? They may not need the full RDA of vitamin D.

2. Iodine: Does your child consume cow's milk? Do you use iodized salt?

3. DHA: Does your child eat eggs or fish more than once a week?

Keep in mind that fully formula-fed babies will not need any supplements from 0 to 12 months unless otherwise directed by your physician.

*Iron is only included in this list for exclusively breastfed babies from 4 to 6 months, per AAP recommendations. After this time, supplementation is only necessary to correct deficiency.

The PB3 Plate

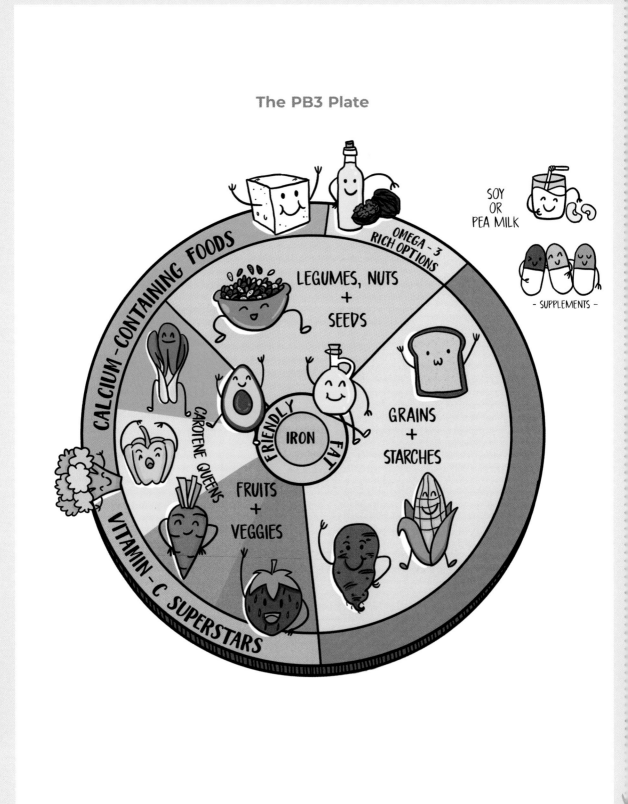

PB3 Plate How-Tos and Staples

If you're going to eat plant-based, there are a few staple recipes, recipe swaps, and cooking how-tos we think every parent should have in their back pocket. These simple tips and tutorials will help round out your meals and make plant-based family eating a breeze.

Staple Recipes:

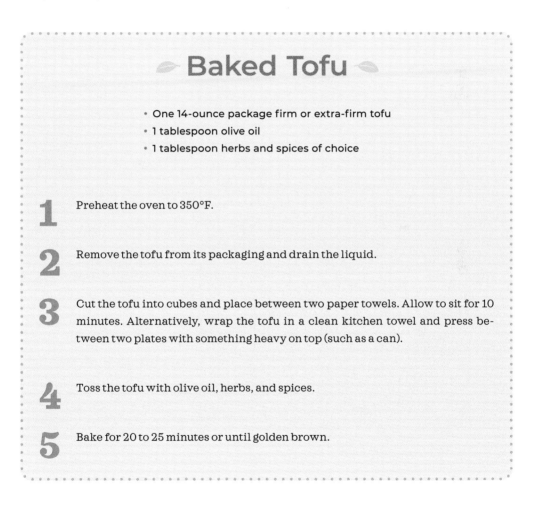

Baked Tofu

- One 14-ounce package firm or extra-firm tofu
- 1 tablespoon olive oil
- 1 tablespoon herbs and spices of choice

1 Preheat the oven to 350°F.

2 Remove the tofu from its packaging and drain the liquid.

3 Cut the tofu into cubes and place between two paper towels. Allow to sit for 10 minutes. Alternatively, wrap the tofu in a clean kitchen towel and press between two plates with something heavy on top (such as a can).

4 Toss the tofu with olive oil, herbs, and spices.

5 Bake for 20 to 25 minutes or until golden brown.

Basic Hummus

- 2 cups canned chickpeas, drained, liquid reserved
- ½ teaspoon salt
- ⅓ cup tahini
- ¼ cup lemon juice
- 3 ice cubes
- 2 tablespoons olive oil, for drizzling

1 Place the chickpeas, 2 tablespoons of the reserved chickpea liquid or water, the salt, tahini, lemon juice, and ice cubes in a food processor or high-powered blender.

2 Process until very smooth, about 3 minutes.

3 Transfer to a serving bowl or container and drizzle with olive oil.

Vegan Parmesan

- 1 cup raw cashews or pepitas
- 1 cup nutritional yeast
- ¼ to ½ teaspoon salt*

1 Place the cashews, nutritional yeast, and salt in a high-powered blender or food processor and pulverize until flaky.

2 Store in an airtight jar in the refrigerator for up to 6 months.

Omit for babies under 12 months and limit under 2 years.

Vegan Cheese Sauce

- 1 cup cashews (preferably raw and unsalted)
- 1 cup low-sodium vegetable broth
- ¼ cup nutritional yeast
- ¼ teaspoon ground turmeric
- 1 tablespoon fresh lemon juice
- 1 tablespoon onion powder
- ¼ to ½ teaspoon salt*

1 Place all the ingredients in a high-speed blender and puree for up to 2 minutes, or until completely smooth, using a spatula to scrape down the sides every 20 seconds or so.

Omit for babies under 12 months and limit under 2 years.

DIY Oat Flour

- 1½ cups rolled oats

1 Place the oats in a high-speed blender or food processor and process until powdery, 30 seconds to 1 minute. Take care not to overprocess, as the flour can clump.

2 Transfer the flour to a jar or container and store up to 1 month unrefrigerated.

Plant-Based Recipe Swaps

If a recipe calls for butter . . .

    . . . swap for an equal amount of pureed fruit (banana, apple, prunes) or vegetable oil (olive, avocado, or coconut)

If a recipe calls for 1 cup of buttermilk . . .

    . . . swap for 1 cup of unsweetened soy milk mixed with 1 tablespoon of lemon juice (let sit for 10 minutes before using)

If a recipe calls for 1 egg . . .

    . . . swap for 1 tablespoon of ground flaxseed or chia seeds mixed with 3 tablespoons of warm water (let sit for 5 minutes before using)

If a recipe calls for ground beef . . .

    . . . swap for an equal amount of cooked lentils or beans. This works best in dishes such as tacos, enchiladas, chili, and stews.

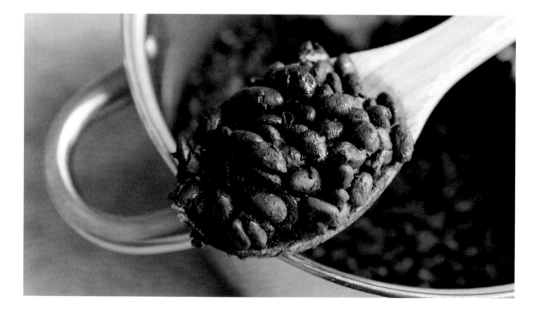

⬲ Dry Beans ⬱

1 In a large bowl, place 1 pound beans and pick out any broken beans, stones, or debris. Cover with a few inches of water. Soak the beans for 10 to 14 hours, or overnight, on the counter or in the refrigerator.

2 Drain the beans and place in a pot. Add fresh water to cover by about 1 inch.

3 Bring the water to a boil, then reduce the heat to a gentle simmer. Cover and cook for 1 to 3 hours depending on age of the beans, size, and variety, stirring occasionally. Add more water as needed to keep the beans fully submerged. Check for doneness after 1 hour.

4 Cool the beans in their cooking liquid. Store with their liquid in an airtight container until ready to use. They will keep in the refrigerator for up to 1 week or in the freezer for up to 3 months.

Pressure Cooker:

1 In a pressure cooker, combine 1 pound of dried beans, 8 cups of water (at least enough to cover the beans by a few inches), 1 to 2 teaspoons of salt depending on age of kids, and 1 tablespoon of oil. The oil helps to reduce foaming, which can clog the pressure valve, so we don't recommend skipping it. Make sure not to fill the cooker more than halfway.

2 Secure the lid in the sealing position. Cook the beans on high pressure according to the table below.

3 Once cooking is complete, let the pressure release naturally on its own. This will allow the beans to retain their shape and limits foaming.

Slow Cooker:

1 Soak the beans for at least 8 hours. Drain.

2 Place the beans in a slow cooker and add any aromatics or seasonings. Cover and cook on low for 6 to 8 hours. When the beans are slightly soft, add salt and continue to cook until done.

TIPS:

Add onion, garlic, or bay leaves at the start of cooking to add flavor.

If adding salt, add once the beans are almost fully cooked, about three-quarters of the way through.

Lentils do not need to be soaked before cooking. See below for cooking instructions.

Slightly undercook the beans if you plan to cook them again in another recipe or soup.

When cooking kidney beans, we recommend boiling them for 10 minutes regardless of which cooking method you choose to finish cooking. This helps neutralize a toxin called phytohemagglutinin.

BEAN TYPE	COOK TIME SOAKED	COOK TIME UNSOAKED (PRESSURE COOKER, NATURAL RELEASE)
Adzuki Beans	45–60 minutes	20–25 minutes
Black Beans	60–90 minutes	20–25 minutes
Black-Eyed Peas	60 minutes	20–25 minutes
Cannellini Beans	60 minutes	35–40 minutes
Chickpeas	1–2 hours	35–40 minutes
Great Northern Beans	60–90 minutes	25–30 minutes
Kidney Beans	60 minutes	25–30 minutes
Lentils	20–25 minutes (unsoaked)	5 minutes
Navy Beans	45–60 minutes	20–25 minutes
Pinto Beans	60–90 minutes	25–30 minutes
Split Peas	25 minutes	6 minutes

Dried Peas and Lentils

1 Rinse and sort lentils, discarding any broken beans, stones, or debris.

2 Add 1½ cups of water or stock to a pot for each cup of dried lentils or peas and bring to a boil.

3 Add the lentils or peas and return to a boil, then reduce the heat and simmer, partially covered, for 30 to 45 minutes.

GRAINS	LIQUID-TO-GRAIN RATIO	COOK TIME
Barley	1:3	45–60 minutes
Brown Rice	1:2	40–60 minutes
Bulgur Wheat	1:2	5 minutes
Couscous	1:1–1 ½	5 minutes
Farro	1:3	25–30 minutes
Millet	1:3	20–25 minutes
Quinoa	1:2	15 minutes
Polenta	1:4	15–20 minutes, whisking often
Steel Cut Oats	1:3	20–25 minutes
Wheat Berries	1:3	60–90 minutes
White Rice	1:2	15–20 minutes

Our favorite ways to use grains:

- As a stuffing for peppers, squash, and tomatoes
- As a filling for enchiladas, fajitas, and tacos
- As a cold grain salad with fresh herbs, beans of choice, chopped vegetables, and a dressing
- Sprinkled into soups or stews to add heft
- As a risotto or stir-fry
- As meat alternatives such as grain burgers, loaves, and stuffings
- For baking quick breads and cookies

AVERAGE NUTRIENT COMPOSITION OF BREAST MILK

Nutrient Amount/Liter (33 oz) in Human Milk	
Calories	65 calories
Macronutrients	
Carbohydrates (Lactose)	72 grams
Protein	10.5 grams
Fat	39 grams
Minerals	
Calcium	280 mg
Phosphorus	140 mg
Magnesium	35 mg
Sodium	180 mg
Potassium	525 mg
Chloride	420 mg
Iron	0.3 mg
Zinc	1.2 mg
Copper	0.25 mg
Iodine	110 mcg
Selenium	20 mcg
Manganese	6 mcg
Fluoride	16 mcg
Chromium	50 mcg
Vitamins	
Vitamin A	670 mcg
Vitamin C	40 mg
Vitamin D	0.55 mcg
Vitamin E	2.3 mg
Vitamin K	2.1 mcg
Thiamin	0.21 mg
Riboflavin	0.35 mg
Niacin	1.5 mg
Vitamin B5	1.8 mg
Vitamin B6	93 mg
Biotin	4 mcg
Folate	85 mcg
Vitamin B12	0.97 mcg

Reference: Nutrition During Lactation. *National Academies Press: OpenBook.* *Accessed April 27, 2020. https://www.nap.edu/read/1577/chapter/7#116.*

Sample Meal Plans

6 MONTHS			
	Breakfast	**Lunch**	**Dinner**
Monday	Sunshine Bowl (page 196)	Breast milk or Formula	Breast milk or Formula
Tuesday	PBJ's Blender Bean Muffins (page 206)	Breast milk or Formula	Breast milk or Formula
Wednesday	Sunshine Bowl	Breast milk or Formula	Breast milk or Formula
Thursday	PBJ's Blender Bean Muffins	Breast milk or Formula	Breast milk or Formula
Friday	Sunshine Bowl	Breast milk or Formula	Breast milk or Formula
Saturday	Breast milk or Formula	Breast milk or Formula	Tofu Marinara (page 218) with Cheezy Broccoli Trees (page 215)
Sunday	BLW Oatmeal Pancakes (page 210)	Breast milk or Formula	Breast milk or Formula

9–12 MONTHS			
	Breakfast	**Lunch**	**Dinner**
Monday	Iron-Optimized Oatmeal (page 57) with strawberries	Green Dragon Smoothie (page 227) with peanut butter toast strips	Breast milk or Formula
Tuesday	Veggie Omelet Cups (page 224) with Sweet Potato Stars (page 212)	Breast milk or Formula	Tex-Mex Millet Meatballs (page 208) with avocado slices
Wednesday	PBJ's Blender Bean Muffins with orange slices	Tex-Mex Millet Meatballs with avocado slices	Breast milk or Formula
Thursday	Veggie Omelet Cups with Sweet Potato Stars	Calcium Creamsicle Smoothie (page 221) with Chewy Granola Bars (page 244)	Breast milk or Formula
Friday	Iron-Optimized Oatmeal with strawberries	PBJ's Blender Bean Muffins with orange slices	Breast milk or Formula
Saturday	Veggie Omelet Cups with Sweet Potato Stars	Breast milk or Formula	Red Lentil Pizza Strips (page 216) with Butternut Squash Fries (page 205)
Sunday	French Toast Fingers with Quick Berry Syrup (page 222)	Red Lentil Pizza Strips with Butternut Squash Fries	Breast milk or Formula

	Breakfast	Snack	Lunch	Snack	Dinner
Monday	Apple Baked Oatmeal (page 230) with peanut butter drizzle	Fortified soy or pea milk with berries	Peanut butter sandwich with avocado and tomato slices	Calcium Creamsicle Smoothie (page 221)	Sheet Pan BBQ Tofu Bowls (page 266)
Tuesday	Creamy Bircher Muesli (page 237)	Fortified soy or pea milk with orange and bell pepper slices	Strawberry Cashew Yogurt (page 240) with hummus sandwich pinwheels	Tropical Chia Pudding (page 243)	Sunflower Mac 'n' Cheese (page 250) with roasted asparagus and blackberries
Wednesday	Apple Baked Oatmeal with peanut butter drizzle	Fortified soy or pea milk with berries	Sunflower Mac 'n' Cheese with roasted asparagus and blackberries	Strawberry Cashew Yogurt (page 240)	Sheet Pan BBQ Tofu Bowls
Thursday	Creamy Bircher Muesli	Fortified soy or pea milk with orange and bell pepper slices	Alphabet Pasta Salad (page 246) with steamed broccoli and blueberries	Tropical Chia Pudding	15-Minute Black Bean Tacos (page 264) with Confetti Guacamole (page 239)
Friday	Apple Baked Oatmeal with peanut butter drizzle	Confetti Guacamole with crackers and fortified soy or pea milk	Peanut butter sandwich with avocado and tomato slices	Green Dragon Smoothie (page 227)	Lentil Sloppy Joes (page 270) with sweet potato fries and roasted cauliflower
Saturday	Simple Breakfast Quinoa Porridge (page 234)	Fortified soy or pea milk with orange and bell pepper slices	Alphabet Pasta Salad with steamed broccoli and blueberries	Strawberry Cashew Yogurt	Lentil Sloppy Joes with sweet potato fries and roasted cauliflower
Sunday	Lemon Chia Waffles (page 233) with berries	Fortified soy or pea milk with berries	Sunflower Mac 'n' Cheese with roasted cauliflower and tomato slices	PB&J Smoothie (page 236)	Tofu Fish Sticks (page 275) with steamed mixed veggies and a side of rice

PBJ's Favorite Feeding Products

Kitchen Tools

Joie Fruit and Vegetable Wavy Chopper
    Knife
LENK Vegetable Cutter Shapes
Guidecraft Kitchen Helper Toddler Stool

Feeding Equipment

Keekaroo Height Right High Chair
OXO Tot Waterproof Silicone Roll Up Bib
phil&teds Lobster Clip-On High Chair
Stokke Tripp Trapp High Chair

Food Storage

LunchBots Stainless Steel Bento Boxes
Stasher 100% Silicone Reusable Food
    Bag
Wakey PQ Snack Cup Collapsible Spill
    Proof Silicone Snack Container

Cups

EcoVessel Insulated Water Bottle
Housavvy Stainless Steel Sippy Cup with
    Lid and Straw
Munchkin Miracle 360° Trainer Cup
Pura Kiki Stainless Steel Insulated Bottle
TalkTools Honey Bear Drinking Cup

Plates/Bowls

BabyBjörn Baby Cup
Béaba Silicone Suction Bowl
Bumkins Silicone Grip Dish

For Baby-Led Weaning:

Bumkins Kids Long Sleeve Smock
ChooMee FlexiDip Baby Starter Spoon
ezpz Mini Bowl
ezpz Mini Mat
eZtotZ Little Dippers Starter Spoon
Paw Legend Washable Highchair Splat
    Floor Mat
NumNum Pre-Spoon GOOtensils

Breastfeeding

Boppy Original Nursing Pillow and
    Positioner
Bravado Designs Ballet Nursing Sleep
    Bra
Haakaa Silicone Breastfeeding Nipple
    Shields
Motherlove Nipple Cream
Kindred Bravely Nursing and Pumping
    Combo Bra

Infant Feeding Supplies

Baby Bottles Boon Grass Countertop
    Drying Rack
Baby Brezza Glass Natural Bottles
Kiinde Kozii Breastmilk and Bottle
    Warmer
Philips Avent Natural Glass Baby
    Bottles
Dr. Brown's Natural Flow Glass Baby
    Bottles

PBJ's Favorite Food Products

Legumes, Nuts, and Seeds:
Banza Chickpea Penne or Elbows
Dr. Praeger's California Veggie Burgers*
Hodo Foods Organic Thai Curry Nuggets*
House Foods Organic Tofu Extra Firm
Modern Table Vegan Mac & Cheese (made with lentils)*
Tolerant Foods Green Lentil Elbows

Grains and Starches:
Bob's Red Mill Whole Wheat Couscous
Cascadian Farm Organic Purely O's
Earth's Best Organic Whole Grain Oatmeal Infant Cereal
Food For Life Sprouted Corn Tortillas
Silver Hills Organic Sprouted Soft Wheat Bread (½ whole wheat, ½ refined)
One Degree Organics Sprouted Oats

Plant-Based Dairy Products:
Lavva Plant-Based Yogurt
Ripple Unsweetened Pea Milk
Silk Organic Unsweetened Soy Milk
365 Everyday Value Organic Unsweetened Soy Milk

Snack Foods:
Annie's Organic Whole Wheat Bunnies*
Lärabar Fruits and Greens
Harvest Snaps

Condiments/Spices:
Bragg Nutritional Yeast
Bragg Organic Sea Kelp Delight Seasoning
Penzeys Salt-Free Seasoning

Best for older tots due to higher sodium or sugar content.

Additional Reading

BOOKS

Books for plant-based babies:
Eating the Alphabet by Lois Ehlert
Mrs. Peanuckle's Vegetable Alphabet by Mrs. Peanuckle and Jessie Ford
A Prayer for the Animals by Daniel Kirk
We All Love by Julie Hausen
N is for Nutrition by Todd Skene and Dr. Amneet Aulakh
Where Does Broccoli Come From? by Arielle D. Lebovitz
Where Do Bananas Come From? by Arielle D. Lebovitz
The Proof Is in the Plants by Simon Hill

On baby-led weaning:
Baby-Led Feeding by Jenna Helwig

On raising plant-based children:
The Smart Parent's Guide to Raising Vegan Kids by Eric C. Lindstrom

Cookbooks for plant-based families:
But My Family Would Never Eat Vegan! by Kristy Turner
Plant-Powered Families by Dreena Burton
Vegan for Everybody by America's Test Kitchen
Isa Does It by Isa Chandra Moskowitz

ONLINE RESOURCES

Delish Knowledge: delishknowledge.com—easy, family-friendly, plant-based recipes
Plant-Based Juniors: plantbasedjuniors.com—our website!
Vegetarian Nutrition: vegetariannutrition.net—consumer website run by the Vegetarian Nutrition

Dietetic Nutrition Group of the Academy of Nutrition and Dietetics, with free informational handouts

Vegan Health: veganhealth.org—informational website run by dietitian Jack Norris

The Vegetarian Resource Group: vrg.org—the Vegetarian Resource Group's website. "Feeding Vegan Kids" article by Reed Mangels, PhD, RD.

Whitney E., RD: whitneyerd.com—information on plant-based nutrition for all life stages, and family-friendly recipes

Acknowledgments

This book was, appropriately, a labor of love and we couldn't have done it without the support and guidance of our village.

To our wonderful editor, Nina, thank you for believing in our mission to help all parents get more plants on their children's plates. To our agent, Coleen, thank you for taking a chance on us and for your expert guidance along the way. To Lorie, Hannah, Laura, and the rest of the team at Avery, thank you for bringing our vision to life.

To Jack Norris and Dr. Ralph Carmel, thank you for your many conversations into the intricacies of B12 absorption and metabolism. To Dr. Mark Messina, thank you for helping us unravel the science behind the unfairly demonized soybean.

To our reviewers Lauren Panoff, Hannah Fried, Kaytee Hadley, Deanne Diorio, Laura Carlos, Laura Lane, and Julia Hadley, thank you for taking the time to share your feedback, questions, and thoughtful notes. Your insight was invaluable in helping us create this book and refine our message.

To our parents and in-laws, thank you for being such supportive rock stars. To Barbara, thanks for recipe testing, your many tasting notes, and washing so many dishes. To the Englishs—Patti for instilling an appreciation of health and nutrition and Scott for broadening your horizons to ingredients you previously didn't consider to be food. To Donna, for being one of PBJs biggest fans, top commenters, and occasional amateur videographer.

To our children: Vander, Caleb, Emery, and Ella. Thank you for being our greatest teachers. You've taught us so much about feeding, patience, and empathy. Thank you for choosing us to be your mamas—we love you so much!

To our incredibly supportive husbands, Bryan and Abe. Thank you for believing in us, giving us the time and space to chase our dreams, and doing the dishes. Bryan, thank you for tracking down study after study after study. Abe, thank you for your legal guidance and papa bear defensiveness of PBJs.

Lastly, thank you to the Plant-Based Junior's community for showing up, sharing your stories, and entrusting us to provide guidance for raising your beautiful babes. But most importantly, thank you for choosing to join us in raising the next generation of compassionate, conscious humans who will change this world. This book is for you!

Notes

Introduction

1. **obesity affects 13.9% of preschool-aged children:** "Childhood Obesity Facts." Last reviewed June 24, 2019. Centers for Disease Control and Prevention. Accessed March 17, 2020. https://www.cdc.gov/obesity/data/childhood.html.

2. **increasing by about 60% since 1990:** de Onis, Mercedes, Monika Blössner, and Elaine Borghi. 2010. "Global Prevalence and Trends of Overweight and Obesity Among Preschool Children." *The American Journal of Clinical Nutrition* 92 (5): 1257–1264. https://doi.org/10.3945/ajcn.2010.29786.

3. **shift in developing countries away from primarily plant-based diets:** Fox, Ashley, Wenhui Feng, and Victor Asal. 2019. "What Is Driving Global Obesity Trends? Globalization Or 'Modernization'?" *Globalization and Health* 15 (1). https://doi.org/10.1186/s12992-019-0457-y.

4. **increased by over 30% and children as young as 10:** "Prevent Type 2 Diabetes in Kids." Last reviewed September 28, 2017. *Centers for Disease Control and Prevention.* Accessed March 17, 2020. https://www.cdc.gov/diabetes/prevent-type-2/type-2-kids.html.

5. **increased by over 30% and children as young as 10:** Hamman, Richard F., Ronny A. Bell, Dana Dabelea, Ralph B. D'Agostino, Lawrence Dolan, Giuseppina Imperatore, and Jean M. Lawrence et al. 2014. "The SEARCH for Diabetes in Youth Study: Rationale, Findings, and Future Directions." *Diabetes Care* 37 (12): 3336–3344. https://doi.org/10.2337/dc14-0574.

6. **two-to-fourfold rise in cases by 2050:** Jensen, Elizabeth T., and Dana Dabelea. 2018. "Type 2 Diabetes in Youth: New Lessons from the SEARCH Study." *Current Diabetes Reports* 18 (6). https://doi.org/10.1007/s11892-018-0997-1.

7. **vegan and vegetarian diets are safe and healthy:** Melina, Vesanto, Winston Craig, and Susan Levin. 2016. "Position of the Academy of Nutrition and Dietetics: Vegetarian Diets." *Journal of the Academy of Nutrition and Dietetics* 116 (12): 1970–1980. https://doi.org/10.1016/j.jand.2016.09.025.

8. **a reduced risk of chronic diseases like diabetes, heart disease, and some cancers:** Orlich, Michael J., Pramil N. Singh, Joan Sabaté, Karen Jaceldo-Siegl, Jing Fan, Synnove Knutsen, W. Lawrence Beeson, and Gary E. Fraser. 2013. "Vegetarian Dietary Patterns and Mortality in Adventist Health Study 2." *JAMA Internal Medicine* 173 (13): 1230. https://doi.org/10.1001/jamainternmed.2013.6473.

9. **between the 25th and 75th percentiles for weight and height:** O'Connell, Joan M., Michael J. Dibley, Janet Sierra, Barbara Wallace, James S. Marks, and Ray Yip. 1989. "Growth of Vegetarian Children: The Farm Study." *Pediatris* 84 (3): 476–481.

10. **lower levels of inflammatory signaling molecules:** Ambroszkiewicz, Jadwiga, Magdalena Chełchowska, Grażyna Rowicka, Witold Klemarczyk, Małgorzata Strucińska, and Joanna Gajewska. 2018. "Anti-Inflammatory and Pro-Inflammatory Adipokine Profiles in Children on Vegetarian and Omnivorous Diets." *Nutrients* 10 (9): 1241. https://doi.org/10.3390/nu10091241.

11. **eat more fruits, vegetables, fiber, and important micronutrients:** Weder, Stine, Morwenna Hoffmann, Katja Becker, Ute Alexy, and Markus Keller. 2019. "Energy, Macronutrient Intake, and Anthropometrics of Vegetarian, Vegan, and Omnivorous Children (1-3 Years) in Germany (VeChi Diet Study)." *Nutrients* 11, no. 4 (December): 832. https://doi.org/10.3390/nu11040832.

12. **Schürmann, S., M. Kersting, and U. Alexy. 2017. "Vegetarian Diets in Children:** A Systematic Review." *European Journal of Nutrition* 56 (5): 1797-1817. https://doi.org/10.1007/s00394-017-1416-0.

13. **fewer unhealthy items like sweets, salty snacks, and saturated fat-rich foods:** Melina, Vesanto, Winston Craig, and Susan Levin. 2016. "Position of the Academy of Nutrition and Dietetics: Vegetarian Diets." *Journal of the Academy of Nutrition and Dietetics* 116 (12): 1970-1980. https://doi.org/10.1016/j.jand.2016.09.025.

14. Stine, Morwenna Hoffmann, Katja Becker, Ute Alexy, and Markus Keller. 2019. "Energy, Macronutrient Intake, and Anthropometrics of Vegetarian, Vegan, and Omnivorous Children (1-3 Years) in Germany (VeChi Diet Study)." *Nutrients* 11, no. 4 (December): 832. https://doi.org/10.3390/nu11040832.

15. **vegetarian moms had just 1%-2% the amount of pollutants:** Wang, Hexing, Chuanxi Tang, Jiaqi Yang, Na Wang, Feng Jiang, Qinghua Xia, Gengsheng He, Yue Chen, and Qingwu Jiang. 2018. "Predictors of Urinary Antibiotics in Children of Shanghai and Health Risk Assessment." *Environment International* 121: 507-514. https://doi.org/10.1016/j.envint.2018.09.032.

16. **IQ scores corresponded with a mental age more than a year higher:** Dwyer, Joanna T., et al. 1980. "Mental Age and I.Q. of Predominantly Vegetarian Children." *Journal of the American Dietetic Association* 76 (2): 142-147.

17. **have linked cow's milk with an increased risk of childhood obesity:** DeBoer, Mark D., Hannah E. Agard, and Rebecca J. Scharf. 2015. "Milk Intake, Height and Body Mass Index in Preschool Children." *Archives of Disease in Childhood* 100 (5): 460-465. https://doi.org/10.1136/archdischild-2014-306958.

18. Berkey, Catherine S., Helaine R. H. Rockett, Walter C. Willett, and Graham A. Colditz. 2005. "Milk, Dairy Fat, Dietary Calcium, and Weight Gain." *Archives of Pediatrics & Adolescent Medicine* 159 (6): 543. https://doi.org/10.1001/archpedi.159.6.543.

19. **associated with an increased risk of obesity later in life:** Michaelsen, Kim F., and Frank R.Greer. 2014. "Protein Needs Early in Life and Long-Term Health." *American Journal of Clinical Nutrition* 99 (3): 718S-722S. https://doi.org/10.3945/ajcn.113.072603.

20. Michaelsen, K. F., A. Larnkjær, and C. Mølgaard. 2012. "Amount and Quality of Dietary Proteins During the First Two Years of Life in Relation to NCD Risk in Adulthood." *Nutrition, Metabolism and Cardiovascular Diseases* 22 (10): 781-786. https://doi.org/10.1016/j.numecd.2012.03.014.

21. **cow's milk is actually a major cause of iron deficiency in toddlers:** Domellöf, Magnus, et al. 2014. "Iron Requirements of Infants and Toddlers." *Journal of Pediatric Gastroenterology and Nutrition* 58 (1): 119-129. https://doi.org/10.1097/mpg.0000000000000206.

22. **linked to an increased risk of type 2 diabetes, heart disease, and some cancers:** Hooda, Jagmohan, Ajit Shah, and Li Zhang. 2014. "Heme, an Essential Nutrient from Dietary Proteins, Critically Impacts Diverse Physiological and Pathological Processes." *Nutrients* 6 (3): 1080-1102. https://doi.org/10.3390/nu6031080.

23. **associated with an increased risk of early menstruation, which has been linked to breast cancer:** Ramezani Tehrani, Fahimeh, Nazanin Moslehi, Golaleh Asghari, Roya Gholami, Parvin Mirmiran, and Fereidoun Azizi. 2013. "Intake of Dairy Products, Calcium, Magnesium, and Phosphorus in Childhood and Age at Menarche in the Tehran Lipid and Glucose Study." *Plos ONE* 8 (2): e57696. https://doi.org/10.1371/journal.pone.0057696.

24. **more than double the risk of early menstruation:** Ramezani Tehrani, Fahimeh, Nazanin Moslehi, Golaleh Asghari, Roya Gholami, Parvin Mirmiran, and Fereidoun Azizi. 2013. "Intake of Dairy Products, Calcium, Magnesium, and Phosphorus in Childhood and Age at Menarche in the Tehran Lipid and Glucose Study." *Plos ONE* 8 (2): e57696. https://doi.org/10.1371/journal.pone.0057696.

25. **had a 14% and 75% increased risk:** Rogers, Imogen S., Kate Northstone, David B. Dunger, Ashley R. Cooper, Andy

R. Ness, and Pauline M. Emmett. 2010. "Diet throughout Childhood and Age at Menarche in a Contemporary Co-hort of British Girls." *Public Health Nutrition* 13 (12): 2052-2063. https://doi.org/10.1017/s1368980010001461.

26. **have been shown to have a more favorable microbial composition:** De Filippo, Carlotta, Duccio Cavalieri, Monica Di Paola, Matteo Ramazzotti, Jean Baptiste Poullet, Sebastien Massart, Silvia Collini, Guiseppe Pieraccini, and Paolo Lionetti. 2010. "Impact of Diet in Shaping Gut Microbiota Revealed by a Comparative Study in Children from Europe and Rural Africa." *Proceedings of the National Academy of Sciences* 107 (33): 14691-14696. https://doi.org/10.1073/pnas.1005963107.

27. **more likely to have a higher proportion of Bacteroides and Bifidobacterium:** Jang, Han Byul, Min-Kyu Choi, Jae Heon Kang, Sang Ick Park, and Hye-Ja Lee. 2017. "Association of Dietary Patterns with the Fecal Microbiota in Korean Adolescents." *BMC Nutrition* 3 (1). https://doi.org/10.1186/s40795-016-0125-z.

28. **some of their B12 needs from bacteria found naturally in soil:** Robbins, William J., Annette Hervey, and Mary E. Stebbins. 1950. "Studies on Euglena and Vitamin B12." *Bulletin of the Torrey Botanical Club* 77, no. 6: 423-441. Accessed March 17, 2020. https://doi.org/10.2307/2482180.

29. **about 20% of older adults in the US:** Langan, Robert C., and Andrew J. Goodbred. 2017. "Vitamin B12 Deficiency: Recognition and Management." *American Family Physician* 96 (6): 384-389. https://www.aafp.org/afp/2017/0915/p384.html.

30. **have a lower risk of B12 deficiency compared to those who eat a lot of meat:** Tucker, Katherine L., Sharron Rich, Irwin Rosenberg, Paul Jacques, Gerard Dallal, Peter W.F.Wilson, and Jacob Selhub. 2000. "Plasma Vitamin B-12 Concentrations Relate to Intake Source in the Framingham Offspring Study." *American Journal of Clinical Nutrition* 71, no. 2 (January): 514-522. https://doi.org/10.1093/ajcn/71.2.514.

31. **show major health benefits over a traditional omnivorous diet:** Orlich, Michael J., Pramil N.Singh, Joan Sabaté, Karen Jaceldo-Siegl, Jing Fan, Synnove Knutsen, W. Lawrence Beeson, and Gary E. Fraser. 2013. "Vegetarian Dietary Patterns and Mortality in Adventist Health Study 2." *JAMA Internal Medicine* 173 (13): 1230. https://doi.org/10.1001/jamainternmed.2013.6473.

32. **save about 8 million lives, reduce food-related greenhouse gas emissions by about two-thirds, and save approximately $1.5 trillion:** Springmann, Marco, H. Charles J. Godfray, Mike Rayner, and Peter Scarborough. 2016. "Analysis and Valuation of the Health and Climate Change Cobenefits of Dietary Change." *Proceedings of the National Academy of Sciences* 113 (15): 4146-4151. https://doi.org/10.1073/pnas.1523119113.

Chapter 1

1. **recommends iron supplementation for all exclusively breastfed babies:** Baker, Robert D., Frank R. Greer, and the Committee on Nutrition. 2010. "Diagnosis and Prevention of Iron Deficiency and Iron-Deficiency Anemia in Infants and Young Children (0-3 Years of Age)." *Pediatrics* 126 (5): 1040-1050. https://doi.org/10.1542/peds.2010-2576.

2. **only 3.7% of the iron found in an egg yolk gets absorbed:** Callender, Sheila T., S. R. Marney, and G. T. Warner. 1970. "Eggs and Iron Absorption." *British Journal of Haematology* 19 (6): 657-666. https://doi.org/10.1111/j.1365-2141.1970.tb07010.x.

3. **can decrease the absorption of other iron-rich foods:** Samaraweera, Himali, Wan-Gang Zhang, Eun Joo Lee, and Dong U. Ahn. 2011. "Egg Yolk Phosvitin and Functional Phosphopeptides-Review." *Journal of Food Science* 76 (7): R143-R150. https://doi.org/10.1111/j.1750-3841.2011.02291.x.

4. **those who are restricted end up eating more:** Savage, Jennifer S., Jennifer Orlet Fisher, and Leann L. Birch. 2007. "Parental Influence on Eating Behavior: Conception to Adolescence." *The Journal of Law, Medicine & Ethics* 35 (1): 22-34. https://doi.org/10.1111/j.1748-720x.2007.00111.x.

5. **higher than that of any other species due to the enormous nutritional demand:** Andreas, Nicholas J., Beate Kampmann, and Kirsty M. Le-Doare. 2015. "Human Breast Milk: A Review on Its Composition and Bioactivity." *Early Human Development* 91 (11): 629-635. https://doi.org/10.1016/j.earlhumdev.2015.08.013.

6. **requirements for plant-based dieters and omnivores are the same:** "Protein and Amino Acids." 2005. In *Dietary Reference Intakes for Energy, Carbohydrate, Fiber, Fat, Fatty Acids, Cholesterol, Protein, and Amino Acids*, 589-768. Washington, DC: National Academies Press. https://www.nap.edu/read/10490/chapter/12.

7. **slightly increased due to lower digestibility:** Messina, Virginia, and Ann Reed Mangels. 2001. "Considerations in Planning Vegan Diets: Children." *Journal of the American Dietetic Association* 101, no. 6: 661–669. https://doi .org/10.1016/s0002-8223(01)00167-5.

8. **children typically eat way more protein than they need:** Weder, Stine, Morwenna Hoffmann, Katja Becker, Ute Alexy, and Markus Keller. 2019. "Energy, Macronutrient Intake, and Anthropometrics of Vegetarian, Vegan, and Omnivorous Children (1–3 Years) in Germany (VeChi Diet Study)." *Nutrients* 11, no. 4 (December): 832. https://doi .org/10.3390/nu11040832.

9. **contain all nine of the essential amino acids:** "Protein and Amino Acids." 2005. In *Dietary Reference Intakes for Energy, Carbohydrate, Fiber, Fat, Fatty Acids, Cholesterol, Protein, and Amino Acids*, 589–768. Washington, DC: National Academies Press. https://www.nap.edu/read/10490/chapter/12.

10. **combine proteins to meet your child's needs:** Young, V. R., and P. L. Pellett. 1994. "Plant Proteins in Relation to Human Protein and Amino Acid Nutrition." *American Journal of Clinical Nutrition* 59 (5): 1203S–1212S. https:// doi.org/10.1093/ajcn/59.5.1203s.

11. **plays a major role in neurological, physical, and behavioral functioning:** Weiser, Michael J., Christopher M. Butt, and M. Hasan Mohajeri. 2016. "Docosahexaenoic Acid and Cognition throughout the Lifespan." *Nutrients* 8 (2): 99. https://doi.org/10.3390/nu8020099.

12. **can be traced back to when man first migrated toward the water:** Bradbury, Joanne. 2011. "Docosahexaenoic Acid (DHA): An Ancient Nutrient for the Modern Human Brain." *Nutrients* 3 (5): 529–554. https://doi.org/10.3390 /nu3050529.

13. **increase birth weight and reduce preterm birth:** Salvig, Jannie Dalby, and Ronald F. Lamont. 2011. "Evidence Regarding an Effect of Marine n-3 Fatty Acids on Preterm Birth: A Systematic Review and Meta-Analysis." *Acta Obstetricia Et Gynecologica Scandinavica* 90 (8): 825–838. https://doi.org/10.1111/j.1600-0412.2011.01171.x.

14. **supplementation in preterm infants has been shown to reduce the risk of mental delays:** Weiser, Michael J., Christopher M. Butt, and M. Hasan Mohajeri. 2016. "Docosahexaenoic Acid and Cognition throughout the Life- span." *Nutrients* 8 (2): 99. https://doi.org/10.3390/nu8020099.

15. **High levels of DHA in breast milk have been associated with:** Weiser, Michael J., Christopher M. Butt, and M. Hasan Mohajeri. 2016. "Docosahexaenoic Acid and Cognition throughout the Lifespan." *Nutrients* 8 (2): 99. https://doi.org/10.3390/nu8020099.

16. **have been reported in children with developmental and behavioral disorders:** Kuratko, Connye N., Erin Cernkovich Barrett, Edward B. Nelson, and Norman Salem. 2013. "The Relationship of Docosahexaenoic Acid (DHA) with Learning and Behavior in Healthy Children: A Review." *Nutrients* 5 (7): 2777–2810. https://doi .org/10.3390/nu5072777.

17. **ALA to DHA is very low—about 1%–10%:** "Essential Fatty Acids." 2019. Linus Pauling Institute. Last modified June 2019. https://lpi.oregonstate.edu/mic/other-nutrients/essential-fatty-acids.

18. **eating ALA does not increase the amount of DHA found in blood or breast milk:** *Fats and Fatty Acids in Human Nutrition: Report of an Expert Consultation.* 2010. Rome: Food and Agriculture Organization of the United Nations. https://www.who.int/nutrition/publications/nutrientrequirements/fatsandfattyacids_humannutri tion/en/.

19. **has the lowest amount of DHA:** *Fats and Fatty Acids in Human Nutrition: Report of an Expert Consultation.* 2010. Rome: Food and Agriculture Organization of the United Nations. https://www.who.int/nutrition/publications /nutrientrequirements/fatsandfattyacids_humannutrition/en/.

20. **just as effective at raising blood levels of DHA:** Arterburn, Linda M., Harry A. Oken, James P. Hoffman, Eileen Bailey-Hall, Gloria Chung, Dror Rom, Jacqueline Hamersley, and Deanna Mccarthy. 2007. "Bioequivalence of Docosahexaenoic Acid from Different Algal Oils in Capsules and in a DHA-Fortified Food." *Lipids* 42 (11): 1011–1024. https://doi.org/10.1007/s11745-007-3098-5.

21. **minimize baby's exposure to toxins found in seafood:** "Contaminants in Fish." n.d. Washington State Depart- ment of Health. Accessed February 7, 2020. https://www.doh.wa.gov/CommunityandEnvironment/Food/Fish /ContaminantsinFish.

22. **ramps up in the third trimester of pregnancy and continues:** Weiser, Michael J., Christopher M. Butt, and

M. Hasan Mohajeri. 2016. "Docosahexaenoic Acid and Cognition throughout the Lifespan." Nutrients 8 (2): 99. https://doi.org/10.3390/nu8020099.

23. **supplement with 200-300 mg of DHA per day:** Eidelman, Arthur I., and Richard J. Schanler. 2012. "Breastfeeding and the Use of Human Milk." Pediatrics 129 (3): e827–e841. https://doi.org/10.1542/peds.2011-3552.

24. **receive 15-20 mg/kg per day of EPA and DHA combined from fish:** "Global Recommendations for EPA and DHA Intake." 2015. The Global Organization for EPA & DHA Omega-3s. Last modified March 2015. https://www.iffo.net/cn/system/files/A%206%20Summary%20GOED%20For%20IADSA%20only%20english.pdf.

25. **raise levels of so-called bad cholesterol:** Sacks, Frank M., et al. 2017. "Dietary Fats and Cardiovascular Disease: A Presidential Advisory from the American Heart Association." Circulation 136, no. 3 (July 18): e1–e23. https://doi.org/10.1161/cir.0000000000000510.

26. **may be healthier than longer-chain fatty acids:** Praagman, Jaike, et al. 2019. "Consumption of Individual Saturated Fatty Acids and the Risk of Myocardial Infarction in a UK and a Danish Cohort." *International Journal of Cardiology* 279: 18–26. https://doi.org/10.1016/j.ijcard.2018.10.064.

27. **50% of the fatty acids found in breast milk:** German, J. Bruce, and Cora J. Dillard. 2010. "Saturated Fats: A Perspective from Lactation and Milk Composition." *Lipids* 45 (10): 915–923. https://doi.org/10.1007/s11745-010-3445-9.

28. **typically consume more iron:** Śliwińska, Aleksandra, Justyna Luty, Ewa Aleksandrowicz-Wrona, and Sylwia Małgorzewicz. 2018. "Iron Status and Dietary Iron Intake in Vegetarians." *Advances in Clinical and Experimental Medicine* 27, no. 10: 1383–1389. https://doi.org/10.17219/acem/70527.

29. **increase the absorption of iron by 2-4 times:** Hallberg, Leif, Mats Brune, and Lena Rossander. 1989. "The Role of Vitamin C in Iron Absorption." *International Journal for Vitamin and Nutrition Research* 30: 103–108. https://www.ncbi.nlm.nih.gov/pubmed/2507689.

30. **poor source due to its extremely low bioavailability:** Bonsmann, S. Storcksdieck genannt, et al. 2007. "Oxalic Acid Does Not Influence Nonhaem Iron Absorption in Humans: A Comparison of Kale and Spinach Meals." *European Journal of Clinical Nutrition*, 62 (3): 336–341. https://doi.org/10.1038/sj.ejcn.1602721.

31. **necessary for normal taste processing:** Yagi, Takakazu, Akihiro Asakawa, Hirotaka Ueda, Satoshi Ikeda, Shouichi Miyawaki, and Akio Inui. 2013. "The Role of Zinc in the Treatment of Taste Disorders." *Recent Patents on Food, Nutrition & Agriculture* 5 (1): 44–51. https://doi.org/10.2174/2212798411305010007.

32. **needs increase around six months of age:** "Zinc." 2001. In *DRI: Dietary Reference Intakes for Vitamin A, Vitamin K, Arsenic, Boron, Chromium, Copper, Iodine, Iron, Manganese, Molybdenum, Nickel, Silicon, Vanadium, and Zinc*, 442–501. Washington, DC: National Academies Press. https://www.ncbi.nlm.nih.gov/books/NBK222317/#ddd00620.

33. **need about 50% more zinc:** "Zinc." 2001. In *DRI: Dietary Reference Intakes for Vitamin A, Vitamin K, Arsenic, Boron, Chromium, Copper, Iodine, Iron, Manganese, Molybdenum, Nickel, Silicon, Vanadium, and Zinc*, 442–501. Washington, DC: National Academies Press. https://www.ncbi.nlm.nih.gov/books/NBK222317/#ddd00620.

34. **higher rate during the first year than at any other time:** "Overview of Calcium." 2011. In *Dietary Reference Intakes for Calcium and Vitamin D*, 35–74. Washington, DC: National Academies Press. https://www.nap.edu/read/13050/chapter/4.

35. **twice as bioavailable from plants as from dairy:** "Calcium." 2017. Linus Pauling Institute. Last modified September 2017. https://lpi.oregonstate.edu/mic/minerals/calcium#food-sources.

36. **most prevalent and preventable cause of mental impairment:** "Micronutrient Deficiencies." 2013. World Health Organization. October 8. https://www.who.int/nutrition/topics/idd/en/.

37. **lower than average IQ and negative performance:** Zimmermann, Michael B. 2009. "Iodine Deficiency." *Endocrine Reviews* 30 (4): 376–408. https://doi.org/10.1210/er.2009-0011.

38. **iodine-based chemicals (iodophors) are used to disinfect cows' udders:** Van der Reijden, Olivia L., et al. 2018. "The Main Determinants of Iodine in Cows' Milk in Switzerland Are Farm Type, Season and Teat Dipping." *British Journal of Nutrition* 119 (5): 559–569. https://doi.org/10.1017/s0007114517003798.

39. **just as harmful as too little iodine and cause goiter:** Zimmermann, Michael B. 2009. "Iodine Deficiency." *Endocrine Reviews* 30 (4): 376–408. https://doi.org/10.1210/er.2009-0011.

40. **lower in iodine while kombu is significantly higher:** Yeh, Tai Sheng, Nu Hui Hung, and Tzu Chun Lin. 2014. "Analysis of Iodine Content in Seaweed by GC-ECD and Estimation of Iodine Intake." *Journal of Food and Drug Analysis* 22 (2): 189–196. https://doi.org/10.1016/j.jfda.2014.01.014.

41. **interfere with the body's production of thyroid hormones:** "Summary." 2001. In *DRI: Dietary Reference Intakes for Vitamin A, Vitamin K, Arsenic, Boron, Chromium, Copper, Iodine, Iron, Manganese, Molybdenum, Nickel, Silicon, Vanadium, and Zinc,* 1–28. Washington, DC: National Academies Press. https://www.nap.edu/read/10026/chapter/2.

42. **lower intakes of selenium compared to omnivores:** Kristensen, Nadja B., et al. 2015. "Intake of Macro- and Micronutrients in Danish Vegans." *Nutrition Journal* 14 (115). https://doi.org/10.1186/s12937-015-0103-3.

43. Sobiecki, Jakub G., Paul N. Appleby, Kathryn E. Bradbury, and Timothy J. Key. 2016. "High Compliance with Dietary Recommendations in a Cohort of Meat Eaters, Fish Eaters, Vegetarians, and Vegans: Results from the European Prospective Investigation into Cancer and Nutrition–Oxford Study." *Nutrition Research* 36 (5): 464–477. https://doi.org/10.1016/j.nutres.2015.12.016.

44. Elorinne, Anna-Liisa, Georg Alfthan, Iris Erlund, Hanna Kivimäki, Annukka Paju, Irma Salminen, Ursula Turpeinen, Sari Voutilainen, and Juha Laakso. 2016. "Food and Nutrient Intake and Nutritional Status of Finnish Vegans and Non-Vegetarians." *Plos One* 11 (2): e0148235. https://doi.org/10.1371/journal.pone.0148235.

45. **selenium intake may be a concern:** World Health Organization and Food and Agricultural Organization of the United Nations. 2004. *Vitamin and Mineral Requirements in Human Nutrition,* 2nd ed. https://apps.who.int/iris/bitstream/handle/10665/42716/9241546123.pdf?sequence=1.

46. **meet the recommendations for selenium intake:** Ganapathy, Seetha N., and Rita Dhanda. 1980. "Selenium Content of Omnivorous and Vegetarian Diets." *Indian Journal of Nutrition and Dietetics* 17 (2): 53–59. http://www.informaticsjournals.com/index.php/ijnd/article/view/12636.

47. **may result in psychomotor and cognitive delays:** Dror, D. K., and L. H. Allen. 2008. "Effect of Vitamin B12 Deficiency on Neurodevelopment in Infants: Current Knowledge and Possible Mechanisms." *Nutrition Reviews* 66 (5): 250–255. https://doi.org/10.1111/j.1753-4887.2008.00031.x.

48. **reported brain shrinkage in infants:** Goraya, Jatinder Singh, Sukhjot Kaur, and Bharat Mehra. 2015. "Neurology of Nutritional Vitamin B12 Deficiency in Infants: Case Series from India and Literature Review." *Journal of Child Neurology* 30 (13): 1831–1837. https://doi.org/10.1177/0883073815583688.

49. **in about 40%–50% of cases, damage was irreversible:** Dror, D. K., and L. H. Allen. 2008. "Effect of Vitamin B12 Deficiency on Neurodevelopment in Infants: Current Knowledge and Possible Mechanisms." *Nutrition Reviews* 66 (5): 250–255. https://doi.org/10.1111/j.1753-4887.2008.00031.x.

50. **still at a high risk of deficiency:** Herrmann, Wolfgang, Heike Schorr, Rima Obeid, and Jürgen Geisel. 2003. "Vitamin B-12 Status, Particularly Holotranscobalamin II and Methylmalonic Acid Concentrations, and Hyperhomocysteinemia in Vegetarians." *American Journal of Clinical Nutrition* 78 (1): 131–136. https://doi.org/10.1093/ajcn/78.1.131.

51. **about 1.5–2 mcg of B12 at a time:** Chanarin, I. 1971. "Absorption of Cobalamins." *Journal of Clinical Pathology* 5: 60–65. https://doi.org/10.1136/jcp.s3-5.1.60.

52. **at least 5 mcg per day:** Baroni, Luciana, et al. 2018. "Vegan Nutrition for Mothers and Children: Practical Tools for Healthcare Providers." *Nutrients* 11, no. (1): 5. https://doi.org/10.3390/nu11010005.

53. **two daily doses of 1 mcg each, which would be absorbed at a higher rate:** Norris, Jack. n.d. "Daily Needs." *Vegan Health.* https://veganhealth.org/daily-needs/#Vitamin-B12.

54. Baroni, Luciana, et al. 2018. "Vegan Nutrition for Mothers and Children: Practical Tools for Healthcare Providers." *Nutrients* 11 (1): 5. https://doi.org/10.3390/nu11010005.

55. **no strong evidence to suggest one form is better:** Obeid, Rima, Sergey N. Fedosov, and Ebba Nexo. 2015. "Cobalamin Coenzyme Forms Are Not Likely to Be Superior to Cyano- and Hydroxyl-Cobalamin in Prevention or Treatment of Cobalamin Deficiency." *Molecular Nutrition & Food Research* 59 (7): 1364–1372. https://doi.org/10.1002/mnfr.201500019.

56. **need to get vitamin D from the diet:** "Overview of Vitamin D." 2011. In *Dietary Reference Intakes for Calcium and Vitamin D,* 75–124. Washington, DC: National Academies Press. https://www.ncbi.nlm.nih.gov/books/NBK56061/.

57. **Breast milk is low in vitamin D:** "Vitamin D." 2019. Drugs and Lactation Database (LactMed) [Internet]. U.S. National Library of Medicine, April 1. https://www.ncbi.nlm.nih.gov/books/NBK500914/.

58. **D3 is more effective at raising blood levels:** Tripkovic, Laura, et al. 2012. "Comparison of Vitamin D2 and Vitamin D3 Supplementation in Raising Serum 25-Hydroxyvitamin D Status: A Systematic Review and Meta-Analysis." *American Journal of Clinical Nutrition* 95 (6): 1357-1364. https://doi.org/10.4016/48110.01.

59. **may cause blindness or thyroid dysfunction:** Zimmermann, Michael B., Wegmüller Rita, Christophe Zeder, Nourredine Chaouki, and Toni Torresani. 2004. "The Effects of Vitamin A Deficiency and Vitamin A Supplementation on Thyroid Function in Goitrous Children." *The Journal of Clinical Endocrinology & Metabolism* 89 (11): 5441-5447. https://doi.org/10.1210/jc.2004-0862.

60. **risk of respiratory infections and diarrhea:** Field, Catherine J., Ian R. Johnson, and Patricia D. Schley. 2002. "Nutrients and Their Role in Host Resistance to Infection." *Journal of Leukocyte Biology* 71 (1): 16-32. https://doi.org/10.1189/jlb.71.1.16.

61. **bodies convert provitamins to the active form:** "Vitamin A." 2001. In *DRI: Dietary Reference Intakes for Vitamin A, Vitamin K, Arsenic, Boron, Chromium, Copper, Iodine, Iron, Manganese, Molybdenum, Nickel, Silicon, Vanadium, and Zinc,* 82-161. Washington, DC: National Academies Press. https://www.nap.edu/read/10026/chapter/6.

62. **significantly lower than that of breast milk:** "Vitamin A." 2001. In *DRI: Dietary Reference Intakes for Vitamin A, Vitamin K, Arsenic, Boron, Chromium, Copper, Iodine, Iron, Manganese, Molybdenum, Nickel, Silicon, Vanadium, and Zinc,* 82-161. Washington, DC: National Academies Press. https://www.nap.edu/read/10026/chapter/6.

63. **no biological need for vitamin A from animal products:** "Vitamin A." 2001. In *DRI: Dietary Reference Intakes for Vitamin A, Vitamin K, Arsenic, Boron, Chromium, Copper, Iodine, Iron, Manganese, Molybdenum, Nickel, Silicon, Vanadium, and Zinc,* 82-161. Washington, D.C.: National Academies Press. https://www.nap.edu/read/10026/chapter/6.

64. **body ensures that mom's milk contains adequate amounts:** Newman, Vicky. 1994. "Vitamin A and Breast-Feeding: A Comparison of Data from Developed and Developing Countries." *Food and Nutrition Bulletin* 15 (2): 1-16. https://doi.org/10.1177/156482659401500201.

65. **more easily converted to the active form:** "Vitamin A." 2001. In *DRI: Dietary Reference Intakes for Vitamin A, Vitamin K, Arsenic, Boron, Chromium, Copper, Iodine, Iron, Manganese, Molybdenum, Nickel, Silicon, Vanadium, and Zinc,* 82-161. Washington, DC: National Academies Press. https://www.nap.edu/read/10026/chapter/6.

66. **creates a molecule known as TMAO that has been associated with heart disease:** Janeiro, Manuel, María Ramírez, Fermin Milagro, J. Martínez, and Maite Solas. 2018. "Implication of Trimethylamine N-Oxide (TMAO) in Disease: Potential Biomarker or New Therapeutic Target?" *Nutrients* 10 (10): 1398. https://doi.org/10.3390/nu10101398.

67. **Mangels, Simply Vegan:** https://www.vrg.org/nutrition/protein.php

68. Wasserman, Debra, and Reed Mangels. *Simply Vegan: Quick Vegetarian Meals.* 5th ed. Baltimore, MD: Vegetarian Resource Group, 2013.

69. **may help protect against neurocognitive and developmental disorders:** Boeke, Caroline E., Matthew W. Gillman, Michael D. Hughes, Sheryl L. Rifas-Shiman, Eduardo Villamor, and Emily Oken. 2013. "Choline Intake During Pregnancy and Child Cognition at Age 7 Years." *American Journal of Epidemiology* 177 (12): 1338-1347. https://doi.org/10.1093/aje/kws395.

70. **had better scores on memory tests at 7:** Boeke, Caroline E., Matthew W. Gillman, Michael D. Hughes, Sheryl L. Rifas-Shiman, Eduardo Villamor, and Emily Oken. 2013. "Choline Intake During Pregnancy and Child Cognition at Age 7 Years." *American Journal of Epidemiology* 177 (12): 1338-1347. https://doi.org/10.1093/aje/kws395.

71. **some showing benefits from supplementation and others showing no benefit:** Cheatham, Carol L., Barbara Davis Goldman, Leslie M. Fischer, Kerry-Ann Da Costa, J. Steven Reznick, and Steven H. Zeisel. 2012. "Phosphatidylcholine Supplementation in Pregnant Women Consuming Moderate-Choline Diets Does Not Enhance Infant Cognitive Function: A Randomized, Double-Blind, Placebo-Controlled Trial." *American Journal of Clinical Nutrition* 96 (6): 1465-1472. https://doi.org/10.3945/ajcn.112.037184. See also Caudill, Marie A., Barbara J. Strupp, Laura Muscalu, Julie E. H. Nevins, and Richard L. Canfield. 2018. "Maternal Choline Supplementation during the Third Trimester of Pregnancy Improves Infant Information Processing Speed: A Randomized, Double-Blind,

Controlled Feeding Study." *FASEB Journal* 32, no. 4 (May): 2172–2180. https://doi.org/10.1096/fj.20170 0692rr.

72. **"a variety of diets can satisfy the need for this nutrient":** Blusztajn, Jan K., Barbara E. Slack, and Tiffany J. Mellott. 2017. "Neuroprotective Actions of Dietary Choline." *Nutrients* 9 (8): 815. https://doi.org/10.3390/nu9080815.

73. **Sample Choline-Rich Menu for 1-to-2-Year-Old:** Patterson, Kristine Y., Seema A. Bhagwat, Juhi R. Williams, Juliette C. Howe, Joanne M. Holden, Steven H. Zeisel, Kerry A. Dacosta, and Mei-Heng Mar. 2008. "USDA Database for the Choline Content of Common Foods Release Two." U.S. Department of Agriculture. https://www.ars.usda .gov/ARSUserFiles/80400525/Data/Choline/Choln02.pdf.

Chapter 2

1. **some may even possess health benefits:** Silva, Elisângela O., and Ana Paula F. R. L. Bracarense. 2016. "Phytic Acid: From Antinutritional to Multiple Protection Factor of Organic Systems." *Journal of Food Science* 81, no. 6 (March). https://doi.org/10.1111/1750-3841.13320.

2. **about 30% and increase the availability of iron and zinc:** Luo, Yuwei, and Weihua Xie. 2014. "Effect of Soaking and Sprouting on Iron and Zinc Availability in Green and White Faba Bean (*Vicia faba* L.)." *Journal of Food Science and Technology* 51, no. 12 (December): 3970–3979. https://doi.org/https://dx.doi.org/10.1007/s13197-012-0921-7.

3. **leach endocrine-disrupting chemicals into food:** Braun, Joe M., and Russ Hauser. 2011. "Bisphenol A and Children's Health." *Current Opinion in Pediatrics* 23 (2): 233–239. https://doi.org/10.1097/mop.0b013e3283445675.

4. **may contain compounds that are structurally similar to BPA:** Horan, Tegan S., Hannah Pulcastro, Crystal Lawson, Roy Gerona, Spencer Martin, Mary C. Gieske, Caroline V. Sartain, and Patricia A. Hunt. 2018. "Replacement Bisphenols Adversely Affect Mouse Gametogenesis with Consequences for Subsequent Generations." *Current Biology* 28 (18): 2948–2954. https://doi.org/10.1016/j.cub.2018.06.070.

5. **higher in phytochemicals and lower in heavy metals:** Barański, Marcin, et al. 2014. "Higher Antioxidant and Lower Cadmium Concentrations and Lower Incidence of Pesticide Residues in Organically Grown Crops: A Systematic Literature Review and Meta-Analyses." *British Journal of Nutrition* 112 (5): 794–811. https://doi.org /10.1017/s0007114514001366.

6. **pesticides on human health are still largely unknown:** Mostafalou, Sara, and Mohammad Abdollahi. 2016. "Pesticides: An Update of Human Exposure and Toxicity." *Archives of Toxicology* 91 (2): 549–599. https://doi .org/10.1007/s00204-016-1849-x.

7. **based on outdated science and that new risk assessments need to be made:** Myers, J. P., M. N. Antoniou, B. Blumberg, L. Carroll, T. Colborn, L. G. Everett, M. Hansen, P. J. Landrigan, B. P. Lanphear, R. Mesnage, L. N. Vandenberg, F. S. vom Saal, W. V. Welshons, and C. M. Benbrook. 2016. "Concerns over Use of Glyphosate-Based Herbicides and Risks Associated with Exposures: A Consensus Statement." *Environmental Health* 15: 19. https://doi .org/10.1186/s12940-016-0117-0.

8. **end up eating less produce overall:** Huang, Yancui, Indika Edirisinghe, and Britt M. Burton-Freeman. 2016. "Low-Income Shoppers and Fruit and Vegetables." *Nutrition Today* 51 (5): 242–250. https://doi.org/10.1097 /nt.0000000000000176.

9. **reduced risk of chronic disease:** Zhan, Jian, Yu-Jian Liu, Long-Biao Cai, Fang-Rong Xu, Tao Xie, and Qi-Qiang He. 2015. "Fruit and Vegetable Consumption and Risk of Cardiovascular Disease: A Meta-Analysis of Prospective Cohort Studies." *Critical Reviews in Food Science and Nutrition* 57 (8): 1650–1663. https://doi.org/10.1080/10408 398.2015.1008980.

10. **detectable levels of the herbicide glyphosate and 26 exceeded the acceptable upper level:** Temkin, Alexis. 2018. "Breakfast With a Dose of Roundup? Weed Killer in $289 Million Cancer Verdict Found in Oat Cereal and Granola Bars." EWG's Children's Health Initiative. Environmental Working Group. August 15. https://www.ewg .org/childrenshealth/glyphosateincereal/.

11. **majority of soy grown is genetically modified:** "Recent Trends in GE Adoption." 2019. United States Department of Agriculture Economic Research Service. United States Department of Agriculture. September 18. https:// www.ers.usda.gov/data-products/adoption-of-genetically-engineered-crops-in-the-us/recent-trends-in-ge -adoption.aspx.

12. **may contain higher pesticide residues:** Benbrook, Charles M. 2016. "Trends in Glyphosate Herbicide Use in the United States and Globally." *Environmental Sciences Europe* 28, no. 1 (February). https://doi.org/10.1186/s12302 -016-0070-0.

13. **pesticides can seep into plants:** Yang, Tianxi, Jeffery Doherty, Bin Zhao, Amanda J. Kinchla, John M. Clark, and Lili He. 2017. "Effectiveness of Commercial and Homemade Washing Agents in Removing Pesticide Residues on and in Apples." *Journal of Agricultural and Food Chemistry* 65 (44): 9744–9752. https://doi.org/10.1021/acs .jafc.7b03118.

14. **biologically programmed to prefer the taste of sweet food:** Ventura, Alison K., and John Worobey. 2013. "Early Influences on the Development of Food Preferences." *Current Biology* 23 (9): R401–R408. https://doi.org/10.1016/j .cub.2013.02.037.

16. **preference for these foods increases:** Liem, Djin Gie, and Cees de Graaf. 2004. "Sweet and Sour Preferences in Young Children and Adults: Role of Repeated Exposure." *Physiology & Behavior* 83 (3): 421–429. https://doi .org/10.1016/j.physbeh.2004.08.028.

17. **high blood pressure in adulthood and increase a child's risk of obesity:** Yang, Quanhe, et al. 2012. "Sodium Intake and Blood Pressure Among US Children and Adolescents." *Pediatrics* 130 (4): 611–619. https://doi .org/10.1542/peds.2011-3870.

18. **alter the body's metabolism of fat:** Ma, Yuan, Feng J. He, and Graham A. Macgregor. 2015. "High Salt Intake: Independent Risk Factor for Obesity?" *Hypertension* 66 (4): 843–849. https://doi.org/10.1161/hypertensio naha.115.05948.

19. **likely beneficial for chronic disease prevention:** Applegate, Catherine C., Joe L. Rowles, Katherine M. Ranard, Sookyoung Jeon, and John W. Erdman. 2018. "Soy Consumption and the Risk of Prostate Cancer: An Updated Systematic Review and Meta-Analysis." *Nutrients* 10 (1): 40. https://doi.org/10.3390/nu10010040.

20. Van Die, M. Diana, Kerry M. Bone, Scott G. Williams, and Marie V. Pirotta. 2014. "Soy and Soy Isoflavones in Prostate Cancer: A Systematic Review and Meta-Analysis of Randomized Controlled Trials." *BJU International* 113 (5b): E119–E130. https://doi.org/10.1111/bju.12435.

21. **Messina, Mark. 2016. "Soy and Health Update:** Evaluation of the Clinical and Epidemiologic Literature." *Nutrients* 8 (12): 754. https://doi.org/10.3390/nu8120754.

22. **consuming soy in early childhood:** Shu, Xiao Ou, Fan D. Jin, Qi H. Dai, Wanqing Wen, John D. Potter, Lawrence H. Kushi, Zhixian Ruan, Yu-Tang Gao, and Wei Zheng. 2001. "Soyfood Intake during Adolescence and Subsequent Risk of Breast Cancer among Chinese Women." *Cancer Epidemiology, Biomarkers, & Prevention* 10 (5): 483–488. https://cebp.aacrjournals.org/content/10/5/483.long.

23. **soy is safe for infants and children:** Testa, Ilaria, Cristina Salvatori, Giuseppe Di Cara, Arianna Latini, Franco Frati, Stefania Troiani, Nicola Principi, and Susanna Esposito. 2018. "Soy-Based Infant Formula: Are Phyto-Oestrogens Still in Doubt?" *Frontiers in Nutrition* 5: 110. https://doi.org/10.3389/fnut.2018.00110.

24. **no differences in endocrine or reproductive functioning:** Strom, Brian L. 2001. "Exposure to Soy-Based Formula in Infancy and Endocrinological and Reproductive Outcomes in Young Adulthood." *JAMA* 286 (7): 807–814. https://doi.org/10.1001/jama.286.7.807.

25. **take up and concentrate arsenic from soil more than other cereal:** "Arsenic." 2018. World Health Organization. February 15. https://www.who.int/news-room/fact-sheets/detail/arsenic.

26. **can cut the arsenic content in half:** Gray, Patrick J., Sean D. Conklin, Todor I. Todorov, and Sasha M. Kasko. 2016. "Cooking Rice in Excess Water Reduces Both Arsenic and Enriched Vitamins in the Cooked Grain." *Food Additives & Contaminants: Part A* 33 (1): 78–85. https://doi.org/10.1080/19440049.2015.1103906.

Chapter 3

1. **twice the activity level of an adult:** American Academy of Pediatrics. 2019. *Caring for Your Baby and Young Child: Birth to Age 5.* 7th ed. New York: Bantam Books.

2. **main source of persistent, bioaccumulative chemicals:** Wang, R. Y., and L. L. Needham. 2007. "Environmental Chemicals: From the Environment to Food, to Breast Milk, to the Infant." *Journal of Toxicology and Environmental Health, Part B* 10 (8): 597–609. https://doi.org/10.1080/10937400701389891.

3. **just 1%–2% of that reported in omnivorous women:** Hergenrather, J., G. Hlady, B. Wallace, and E. Savage. 1981. "Pollutants in Breast Milk of Vegetarians." *New England Journal of Medicine* 304 (13): 792. https://doi.org/10.1056/nejm198103263041321.

4. **showed fewer negative facial expressions:** Mennella, Julie A., Coren P. Jagnow, and Gary K. Beauchamp. 2001. "Prenatal and Postnatal Flavor Learning by Human Infants." *Pediatrics* 107 (6): e88. https://doi.org/10.1542/peds.107.6.e88.

5. **eats more fruits and vegetables:** Orlich, Michael J., Karen Jaceldo-Siegl, Joan Sabaté, Jing Fan, Pramil N. Singh, and Gary E. Fraser. 2014. "Patterns of Food Consumption among Vegetarians and Non-Vegetarians." *British Journal of Nutrition* 112 (10): 1644–1653. https://doi.org/10.1017/s000711451400261x.

6. **Average Intake (Table):** American Academy of Pediatrics. 2019. *Caring for Your Baby and Young Child: Birth to Age 5.* 7th ed. New York: Bantam Books.

7. **about 3 times each night:** Goodlin-Jones, Beth L., Melissa M. Burnham, Erika E. Gaylor, and Thomas F. Anders. 2001. "Night Waking, Sleep-Wake Organization, and Self-Soothing in the First Year of Life." *Journal of Developmental & Behavioral Pediatrics* 22 (4): 226–233. https://doi.org/10.1097/00004703-200108000-00003.

8. **do not need middle-of-the-night feeds:** American Academy of Pediatrics. 2019. *Caring for Your Baby and Young Child: Birth to Age 5.* 7th ed. New York: Bantam Books.

9. **scored 4 points lower on IQ tests at age 8:** Lacovou, Maria, and Almudena Sevilla. 2013. "Infant Feeding: The Effects of Scheduled vs. On-Demand Feeding on Mothers' Wellbeing and Children's Cognitive Development." *European Journal of Public Health* 23 (1): 13–19. https://doi.org/10.1093/eurpub/cks012.

10. **Average Weight Gain (Table):** AAP Committee on Nutrition. 2014. *Pediatric Nutrition.* Edited by Ronald E. Kleinman and Frank R. Greer. 7th ed. Elk Grove Village, IL: American Academy of Pediatrics.

11. **Adequate Output* (Table):** AAP Committee on Nutrition. 2014. *Pediatric Nutrition.* Edited by Ronald E. Kleinman and Frank R. Greer. 7th ed. Elk Grove Village, IL: American Academy of Pediatrics.

12. **higher during the first few months of life, then levels out:** Mosca, Fabio, and Maria Lorella Giannì. 2017. "Human Milk: Composition and Health Benefits." *La Pediatria Medica e Chirurgica* 39 (2): 155. https://doi.org/10.4081/pmc.2017.155.

13. **increasing toward the end of a feed:** Mosca, Fabio, and Maria Lorella Giannì. 2017. "Human Milk: Composition and Health Benefits." *La Pediatria Medica e Chirurgica* 39 (2): 155. https://doi.org/10.4081/pmc.2017.155.

14. **32% reduced risk of type 2 diabetes:** Chowdhury, Ranadip, Bireshwar Sinha, Mari Jeeva Sankar, Sunita Taneja, Nita Bhandari, Nigel Rollins, Rajiv Bahl, and Jose Martines. 2015. "Breastfeeding and Maternal Health Outcomes: A Systematic Review and Meta-Analysis." *Acta Paediatrica* 104 (467): 96–113. https://doi.org/10.1111/apa.13102.

15. **return to a healthy weight postpartum:** Baker, Jennifer L., Michael Gamborg, Berit L. Heitmann, Lauren Lissner, Thorkild I. Sørensen, and Kathleen M. Rasmussen. 2008. "Breastfeeding Reduces Postpartum Weight Retention." *American Journal of Clinical Nutrition* 88 (6): 1543–1551. https://doi.org/10.3945/ajcn.2008.26379.

16. **significantly reduced rates of ear, throat, and nasal infections:** Li, Ruowei, Deborah Dee, Chuan-Ming Li, Howard J. Hoffman, and Laurence M. Grummer-Strawn. 2014. "Breastfeeding and Risk of Infections at 6 Years." *Pediatrics* 134 (Suppl 1): S13–S20. https://doi.org/10.1542/peds.2014-0646d.

17. **higher levels of the hunger hormone ghrelin:** Savino, Francesco, Maria F. Fissore, Stefania A. Liguori, and Roberto Oggero. 2009. "Can Hormones Contained in Mothers' Milk Account for the Beneficial Effect of Breast-Feeding on Obesity in Children?" *Clinical Endocrinology* 71 (6): 757–765. https://doi.org/10.1111/j.1365-2265.2009.03585.x.

18. **greater food acceptance and more adventurous eating:** Ventura, Alison K. 2017. "Does Breastfeeding Shape Food Preferences? Links to Obesity." *Annals of Nutrition and Metabolism* 70 (Suppl 3): 8–15. https://doi.org/10.1159/000478757.

19. **better self-regulation of milk intake:** Li, Ruowei, Sara B. Fein, and Laurence M. Grummer-Strawn. 2010. "Do Infants Fed from Bottles Lack Self-Regulation of Milk Intake Compared with Directly Breastfed Infants?" *Pediatrics* 125 (6): e1386–e1393. https://doi.org/10.1542/peds.2009-2549.

20. **39% risk reduction compared to formula-fed infants and had lower levels of insulin:** Owen, Christopher G., Richard M. Martin, Peter H. Whincup, George Davey Smith, and Derek G. Cook. 2006. "Does Breastfeeding Influ-

ence Risk of Type 2 Diabetes in Later Life? A Quantitative Analysis of Published Evidence." *American Journal of Clinical Nutrition* 84 (5): 1043-1054. https://doi.org/10.1093/ajcn/84.5.1043.

21. **higher IQ scores in children:** Kramer, Michael S., et al. 2008. "Breastfeeding and Child Cognitive Development: New Evidence from a Large Randomized Trial." *Archives of General Psychiatry* 65 (5): 578-584. https://doi .org/10.1001/archpsyc.65.5.578.

22. **may reduce the risk of childhood cancers:** Kwan, Marilyn L., Patricia A. Buffler, Barbara Abrams, and Vincent A. Kiley. 2004. "Breastfeeding and the Risk of Childhood Leukemia: A Meta-Analysis." *Public Health Reports* 119 (6): 521-535. https://doi.org/10.1016/j.phr.2004.09.002.

23. Bener, Abdulbari F., G. I. Hoffmann, Z. Afify, Kakil Rasul, and I. Tewfik. 2008. "Does Prolonged Breastfeeding Reduce the Risk for Childhood Leukemia and Lymphomas?" *Minerva Pediatrica* 60 (2): 155-161. https://www .ncbi.nlm.nih.gov/pubmed/18449131.

24. **14% to 19% of childhood leukemia cases could be prevented:** Amitay, Efrat L., and Lital Keinan-Boker. 2015. "Breastfeeding and Childhood Leukemia Incidence: A Meta-Analysis and Systematic Review." *JAMA Pediatrics* 169 (6). https://doi.org/10.1001/jamapediatrics.2015.1025.

25. **more easily aroused from sleep:** Horne, R. S.C., P. M. Parslow, D. Ferens, A-M Watts, and T. M. Adamson. 2004. "Comparison of Evoked Arousability in Breast and Formula Fed Infants." *Archives of Disease in Childhood* 89 (1): 22-25. https://www.ncbi.nlm.nih.gov/pmc/articles/PMC1755888/2=tf_ipsecsha.

26. **essential compounds required for immunity:** Kinney, Hannah C., Betty Ann Brody, Dianne M. Finkelstein, Gordon F. Vawter, Frederick Mandell, and Floyd H. Gillies. 1991. "Delayed Central Nervous System Myelination in the Sudden Infant Death Syndrome." *Journal of Neuropathology & Experimental Neurology* 50 (1): 29-48. https:// doi.org/10.1097/00005072-199101000-00003.

27. *any* **breastfeeding cut SIDS risk in half:** Thompson, John M. D., Kawai Tanabe, Rachel Y. Moon, Edwin A. Mitchell, Cliona Mcgarvey, David Tappin, Peter S. Blair, and Fern R. Hauck. 2017. "Duration of Breastfeeding and Risk of SIDS: An Individual Participant Data Meta-Analysis." *Pediatrics* 140 (5). https://doi.org/10.1542/peds.2017-1324.

28. **factors that have been tied to SIDS risk or protection:** Thompson, John M. D., Kawai Tanabe, Rachel Y. Moon, Edwin A. Mitchell, Cliona Mcgarvey, David Tappin, Peter S. Blair, and Fern R. Hauck. 2017. "Duration of Breastfeeding and Risk of SIDS: An Individual Participant Data Meta-Analysis." *Pediatrics* 140 (5). https://doi .org/10.1542/peds.2017-1324.

29. **continued breastfeeding along with complementary foods:** "Breastfeeding." n.d. World Health Organization. https://www.who.int/health-topics/breastfeeding#tab=tab_1.

30. **Breastfeeding continues until age 6:** Piovanetti, Yvette. 2001. "Breastfeeding Beyond 12 Months: An Historical Perspective." *Pediatric Clinics of North America* 48 (1): 199-206. https://doi.org/10.1016/s0031-3955(05)70294-7.

31. **maintained in high concentrations throughout the second year:** Piovanetti, Yvette. 2001. "Breastfeeding Beyond 12 Months: An Historical Perspective." *Pediatric Clinics of North America* 48 (1): 199-206. https://doi .org/10.1016/s0031-3955(05)70294-7.

32. **won't be able to meet the high nutrient demands:** Institute of Medicine (US) Committee on Nutritional Status During Pregnancy and Lactation. 1991. "Meeting Maternal Nutrient Needs During Lactation." In *Nutrition During Lactation.* Washington, DC: National Academies Press. https://www.ncbi.nlm.nih.gov/books/NBK235579/.

33. **have higher amounts of these fatty acids:** Bravi, Francesca, Frank Wiens, Adriano Decarli, Alessia Dal Pont, Carlo Agostoni, and Monica Ferraroni. 2016. "Impact of Maternal Nutrition on Breast-Milk Composition: A Systematic Review." *American Journal of Clinical Nutrition* 104 (3): 646-662. https://doi.org/10.3945/ajcn.115.120881.

34. **more likely to have higher levels of saturated fat:** Mosca, Fabio, and Maria Lorella Giannì. 2017. "Human Milk: Composition and Health Benefits." *La Pediatria Medica e Chirurgica* 39 (2): 155. https://doi.org/10.4081/pmc .2017.155.

35. **infants born at < 33 weeks had increased visual acuity at 4 months:** Smithers, Lisa G., Robert A. Gibson, Andrew Mcphee, and Maria Makrides. 2008. "Higher Dose of Docosahexaenoic Acid in the Neonatal Period Improves Visual Acuity of Preterm Infants: Results of a Randomized Controlled Trial." *American Journal of Clinical Nutrition* 88 (4): 1049-1056. https://doi.org/10.1093/ajcn/88.4.1049.

36. **20% of vegan, vegetarian, and non-vegetarian women had inadequate levels:** Pawlak, Roman, Paul Vos, Setareh Shahab-Ferdows, Daniela Hampel, Lindsay H. Allen, and Maryanne Tigchelaar Perrin. 2018. "Vitamin B-12 Content in Breast Milk of Vegan, Vegetarian, and Nonvegetarian Lactating Women in the United States." *American Journal of Clinical Nutrition* 108 (3): 525–531. https://doi.org/10.1093/ajcn/nqy104.

37. **wide variations in the amount of choline in breast milk:** Ilcol, Yeşim Ozarda, Resul Ozbek, Emre Hamurtekin, and Ismail Ulus. 2005. "Choline Status in Newborns, Infants, Children, Breast-Feeding Women, Breast-Fed Infants and Human Breast Milk." *Journal of Nutritional Biochemistry* 16 (8): 489–499. https://doi.org/10.1016/j.jnutbio.2005.01.011.

38. **showed no significant difference:** Wiedeman, Alejandra M., et al. 2018. "Concentrations of Water-Soluble Forms of Choline in Human Milk from Lactating Women in Canada and Cambodia." *Nutrients* 10 (3): 381. https://doi.org/10.3390/nu10030381.

39. **only a 20% increase in breast milk choline:** Fischer, L. M., K. A. da Costa, J. Galanko, W. Sha, B. Stephenson, J. Vick, and S. H. Zeisel. 2010. "Choline Intake and Genetic Polymorphisms Influence Choline Metabolite Concentrations in Human Breast Milk and Plasma." *American Journal of Clinical Nutrition*, 92 (2): 336–346. https://doi.org/10.3945/ajcn.2010.29459.

40. **synthesis in the liver may be a larger contributor:** Ilcol, Yeşim Ozarda, Resul Ozbek, Emre Hamurtekin, and Ismail Ulus. 2005. "Choline Status in Newborns, Infants, Children, Breast-Feeding Women, Breast-Fed Infants and Human Breast Milk." *The Journal of Nutritional Biochemistry* 16 (8): 489–499. https://doi.org/10.1016/j.jnutbio.2005.01.011.

41. **benefits for treating and preventing clogged ducts:** "Lecithin." 2019. Drugs and Lactation Database (LactMed) [Internet]. U.S. National Library of Medicine, October 23. https://www.ncbi.nlm.nih.gov/books/NBK501772/.

42. **2.7 liters per day pre-pregnancy to 3.8 liters per day:** *Dietary Reference Intakes for Water, Potassium, Sodium, Chloride, and Sulfate.* 2005. Washington, DC: National Academies Press. https://www.nap.edu/read/10925/chapter/1.

43. **only 2%–6% of the maternal dose ends up in baby's bloodstream:** Haastrup, M. B., A. Pottegård, and P. Damkier. 2014. "Alcohol and Breastfeeding." *Basic & Clinical Pharmacology & Toxicology*, 114 (2): 168–173. https://doi.org/10.1111/bcpt.12149.

44. **only 2%–6% of the maternal dose ends up in baby's bloodstream:** Mennella, Julie. 2001. "Alcohol's Effect on Lactation." *Alcohol Research: Current Reviews* 25 (3): 230–234. https://www.ncbi.nlm.nih.gov/pmc/articles/PMC6707164/.

45. **expressed 9.3% less breast milk in the next 2 hours:** Mennella, Julie A. 1998. "Short-Term Effects of Maternal Alcohol Consumption on Lactational Performance." *Alcoholism: Clinical and Experimental Research* 22 (7): 1389–1392. https://doi.org/10.1111/j.1530-0277.1998.tb03924.x.

46. **given directly to preterm babies:** Abdel-Hady, Hesham, Nehad Nasef, Abd Elazeez Shabaan, and Islam Nour. 2015. "Caffeine Therapy in Preterm Infants." *World Journal of Clinical Pediatrics* 4 (4): 81–93. https://doi.org/10.5409/wjcp.v4.i4.81.

47. **no difference in an infant's heart rate:** Santos, Iná S., Alicia Matijasevich, and Marlos R. Domingues. 2012. "Maternal Caffeine Consumption and Infant Nighttime Waking: Prospective Cohort Study." *Pediatrics* 129 (5): 860–868. https://doi.org/10.1542/peds.2011-1773d.

48. **no difference in an infant's heart rate:** Ryu, Jacqueline E. 1985. "Effect of Maternal Caffeine Consumption on Heart Rate and Sleep Time of Breast-Fed Infants." *Developmental Pharmacology and Therapeutics* 8 (6): 355–363. https://doi.org/10.1159/000457060.

49. **5%–15% of women suffer:** Hurst, Nancy M. 2007. "Recognizing and Treating Delayed or Failed Lactogenesis II." *Journal of Midwifery & Women's Health* 52 (6): 588–594. https://doi.org/10.1016/j.jmwh.2007.05.005.

50. **Signs of Ineffective Breastfeeding (Table):** Hurst, Nancy M. 2007. "Recognizing and Treating Delayed or Failed Lactogenesis II." *Journal of Midwifery & Women's Health* 52 (6): 588–594. https://doi.org/10.1016/j.jmwh.2007.05.005.

51. **research on the benefits of supplements:** Bazzano, Alessandra N., Rebecca Hofer, Shelley Thibeau, Veronica

Gillispie, Marni Jacobs, and Katherine P. Theall. 2016. "A Review of Herbal and Pharmaceutical Galactagogues for Breast-Feeding." *Ochsner Journal* 16 (4): 511–524. https://www.ncbi.nlm.nih.gov/pmc/articles/PMC5158159/.

52. **fenugreek tea was shown to increase milk volume:** Turkyılmaz, Canan, Esra Onal, Ibrahim Murat Hirfanoglu, Ozden Turan, Esin Koç, Ebru Ergenekon, and Yıldız Atalay. 2011. "The Effect of Galactagogue Herbal Tea on Breast Milk Production and Short-Term Catch-Up of Birth Weight in the First Week of Life." *Journal of Alternative and Complementary Medicine* 17 (2): 139–142. https://doi.org/10.1089/acm.2010.0090.

53. **1000–1500 mg 3x/day:** Hurst, Nancy M. 2007. "Recognizing and Treating Delayed or Failed Lactogenesis II." *Journal of Midwifery & Women's Health* 52 (6): 588–594. https://doi.org/10.1016/j.jmwh.2007.05.005.

54. **linked to poor milk production:** Henly, Susan J., Cindy M. Anderson, Melissa D. Avery, Sharon G. Hills-Bonczyk, Susan Potter, and Laura J. Duckett. 1995. "Anemia and Insufficient Milk in First-Time Mothers." *Birth* 22 (2): 87–92. https://doi.org/10.1111/j.1523-536x.1995.tb00565.x.

55. **1200 mg of soy or sunflower lecithin up to 4 times a day:** "Lecithin." Drugs and Lactation Database (LactMed) [Internet]. U.S. National Library of Medicine, October 23, 2019. https://www.ncbi.nlm.nih.gov/books/NBK 501772/.

56. **10% of moms will suffer from mastitis:** Spencer, Jeanne P. 2008. "Management of Mastitis in Breastfeeding Women." *American Family Physician* 78 (6): 727–731. https://www.aafp.org/afp/2008/0915/p727.html.

57. **more improvement and a lower rate of recurrence:** Arroyo, Rebeca, Virginia Martín, Antonio Maldonado, Esther Jiménez, Leónides Fernández, and Juan Miguel Rodríguez. 2010. "Treatment of Infectious Mastitis during Lactation: Antibiotics versus Oral Administration of Lactobacilli Isolated from Breast Milk." *Clinical Infectious Diseases* 50 (12): 1551–1558. https://doi.org/10.1086/652763.

58. **between 0.4 and 0.5 grams of protein/ounce, which is about 50% more protein:** Kleinman, Ronald E. and Frank R. Greer, eds. 2014. American Academy of Pediatrics Committee on Nutrition. *Pediatric Nutrition*. 7th ed. Elk Grove Village, IL: American Academy of Pediatrics.

59. **contains 80% casein while breast milk is only 40%:** Rafiq, Saima, Nuzhat Huma, Imran Pasha, Aysha Sameen, Omer Mukhtar, and Muhammad Issa Khan. 2015. "Chemical Composition, Nitrogen Fractions and Amino Acids Profile of Milk from Different Animal Species." *Asian-Australasian Journal of Animal Sciences* 29, no. 7 (May): 1022–1028. https://doi.org/10.5713/ajas.15.0452.

60. **oils are better absorbed than the fat from cow's milk:** Kleinman, Robert E. and Frank R. Greer, eds. 2014. American Academy of Pediatrics Committee on Nutrition. *Pediatric Nutrition*. 7th ed. Elk Grove Village, IL: American Academy of Pediatrics.

61. **similar rates of growth, energy intake, and bone mineralization:** Bhatia, Jatinder, and Frank Greer. 2008. "Use of Soy Protein-Based Formulas in Infant Feeding." *Pediatrics* 121 (5): 1062–1068. https://doi.org/10.1542/peds .2008-0564.

62. **given to infants for centuries:** Bhatia, Jatinder, and Frank Greer. 2008. "Use of Soy Protein-Based Formulas in Infant Feeding." *Pediatrics* 121 (5): 1062–1068. https://doi.org/10.1542/peds.2008-0564.

63. **lowest rates of hormone-dependent cancers:** Adlercreutz, Herman, Teiichi Yamada, Kristiina Wähälä, and Shaw Watanabe. 1999. "Maternal and Neonatal Phytoestrogens in Japanese Women during Birth." *American Journal of Obstetrics and Gynecology* 180 (3): 737–743. https://doi.org/10.1016/s0002-9378(99)70281-4.

64. **no demonstrated increased risk of feminization:** Bhatia, Jatinder, and Frank Greer. 2008. "Use of Soy Protein-Based Formulas in Infant Feeding." *Pediatrics* 121 (5): 1062–1068. https://doi.org/10.1542/peds.2008-0564.

65. **no differences in endocrine and reproductive functioning:** Strom, Brian L., Rita Schinnar, Ekhard E. Ziegler, Kurt T. Barnhart, Mary D. Sammel, George A. Macones, Virginia A. Stallings, Jean M. Drulis, Steven E. Nelson, and Sandra A. Hanson. 2001. "Exposure to Soy-Based Formula in Infancy and Endocrinological and Reproductive Outcomes in Young Adulthood." *JAMA* 286 (7): 807–814. https://doi.org/10.1001/jama.286.7.807.

66. **longer duration of menstrual bleeding:** Strom, Brian L., Rita Schinnar, Ekhard E. Ziegler, Kurt T. Barnhart, Mary D. Sammel, George A. Macones, Virginia A. Stallings, Jean M. Drulis, Steven E. Nelson, and Sandra A. Hanson. 2001. "Exposure to Soy-Based Formula in Infancy and Endocrinological and Reproductive Outcomes in Young Adulthood." *JAMA* 286 (7): 807–814. https://doi.org/10.1001/jama.286.7.807.

67. **higher than cow's milk or breast milk:** Bhatia, Jatinder, and Frank Greer. 2008. "Use of Soy Protein-Based Formulas in Infant Feeding." *Pediatrics* 121 (5): 1062-1068. https://doi.org/10.1542/peds.2008-0564.

68. **falls below established safety limits:** Risk Assessment Studies Report No. 35. Chemical Hazard Evaluation: Aluminium in food (2009). https://www.cfs.gov.hk/english/programme/programme_rafs/files/RA35_Aluminium_in_Food_e.pdf.

69. Litov, Richard E., Virginia S. Sickles, Gary M. Chan, Mary A. Springer, and Angel Cordano. 1989. "Plasma Aluminum Measurements in Term Infants Fed Human Milk or a Soy-Based Infant Formula." *Pediatrics* 84 (6): 1105-1107. https://www.ncbi.nlm.nih.gov/pubmed/2587141.

70. **potential to reduce infections:** Andres, Aline, Sharon M. Donovan, Theresa B. Kuhlenschmidt, and Mark S. Kuhlenschmidt. 2007. "Isoflavones at Concentrations Present in Soy Infant Formula Inhibit Rotavirus Infection in Vitro." *Journal of Nutrition* 137 (9): 2068-2073. https://doi.org/10.1093/jn/137.9.2068.

71. **potential to reduce infections:** Donovan, Sharon M., Aline Andres, Rose Ann Mathai, Theresa B. Kuhlenschmidt, and Mark S. Kuhlenschmidt. 2009. "Soy Formula and Isoflavones and the Developing Intestine." *Nutrition Reviews* 67 (2): 192-200. https://doi.org/10.1111/j.1753-4887.2009.00240.x.

72. **reduce the viral activity by 66%-74%:** Andres, Aline, Sharon M. Donovan, Theresa B. Kuhlenschmidt, and Mark S. Kuhlenschmidt. 2007. "Isoflavones at Concentrations Present in Soy Infant Formula Inhibit Rotavirus Infection in Vitro." *Journal of Nutrition* 137 (9): 2068-2073. https://doi.org/10.1093/jn/137.9.2068.

73. **interfere with the absorption of medication:** Conrad, S. C., H. Chiu, and B. L. Silverman. 2004. "Soy Formula Complicates Management of Congenital Hypothyroidism." *Archives of Disease in Childhood* 89 (1): 37-40. https://doi.org/10.1136/adc.2002.009365.

74. **greater risk of osteopenia:** Bhatia, Jatinder, and Frank Greer. 2008. "Use of Soy Protein-Based Formulas in Infant Feeding." *Pediatrics* 121 (5): 1062-1068. https://doi.org/10.1542/peds.2008-0564.

75. **found in higher amounts in soy formula:** Li, Xinwei, Chongwei Hu, Yanzhu Zhu, Hao Sun, Yanfei Li, and Zhigang Zhang. 2011. "Effects of Aluminum Exposure on Bone Mineral Density, Mineral, and Trace Elements in Rats." *Biological Trace Element Research* 143 (1): 378-385. https://doi.org/10.1007/s12011-010-8861-4.

76. **protection of both pre-eruptive and post-eruptive teeth:** Dreyer, Benard P. "Harvard Public Health." *Harvard Public Health.* Accessed April 4, 2020. https://cdn1.sph.harvard.edu/wp-content/uploads/sites/2½016/04/Fluoride-letter-APA.pdf.

77. **Using a pacifier will not jeopardize:** O'Connor, Nina R., Kawai O. Tanabe, Mir S. Siadaty, and Fern R. Hauck. 2009. "Pacifiers and Breastfeeding: A Systematic Review." *Archives of Pediatrics & Adolescent Medicine* 163 (4): 378-382. https://doi.org/10.1001/archpediatrics.2008.578.

78. **30%-64% of infants with cow's milk protein intolerance:** Bhatia, Jatinder, and Frank Greer. 2008. "Use of Soy Protein-Based Formulas in Infant Feeding." *Pediatrics* 121 (5): 1062-1068. https://doi.org/10.1542/peds.2008-0564.

79. **age-dependent and most children outgrow them by age 5:** Bhatia, Jatinder, and Frank Greer. 2008. "Use of Soy Protein-Based Formulas in Infant Feeding." *Pediatrics* 121 (5): 1062-1068. https://doi.org/10.1542/peds.2008-0564.

80. **benefit these infants by shortening crying times:** Anabrees, Jasim, Flavia Indrio, Bosco Paes, and Khalid Alfaleh. 2013. "Probiotics for Infantile Colic: A Systematic Review." *BMC Pediatrics* 13 (1): 186. https://doi.org/10.1186/1471-2431-13-186.

81. **reduce the risk of necrotizing enterocolitis:** Alfaleh, Khalid, and Jasim Anabrees. 2014. "Probiotics for Prevention of Necrotizing Enterocolitis in Preterm Infants." *Cochrane Database of Systematic Review* 9 (4): 584-671. https://doi.org/10.1002/ebch.1976.

Chapter 4

1. **more satiety-responsive:** Brown, A., and M. D. Lee. "Early Influences on Child Satiety-Responsiveness: The Role of Weaning Style." *Pediatric Obesity* 10, no. 1 (2013): 57-66. https://doi.org/10.1111/j.2047-6310.2013.00207.x.

2. **significantly heavier at 18-24 months:** Brown, A., and M. D. Lee. "Early Influences on Child Satiety-

Responsiveness: The Role of Weaning Style." *Pediatric Obesity* 10, no. 1 (2013): 57–66. https://doi.org/10 .1111/j.2047-6310.2013.00207.x.

3. **significantly heavier at 18–24 months:** Brown, Amy, Sara Wyn Jones, and Hannah Rowan. "Baby-Led Weaning: The Evidence to Date." *Current Nutrition Reports* 6, no. 2 (2017): 148–156. https://doi.org/10.1007/s13668-017 -0201-2.

4. **significantly less picky than their spoon-fed peers:** Brown, A., and M. D. Lee. "Early Influences on Child Satiety-Responsiveness: The Role of Weaning Style." *Pediatric Obesity* 10, no. 1 (2013): 57–66. https://doi .org/10.1111/j.2047-6310.2013.00207.x.

5. **preference for carbohydrate-based foods:** Townsend, Ellen, and Nicola J. Pitchford. 2012. "Baby Knows Best? The Impact of Weaning Style on Food Preferences and Body Mass Index in Early Childhood in a Case-Controlled Sample." *BMJ Open* 2, no. 1. https://doi.org/10.1136/bmjopen-2011-000298.

6. **higher incidences of eczema, obesity, and type 1 diabetes:** Frederiksen, Brittni, Miranda Kroehl, Molly M. Lamb, Jennifer Seifert, Katherine Barriga, George S. Eisenbarth, Marian Rewers, and Jill M. Norris. "Infant Ex- posures and Development of Type 1 Diabetes Mellitus." *JAMA Pediatrics* 167, no. 9 (January 2013): 808. https:// doi.org/10.1001/jamapediatrics.2013.317.

7. **higher incidences of eczema, obesity, and type 1 diabetes:** Fergusson, D. M., and L. J. Horwood. 1994. "Early Solid Food Diet and Eczema in Childhood: A 10-Year Longitudinal Study." *Pediatric Allergy and Immunology* 5, no. S5: 44–47. https://doi.org/10.1111/j.1399-3038.1994.tb00347.x.

8. **higher incidences of eczema, obesity, and type 1 diabetes:** Morgan, J. 2004. "Eczema and Early Solid Feeding in Preterm Infants." *Archives of Disease in Childhood* 89, no. 4 (January): 309–314. https://doi.org/10.1136/adc .2002.020065.

9. **increase food acceptance and potentially lead to a more adventurous palate:** Mennella, Julie A., Ashley R. Reiter, and Loran M. Daniels. 2016. "Vegetable and Fruit Acceptance during Infancy: Impact of Ontogeny, Genetics, and Early Experiences." *Advances in Nutrition* 7 (1): 211S–219S. https://doi.org/10.3945/an.115 .008649.

10. **no difference in the likelihood of choking events:** D'Auria, Enza, Marcello Bergamini, Annamaria Staiano, Gi- useppe Banderali, Erica Pendezza, Francesca Penagini, Gian Vincenzo Zuccotti, and Diego Giampietro Peroni. 2018. "Baby-Led Weaning: What a Systematic Review of the Literature Adds On." Italian Journal of Pediatrics 44, no. 1 (March). https://doi.org/10.1186/s13052-018-0487-8.

11. **fruit has an anti-obesity effect:** Sharma, Satya, Hea Chung, Hyeon Kim, and Seong Hong. 2016. "Paradoxical Effects of Fruit on Obesity." *Nutrients* 8 (10): 633. https://doi.org/10.3390/nu8100633.

12. **promote mature drinking skills:** Morris, Suzanne Evans, and Marsha Dunn Klein. 2000. *Pre-Feeding Skills: A Comprehensive Resource for Mealtime Development.* Tucson, AZ: Therapy Skill Builders.

13. **may impact oral development:** Morris, Suzanne Evans, and Marsha Dunn Klein. 2000. *Pre-Feeding Skills: A Com- prehensive Resource for Mealtime Development.* Tucson, AZ: Therapy Skill Builders.

14. **10% of the population is affected by food allergies:** Sicherer, Scott H., and Hugh A. Sampson. 2018. "Food Al- lergy: A Review and Update on Epidemiology, Pathogenesis, Diagnosis, Prevention, and Management." *Journal of Allergy and Clinical Immunology* 141 (1): 41–58. https://doi.org/https://doi.org/10.1016/j.jaci.2017.11.003.

15. **often last for life:** Iweala, Onyinye I., Shailesh K. Choudhary, and Scott P. Commins. 2018. "Food Allergy." *Cur- rent Gastroenterology Reports* 20 (5): 17. https://doi.org/10.1007/s11894-018-0624-y.

16. **account for approximately 90% of all food allergies:** Greer, Frank R., Scott H. Sicherer, A. Wesley Burks, Com- mittee on Nutrition, and Section on Allergy and Immunology. 2019. "The Effects of Early Nutritional Interven- tions on the Development of Atopic Disease in Infants and Children: The Role of Maternal Dietary Restriction, Breastfeeding, Hydrolyzed Formulas, and Timing of Introduction of Allergenic Complementary Foods." *Pediat- rics* 143 (4). https://doi.org/10.1542/peds.2019-0281.

17. **actually increase children's risk:** Greer, Frank R., Scott H. Sicherer, A. Wesley Burks, Committee on Nutrition, and Section on Allergy and Immunology. 2019. "The Effects of Early Nutritional Interventions on the Develop- ment of Atopic Disease in Infants and Children: The Role of Maternal Dietary Restriction, Breastfeeding, Hydro-

lyzed Formulas, and Timing of Introduction of Allergenic Complementary Foods." *Pediatrics* 143 (4). https://doi
.org/10.1542/peds.2019-0281.

18. **reduce the risk of allergy by about 71% and 44%:** Greer, Frank R., Scott H. Sicherer, A. Wesley Burks, Committee
on Nutrition, and Section on Allergy and Immunology. 2019. "The Effects of Early Nutritional Interventions on
the Development of Atopic Disease in Infants and Children: The Role of Maternal Dietary Restriction, Breastfeeding, Hydrolyzed Formulas, and Timing of Introduction of Allergenic Complementary Foods." *Pediatrics* 143
(4). https://doi.org/10.1542/peds.2019-0281.

19. **at least 3 times per week:** Togias, Alkis, et al. 2017. "Addendum Guidelines for the Prevention of Peanut Allergy
in the United States." *Journal of Clinical Immunology* 139 (1): 29–44. https://doi.org/10.1016/j.jaci.2016.10.010.

20. **more likely to accept carrots:** Gerrish, Carolyn J., and Julie A. Mennella. 2001. "Flavor Variety Enhances Food
Acceptance in Formula-Fed Infants." *American Journal of Clinical Nutrition* 73 (6): 1080–1085. https://doi
.org/10.1093/ajcn/73.6.1080.

21. **can take up to 15 exposures:** Lafraire, Jérémie, Camille Rioux, Agnès Giboreau, and Delphine Picard. 2016.
"Food Rejections in Children: Cognitive and Social/Environmental Factors Involved in Food Neophobia and
Picky/Fussy Eating Behavior." *Appetite* 96: 347-357. https://doi.org/10.1016/j.appet.2016.02.121.

Chapter 5

1. **positive effect on bone health and bone mineralization:** Kouvelioti, Rozalia, Andrea R. Josse, and Panagiota
Klentrou. 2017. "Effects of Dairy Consumption on Body Composition and Bone Properties in Youth: A Systematic
Review." *Current Developments in Nutrition* 1 (8). https://doi.org/10.3945/cdn.117.001214.

2. **associated with greater height:** Berkey, Catherine S., Graham A. Colditz, Helaine R. H. Rockett, A. Lindsay
Frazier, and Walter C. Willett. 2009. "Dairy Consumption and Female Height Growth: Prospective Cohort Study."
Cancer Epidemiology Biomarkers & Prevention 18 (6): 1881-1887. https://doi.org/10.1158/1055-9965.epi-08
-1163.

3. Okada, Tomoo. 2004. "Effect of Cow Milk Consumption on Longitudinal Height Gain in Children." *American
Journal of Clinical Nutrition* 80 (4): 1088-1089. https://doi.org/10.1093/ajcn/80.4.1088a.

4. **smaller stature and lower bone mineral density:** Black, Ruth E., Sheila M. Williams, Ianthe E. Jones, and Ailsa
Goulding. 2002. "Children Who Avoid Drinking Cow Milk Have Low Dietary Calcium Intakes and Poor Bone
Health." *American Journal of Clinical Nutrition* 76 (3): 675-680. https://doi.org/10.1093/ajcn/76.3.675.

5. **higher bone mineral density:** Black, Ruth E., Sheila M. Williams, Ianthe E. Jones, and Ailsa Goulding. 2002.
"Children Who Avoid Drinking Cow Milk Have Low Dietary Calcium Intakes and Poor Bone Health." *American
Journal of Clinical Nutrition* 76 (3): 675-680. https://doi.org/10.1093/ajcn/76.3.675.

6. **supplementing calcium improves bone density:** Johnston, C. Conrad, Judy Z. Miller, Charles W. Slemenda, Te-
resa K. Reister, Siu Hui, Joe C. Christian, and Munro Peacock. 1992. "Calcium Supplementation and Increases in
Bone Mineral Density in Children." *New England Journal of Medicine* 327 (2): 82-87. https://doi.org/10.1056
/nejm199207093270204.

7. **associated with higher levels:** M. K. Javaid, S. R. Crozier, N. C. Harvey, C. R. Gale, E. M. Dennison, B. J. Boucher,
N. K. Arden, K. M. Godfrey, and C. Cooper. 2006. "Maternal Vitamin D Status during Pregnancy and Childhood
Bone Mass at Age 9 Years: A Longitudinal Study." *The Lancet* 367 (9504): 36-43. https://doi.org/10.1016/s0140
-6736(06)67922-1.

8. **one of the most important factors:** Davies, J. H. 2005. "Bone Mass Acquisition in Healthy Children." *Archives of
Disease in Childhood* 90 (4): 373-378. https://doi.org/10.1136/adc.2004.053553.

9. **does not decrease fracture risk:** Feskanich, Diane, Walter C. Willett, and Graham A. Colditz. 2003. "Calcium,
Vitamin D, Milk Consumption, and Hip Fractures: A Prospective Study among Postmenopausal Women." *American Journal of Clinical Nutrition* 77 (2): 504-511. https://doi.org/10.1093/ajcn/77.2.504.

10. **increased fracture risk with high dairy intake:** Michaëlsson, Karl, Alicja Wolk, Sophie Langenskiöld, Samar
Basu, Eva Warensjö Lemming, Håkan Melhus, and Liisa Byberg. 2014. "Milk Intake and Risk of Mortality and
Fractures in Women and Men: Cohort Studies." *BMJ* 349. https://doi.org/10.1136/bmj.g6015.

11. **began consuming dairy roughly 10,000 years ago:** Scerri, Eleanor M. L., et al. 2018. "Did Our Species Evolve in

Subdivided Populations across Africa, and Why Does It Matter?" *Trends in Ecology & Evolution* 33 (8): 582–594. https://doi.org/10.1016/j.tree.2018.05.005.

12. **began consuming dairy roughly 10,000 years ago:** Pitt, Daniel, Natalia Sevane, Ezequiel L. Nicolazzi, David E. Machugh, Stephen D. E. Park, Licia Colli, Rodrigo Martinez, Michael W. Bruford, and Pablo Orozco-terWengel. 2019. "Domestication of Cattle: Two or Three Events?" *Evolutionary Applications* 12 (1): 123–136. https://doi .org/10.1111/eva.12674.

13. **generally lasted from 2 to 4 years:** Piovanetti, Yvette. 2001. "Breastfeeding Beyond 12 Months." *Pediatric Clinics of North America* 48 (1): 199–206. https://doi.org/10.1016/s0031-3955(05)70294-7.

14. **as early as the 1500s:** Stevens, Emily E., Thelma E. Patrick, and Rita Pickler. 2009. "A History of Infant Feeding." *Journal of Perinatal Education* 18 (2): 32–39. https://doi.org/10.1624/105812409x426314.

15. **anemia and an increased risk of type 1 diabetes:** Leung, Alexander K. C., and Reginald S. Sauve. 2003. "Whole Cow's Milk in Infancy." *Paediatrics & Child Health*. Pulsus Group Inc, September. https://www.ncbi.nlm.nih.gov /pmc/articles/PMC2791650/.

16. **average age of breastfeeding was only 12 months:** Piovanetti, Yvette. 2001. "Breastfeeding Beyond 12 Months." *Pediatric Clinics of North America* 48 (1): 199–206. https://doi.org/10.1016/s0031-3955(05)70294-7.

17. **did not occur for roughly 60%–65%:** Silanikove, Nissim, Gabriel Leitner, and Uzi Merin. 2015. "The Interrelationships between Lactose Intolerance and the Modern Dairy Industry: Global Perspectives in Evolutional and Historical Backgrounds." *Nutrients* 7 (9): 7312–7331. https://doi.org/10.3390/nu7095340.

18. **7.8 years longer than the average non-Hispanic:** Acciai, Francesco, Aggie J. Noah, and Glenn Firebaugh. 2015. "Pinpointing the Sources of the Asian Mortality Advantage in the USA." *Journal of Epidemiology and Community Health* 69 (10): 1006–1011. https://doi.org/10.1136/jech-2015-205623.

19. **three times the total protein of human milk:** Malacarne M., F. Martuzzi, A. Summer, and P. Mariani. 2002. "Protein and Fat Composition of Mare's Milk: Some Nutritional Remarks with Reference to Human and Cow's Milk." *International Dairy Journal* 12 (11): 869–877. https://doi.org/10.1016/s0958-6946(02)00120-6.

20. **28% of children with chronic constipation experienced relief:** Daher, S., S. Tahan, D. Solé, C. K. Naspitz, F. R. Da Silva Patrício, U. F. Neto, and M. B. De Morais. 2001. "Cow's Milk Protein Intolerance and Chronic Constipation in Children." *Pediatric Allergy and Immunology: Official Publication of the European Society of Pediatric Allergy and Immunology* 12 (6): 339–342. https://doi.org/10.1034/j.1399-3038.2001.0o057.x.

21. **increased risk of prostate cancer:** Gao, Xiang, Michael P. Lavalley, and Katherine L. Tucker. 2005. "Prospective Studies of Dairy Product and Calcium Intakes and Prostate Cancer Risk: A Meta-Analysis." *JNCI: Journal of the National Cancer Institute* 97 (23): 1768–1777. https://doi.org/10.1093/jnci/dji402.

22. **increased risk of prostate cancer:** Lu, Wei, Hanwen Chen, Yuequn Niu, Han Wu, Dajing Xia, and Yihua Wu. 2016. "Dairy Products Intake and Cancer Mortality Risk: A Meta-Analysis of 11 Population-Based Cohort Studies." *Nutrition Journal* 15 (1): 91. https://doi.org/10.1186/s12937-016-0210-9.

23. **earlier age of menstruation:** Rogers, Imogen S., Kate Northstone, David B. Dunger, Ashley R. Cooper, Andy R. Ness, and Pauline M. Emmett. 2010. "Diet throughout Childhood and Age at Menarche in a Contemporary Cohort of British Girls." *Public Health Nutrition* 13 (12): 2052–2063. https://doi.org/10.1017/s1368980010001461.

24. **risk factor for breast cancer, cardiovascular disease, and diabetes:** Tehrani, Fahimeh Ramezani, Nazanin Moslehi, Golaleh Asghari, Roya Gholami, Parvin Mirmiran, and Fereidoun Azizi. 2013. "Intake of Dairy Products, Calcium, Magnesium, and Phosphorus in Childhood and Age at Menarche in the Tehran Lipid and Glucose Study." *PLoS ONE* 8 (2). https://doi.org/10.1371/journal.pone.0057696.

25. **3 cups a day has also been associated with childhood obesity:** Berkey, Catherine S., Helaine R. H. Rockett, Walter C. Willett, and Graham A. Colditz. 2005. "Milk, Dairy Fat, Dietary Calcium, and Weight Gain." *Archives of Pediatrics & Adolescent Medicine* 159 (6): 543–550. https://doi.org/10.1001/archpedi.159.6.543.

26. **3 cups a day has also been associated with childhood obesity:** Deboer, Mark D., Hannah E. Agard, and Rebecca J. Scharf. 2015. "Milk Intake, Height and Body Mass Index in Preschool Children." *Archives of Disease in Childhood* 100 (5): 460–465. https://doi.org/10.1136/archdischild-2014-306958.

27. **whole milk has a lower risk:** Vanderhout, Shelley M., Mary Aglipay, Nazi Torabi, Peter Jüni, Bruno R. Da Costa, Catherine S. Birken, Deborah L. O'Connor, Kevin E. Thorpe, and Jonathon L. Maguire. 2020. "Whole Milk Com-

pared with Reduced-Fat Milk and Childhood Overweight: A Systematic Review and Meta-Analysis." *American Journal of Clinical Nutrition* 111 (2): 266–279. https://doi.org/10.1093/ajcn/nqz276.

28. **20%–30% higher than non-milk drinkers:** Rich-Edwards, Janet W., Davaasambuu Ganmaa, Michael N. Pollak, Erika K. Nakamoto, Ken Kleinman, Uush Tserendolgor, Walter C. Willett, and A. Lindsay Frazier. 2007. "Milk Consumption and the Prepubertal Somatotropic Axis." *Nutrition Journal* 6: 28. https://doi.org/10.1186/1475 -2891-6-28.

29. **increased their levels of IGF-1:** Hoppe, C., C. Mølgaard, A. Juul, and K. F. Michaelsen. 2004. "High Intakes of Skimmed Milk, but Not Meat, Increase Serum IGF-I and IGFBP-3 in Eight-Year-Old Boys." *European Journal of Clinical Nutrition* 58 (9): 1211–1216. https://doi.org/10.1038/sj.ejcn.1601948.

30. **type 2 diabetes, Alzheimer's disease, and certain cancers:** Zoncu, Roberto, Alejo Efeyan, and David M. Sabatini. 2011. "mTOR: From Growth Signal Integration to Cancer, Diabetes and Ageing." *Nature Reviews Molecular Cell Biology* 12 (1): 21–35. https://doi.org/10.1038/nrm3025.

31. **High IGF-1 levels have also been linked to acne:** Melnik, Bodo C., and Christos C. Zouboulis. 2013. "Potential Role of FoxO1 and mTORC1 in the Pathogenesis of Western Diet-Induced Acne." *Experimental Dermatology* 22 (5): 311–315. https://doi.org/10.1111/exd.12142.

32. **obesity:** Melnik, Bodo C. 2012. "Excessive Leucine-mTORC1-Signalling of Cow Milk-Based Infant Formula: The Missing Link to Understand Early Childhood Obesity." *Journal of Obesity* 2012. https://doi.org/10.1155 /2012/197653.

33. **Alzheimer's disease:** Oddo, Salvatore. 2012. "The Role of MTOR Signaling in Alzheimer Disease." *Frontiers in Bioscience* S4: 941–52. https://doi.org/10.2741/s310.

34. **certain cancers, especially prostate cancer:** Hsieh, Andrew C., et al. 2012. "The Translational Landscape of MTOR Signalling Steers Cancer Initiation and Metastasis." *Nature* 485 (7396): 55–61. https://doi.org/10.1038 /nature10912.

35. **85 pounds at birth to 600 pounds:** "Calf Growth Observations of May vs. March Calving." *Drovers,* March 15, 2016. https://www.drovers.com/article/beeftalk-calf-growth-observations-may-vs-march-calving.

36. **lead to early life programming of the IGF-1 axis:** Melnik, Bodo C., Swen Malte John, and Gerd Schmitz. 2013. "Milk Is Not Just Food but Most Likely a Genetic Transfection System Activating mTORC1 Signaling for Postnatal Growth." *Nutrition Journal* 12: 103. https://doi.org/10.1186/1475-2891-12-103.

37. **absorbed intact upon consumption:** Rich-Edwards, Janet W., Davaasambuu Ganmaa, Michael N. Pollak, Er-ika K. Nakamoto, Ken Kleinman, Uush Tserendolgor, Walter C. Willett, and A. Lindsay Frazier. 2007. "Milk Consumption and the Prepubertal Somatotropic Axis." *Nutrition Journal* 6: 28. https://doi.org/10.1186/1475-2891-6-28.

38. **fall far below the RDA:** Fulton, J. R., C. W. Hutton, and K. R. Stitt. 1980. "Preschool Vegetarian Children. Dietary and Anthropometric Data." *Journal of the American Dietetic Association*, 76 (4): 360–365.

39. **were about 1.5 centimeters shorter:** Morency, Marie-Elssa, Catherine S. Birken, Gerald Lebovic, Yang Chen, Mary L'Abbé, Grace J. Lee, and Jonathon L. Maguire. 2017. "Association between Noncow Milk Beverage Consumption and Childhood Height." *American Journal of Clinical Nutrition* 106 (2): 597–602. https://doi.org/10.3945 /ajcn.117.156877.

40. **may be harmful to the gut:** David, Shlomit, Carmit Shani Levi, Lulu Fahoum, Yael Ungar, Esther G. Meyron-Holtz, Avi Shpigelman, and Uri Lesmes. 2018. "Revisiting the Carrageenan Controversy: Do We Really Understand the Digestive Fate and Safety of Carrageenan in Our Foods?" *Food & Function* 9 (3): 1344–1352. https://doi.org/10.1039 /c7fo01721a.

41. **vegetarians are still at an increased risk:** Herrmann, Wolfgang, Heike Schorr, Rima Obeid, and Jürgen Geisel. 2003. "Vitamin B-12 Status, Particularly Holotranscobalamin II and Methylmalonic Acid Concentrations, and Hyperhomocysteinemia in Vegetarians." *The American Journal of Clinical Nutrition* 78 (1): 131–136. https://doi .org/10.1093/ajcn/78.1.131.

42. **increased risk for iron deficiency anemia:** Levy-Costa, Renata Bertazzi, and Carlos Augusto Monteiro. 2004. "Cow's Milk Consumption and Childhood Anemia in the City of São Paulo, Southern Brazil." *Revista de Saude Publica.* https://www.scielosp.org/article/rsp/2004.v38n⁶⁄₇₉₇-803/en/.

43. **contains about 37 mcg/gram:** Yeh, Tai Sheng, Nu Hui Hung, and Tzu Chun Lin. 2014. "Analysis of Iodine Content

in Seaweed by GC-ECD and Estimation of Iodine Intake." *Journal of Food and Drug Analysis* 22 (2): 189–196. https://doi.org/10.1016/j.jfda.2014.01.014.

44. **reduced risk of childhood obesity:** Johnson, Rachel, Greg Welk, Pedro F. Saint-Maurice, and Michelle Ihmels. 2012. "Parenting Styles and Home Obesogenic Environments." *International Journal of Environmental Research and Public Health* 9 (4): 1411–1426. https://doi.org/10.3390/ijerph9041411.

45. **reduced risk of childhood obesity:** Olvera, N., and T. G. Power. 2010. "Brief Report: Parenting Styles and Obesity in Mexican American Children: A Longitudinal Study." *Journal of Pediatric Psychology* 35 (3): 243–249. https://doi.org/10.1093/jpepsy/jsp071.

46. **reduced risk of childhood obesity:** Taylor, A., C. Wilson, A. Slater, and P. Mohr. 2011. "Parent- and Child-Reported Parenting. Associations with Child Weight-Related Outcomes." *Appetite* 57 (3): 700–706. https://doi.org/10.1016/j.appet.2011.08.014.

47. **increased risk of childhood obesity:** Sleddens, Ester F. C., Sanne M. P. L. Gerards, Carel Thijs, Nanne K. de Vries, and Stef P. J. Kremers. 2011. "General Parenting, Childhood Overweight and Obesity-Inducing Behaviors: A Review." *International Journal of Pediatric Obesity* 6 (2-2): e12–e27. https://doi.org/10.3109/17477166.2011.566339.

48. **increased physical activity and healthy eating:** Berge, J. M., M. Wall, K. Loth, and D. Neumark-Sztainer. 2010. "Parenting Style as a Predictor of Adolescent Weight and Weight-Related Behaviors." *Journal of Adolescent Health: Official Publication of the Society for Adolescent Medicine* 46 (4): 331–338. https://doi.org/10.1016/j.jadohealth.2009.08.004.

49. **increased physical activity and healthy eating:** Topham, G. L., L. Hubbs-Tait, J. M. Rutledge, M. C. Page, T. S. Kennedy, L. H. Shriver, and A. W. Harrist. 2011. "Parenting Styles, Parental Response to Child Emotion, and Family Emotional Responsiveness Are Related to Child Emotional Eating." *Appetite* 56 (2): 261–264. https://doi.org/10.1016/j.appet.2011.01.007.

50. **typically eat fewer fruits and vegetables:** Hughes, S. O., T. G. Power, J. Orlet Fisher, S. Mueller, and T. A. Nicklas. 2005. "Revisiting a Neglected Construct: Parenting Styles in a Child-Feeding Context." *Appetite* 44 (1): 83–92. https://doi.org/10.1016/j.appet.2004.08.007.

51. **higher risk of childhood obesity:** Sleddens, Ester F. C., Sanne M. P. L. Gerards, Carel Thijs, Nanne K. de Vries, and Stef P. J. Kremers. 2011. "General Parenting, Childhood Overweight and Obesity-Inducing Behaviors: A Review." *International Journal of Pediatric Obesity* 6 (2-2): e12–e27. https://doi.org/10.3109/17477166.2011.566339.

52. **eat more junk and processed food:** Burdette, H. L., R. C. Whitaker, W. C. Hall, and S. R. Daniels. 2006. "Maternal Infant-Feeding Style and Children's Adiposity at 5 Years of Age." *Archives of Pediatrics & Adolescent Medicine* 160 (5): 513–520. https://doi.org/10.1001/archpedi.160.5.513.

53. **when kids do ask for food, they aren't supported:** Shloim, N., L. R. Edelson, N. Martin, and M. M. Hetherington. 2015. "Parenting Styles, Feeding Styles, Feeding Practices, and Weight Status in 4-12 Year-Old Children: A Systematic Review of the Literature." *Frontiers in Psychology* 6: 1849. https://doi.org/10.3389/fpsyg.2015.01849.

54. **Exposure is the number one factor:** Sullivan, S. A., and L. L. Birch. 1994. "Infant Dietary Experience and Acceptance of Solid Foods." *Pediatrics* 93 (2): 271–277. https://www.ncbi.nlm.nih.gov/pubmed/8121740.

55. **same food on your child's plate a dozen times:** Lam, Jason. 2015. "Picky Eating in Children." *Frontiers in Pediatrics* 3. https://doi.org/10.3389/fped.2015.00041.

56. **encourages kids to try foods that are similar:** Fishbein, M., S. Cox, C. Swenny, C. Mogren, L. Walbert, C. Fraker. 2006. "Food Chaining: A Systematic Approach for the Treatment of Children with Feeding Aversion." *Nutrition in Clinical Practice* (2): 182–184. https://doi.org/10.1177/0115426506021002182.

Chapter 6

1. **they will likely eat more:** Savage, Jennifer S., Jennifer Orlet Fisher, and Leann L. Birch. 2008. "Parental Influence on Eating Behavior: Conception to Adolescence." *Journal of Law, Medicine & Ethics* 35 (1): 22–34. https://doi.org/10.1111/j.1748-720x.2007.00111.x.

2. **lead to emotional eating:** Roberts, Lindsey, Jenna M. Marx, and Dara R. Musher-Eizenman. 2018. "Using Food As a Reward: An Examination of Parental Reward Practices." *Appetite* 120: 318–326. https://doi.org/10.1016/j.appet.2017.09.024.

3. **eat more of them:** Rollins, B. Y., E. Loken, J. S. Savage, and L. L. Birch. 2014. "Effects of Restriction on Children's Intake Differ by Child Temperament, Food Reinforcement, and Parent's Chronic Use of Restriction." *Appetite* 73: 31–39. https://doi.org/10.1016/j.appet.2013.10.005.

4. **Birch, Leann L., Jennifer Orlet Fisher, and Kirsten Krahnstoever Davison. 2003. "Learning to Overeat:** Maternal Use of Restrictive Feeding Practices Promotes Girls' Eating in the Absence of Hunger." *American Journal of Clinical Nutrition* 78 (2): 215–220. https://doi.org/10.1093/ajcn/78.2.215.

5. **increased their intake of that food:** Fisher, J. O., and L. L. Birch. 1999. "Restricting Access to Foods and Children's Eating." *Appetite* 32 (3): 405–419. https://doi.org/10.1006/appe.1999.0231.

6. **greater behavioral regulation and academic achievement:** Rollins, B. Y., E. Loken, J. S. Savage, and L. L. Birch. 2014. "Effects of Restriction on Children's Intake Differ by Child Temperament, Food Reinforcement, and Parent's Chronic Use of Restriction." *Appetite* 73: 31–39. https://doi.org/10.1016/j.appet.2013.10.005.

7. **Restrictive Feeding versus Structured Feeding (Table):** Grolnick, Wendy S., and Eva M. Pomerantz. 2009. "Issues and Challenges in Studying Parental Control: Toward a New Conceptualization." *Child Development Perspectives* 3 (3): 165–170. https://doi.org/10.1111/j.1750-8606.2009.00099.x.

8. **associated with a higher intake:** Martin-Biggers, Jennifer, Kim Spaccarotella, Amanda Berhaupt-Glickstein, Nobuko Hongu, John Worobey, and Carol Byrd-Bredbenner. 2014. "Come and Get It! A Discussion of Family Mealtime Literature and Factors Affecting Obesity Risk 1–3." *Advances in Nutrition* 5 (3): 235–247. https://doi.org/10.3945/an.113.005116.

9. **5 nights a week had a 23%–25% reduced risk:** Anderson, S. E., and R. C. Whitaker. 2010. "Household Routines and Obesity in US Preschool-Aged Children." *Pediatrics* 125 (3): 420–428. https://doi.org/10.1542/peds.2009-0417.

10. **fewer family meals increased the risk:** Gable, Sara, Yiting Chang, and Jennifer L. Krull. 2007. "Television Watching and Frequency of Family Meals Are Predictive of Overweight Onset and Persistence in a National Sample of School-Aged Children." *Journal of the American Dietetic Association* 107 (1): 53–61. https://doi.org/10.1016/j.jada.2006.10.010.

11. **more likely to consume at least five servings:** Andaya, Abegail A., Elva M. Arredondo, John E. Alcaraz, Suzanne P. Lindsay, and John P. Elder. 2011. "The Association between Family Meals, TV Viewing during Meals, and Fruit, Vegetables, Soda, and Chips Intake among Latino Children." *Journal of Nutrition Education and Behavior* 43 (5): 308–315. https://doi.org/10.1016/j.jneb.2009.11.005.

12. **studies have linked their consumption in children:** McCann, Donna, et al. 2007. "Food Additives and Hyperactive Behaviour in 3-Year-Old and 8/9-Year-Old Children in the Community: A Randomised, Double-Blinded, Placebo-Controlled Trial." *The Lancet* 370 (9598): 1560–1567. https://doi.org/10.1016/s0140-6736(07)61306-3.

13. **studies have linked their consumption in children:** Nigg, Joel T., Kara Lewis, Tracy Edinger, and Michael Falk. 2012. "Meta-Analysis of Attention-Deficit/Hyperactivity Disorder or Attention-Deficit/Hyperactivity Disorder Symptoms, Restriction Diet, and Synthetic Food Color Additives." *Journal of the American Academy of Child & Adolescent Psychiatry* 51 (1): 86–97.e8. https://doi.org/10.1016/j.jaac.2011.10.015.

14. **"May have an adverse effect on activity and attention":** "Food Additives." 2020. *Food Standards Agency.* https://www.food.gov.uk/safety-hygiene/food-additives.

15. **more likely to have an eating disorder:** Barthels, Friederike, Saskia Poerschke, Romina Müller, and Reinhard Pietrowsky. 2019. "Orthorexic Eating Behavior in Vegans Is Linked to Health, Not to Animal Welfare." *Eating and Weight Disorders—Studies on Anorexia, Bulimia and Obesity.* https://doi.org/10.1007/s40519-019-00679-8.

Chapter 7

1. **has been shown to induce liver damage:** "Toxicology and Risk Assessment of Coumarin: Focus on Human Data." *Risk Assessment of Phytochemicals in Food,* 2010, 272–360. https://doi.org/10.1002/9783527634705.ch3c.

Index

Note: Page numbers in *italics* refer to illustrations.

vitamin B12 recommendations for, 34, 35, 36, 287

vitamin D recommendations for, 36, 149–50

zinc recommendations for, 27

See also picky eaters

baby-led weaning, 105–17

and allergic reactions/intolerances, 114–15

benefits of, 105–7

and choking risks, 115–17

and food preparation, *109–10*, 111–14

and food progression, 114–15

and getting adequate amounts of food, 115

guidelines for, 117

how to start, 108, *109–10*, 111

and portion sizes, 126

and purees, 136

with runny/slippery foods, 136, 137

signs of readiness for, 107–8

and slow process of learning to eat, 111, 126

when to begin, 134

Bacteroides, 6

Baked Tofu recipe, 289

balls: Blueberry Oat Balls recipe, 257

bananas

and baby-led weaning, 112

Blender Mini Muffins recipe, 228–29

and constipation, 164

organic vs. conventional, 67

rolled in hemp seeds, 58, 66

banging cups and utensils, 182

barley, 50, 295

bars: Quinoa Prune Bars recipe, 211

batch prepping/cooking, 61–62

BBQ tofu bowl recipe, 266–67

beans

and baby-led weaning, 113

batch prepping, 62

Bean and Corn Taquitos recipe, 252–53

benefits of, 52

as calcium source, 29, 58

as choline source, 41

cooking, 293–94

as iron source, 56

macronutrients in, 15

Pasta Fagioli recipe, 262–63

as protein source, 17, 18, 52

serving sizes for, 53

soaking, 54

sprouting, 54

See also legumes

beets

and baby-led weaning, *109*, *110*, 111

Beets + Sweets Mash recipe, 202

organic vs. conventional, 67

behavioral disorders, 20

bell peppers, 57, 58, 111

berries

and baby-led weaning, 112

batch prepping, 62

French Toast Fingers with Quick Berry Syrup recipe, 222–23

in snack combos, 66

Bifidobacterium, 6

bioaccumulative chemicals, 4, 20–21, 66, 74

Bircher muesli recipe, 237

birthday parties, 175–76

birth weight, 19, 24

black beans

and baby-led weaning, *110*

cooking, 294

Cubano Bowl recipe, 195

15-Minute Black Bean Tacos recipe, 264–65

as iron source, 57

serving sizes for, 53

Tex-Mex Millet Meatballs recipe, 208–9

black-eye peas, 294

Blender Mini Muffins recipe, 228–29

BLISS (baby-lead introduction to solids) study, 106

blueberries

Blueberry Muffin Mix recipe, 194

Blueberry Oat Balls recipe, 257

PB&J Smoothie recipe, 236

BLW Oatmeal Pancakes recipe, 210

bok choy, 29

bone health, 29, 37, 38, 48, 141–42

bowel movements (outputs), 78, 79

BPA (bisphenol-A), 63

brain health/development

and breast milk, 16

and choline, 40, 42

and DHA levels, 19

in first six months, 74

and iron, 23

nutrients needed for, 7

and olive oil, 55

and vitamin B12, 34

bran flakes as zinc source, 28

butternut squash
    and baby-led weaning, 111
    Butternut Squash Fries recipe, 205
    multiple benefits of, 7
    organic vs. conventional, 67
    as vitamin A source, 39, 59
B vitamins, 49

caffeine, 89, 90
calcium
    and breastfeeding, 86-87
    Calcium Creamsicle Smoothie recipe, 221
    and cow's milk, 29, 141-42
    foods rich in, 58
    from fruits and vegetables, 48
    and iron absorption, 25, 30, 58, 149
    legumes, nuts, seeds as sources of, 52
    from plant-based milks, 29, 58, 141, 147, 149
    recommendations for, 28-30, 286
    in the second year, 149
    supplementation of, 87
    and zinc absorption, 28, 30
Calcium Creamsicle Smoothie recipe, 221
caloric requirements, 14-15, 286
calzone recipe, 278-79
Canadian Paediatric Society, 3
cancer
    and benefits of breastfeeding, 80, 81-82
    and health benefits of plant-based diets, 3
    and iron from animal sources, 5
    and milk consumption, 144
    and soy formulas, 98
    and soy's protective function, 71
    and whole grains, 49
cannellini beans, 294
cantaloupe, 39, 67
carbohydrates, 15-16, 52, 286
cardiovascular disease, 5
carotene, 59-60
carrageenan, 147
carrots
    and baby-led weaning, *109*, *110*
    batch prepping, 62
    organic vs. conventional, 67
    as vitamin A source, 39, 59
cashew milk, 60, 146
cashews
    Cheezy Broccoli Trees recipe, 215
    mac and cheeze with, 55

and parmesan recipe, 290
    serving sizes for, 53
    and Vegan Cheese Sauce recipe, 291
cashew yogurt, 66, 240
cassava, 32
Caterpillar Pasta recipe, 272-73
cauliflower, 57, 111, 201
celiac disease, 70-71
cell growth, 48
Centers for Disease Control and Prevention (CDC), 100
cereal, iron fortified, 25, 27, 56, 57, 121, 148-49
cheese, 123
Cheesy Broccoli Cauliflower Mash recipe, 201
Cheezy Broccoli Trees recipe, 215
chemical and toxin exposures, 4, 20-21, 66, 74
Cherry Chia Popsicle recipe, 256
Chewy Granola Bars recipe, 244-45
chia seeds
    ALA in, 58
    Cherry Chia Popsicle recipe, 256
    chia jam, 66
    as iron source, 56
    Lemon Chia Waffles recipe, 233
    omega-3 fatty acids in, 19
    as protein source, 17
    as selenium source, 33
    serving sizes for, 53
    as source of good fat, 55
    Tropical Chia Pudding recipe, 243
chickpeas
    Chickpea Coconut Curry recipe, 274
    Chicks 'n' Grits recipe, 193
    cooking, 294
    pastas made of, 56
    PBJ's Blender Bean Muffins recipe, 206-7
    serving sizes for, 53
    as zinc source, 28
Chicks 'n' Grits recipe, 193
China, 33
chocolate, 22
choking risks, 115-17
cholesterol levels, 4, 22
choline, 7, 40-42, 84-85, 90, 146, 286
chronic disease
    risks of, 5, 6, 48, 80, 144-45
    and soy's protective function, 71
citrus, 57, 123
climate change, 10
coconut, 22

fruits
    and baby-led weaning, 111–13, 114, 135
    batch prepping, 62
    benefits of, 47–48, 66–67, 124–25
    as calcium source, 29
    cleaning, 68
    and composition of PB3 Plate, 46, *47*
    and constipation, 164
    consumption of, among plant-based children,
        3, 4
    dark-colored, 39
    eating a variety of colors of, 48
    as fiber source, 48
    and food preparation techniques, 159
    and juices, 68
    and obesity, 124
    organic vs. conventional, 66–67
    phytochemicals in, 48
fullness cues of children, 129
fussy babies, 101

gagging vs. choking, 116–17
galactagogues, 91–93
gastrointestinal issues, 24, 100
genetically modified organisms (GMOs), 67
ghrelin, 81
ginger, 67
gluten, 70–71
goiters, 31
goitrogens, 32
grains, 49–52
    and anti-nutrients, 54
    babies' abilities to digest, 137
    batch prepping, 62
    benefits of, 7, 49
    and composition of PB3 Plate, 46, *47*
    cooking, 295
    favorite uses for, 295
    and fiber, 49, 51–52
    and gluten, 70–71
    and gut microbiome, 6
    and iron, 24, 25, 56
    organic vs. conventional, 67
    as protein source, 17, 18, 50
    refined grains, 51, 52, 56
    serving sizes for, 50
    sprouted grains, 25, 54, 56
    whole grains, 6, 7, 51–52
    as zinc source, 28

grandparents, 184
granola bars recipe, 244–45
grapes, 112
grazing behaviors, 158, 176–78
great northern beans, 294
green beans, 112
Green Dragon Smoothie recipe, 227
greenhouse gas emissions, 10
ground beef, recipe swaps for, 292
growth of children
    carbohydrates' role in, 16
    as infants, 14
    and monitoring food intake, 78
    slowing of, in second year, 152–53
    and small appetites, 163
guacamole recipe, 239

Health Council of the Netherlands, 21
heart disease, 3, 5, 49, 144
heart health, 55
heavy metals, 66
height of children, 3, 141, 146
hemp seeds, 52, 53, 55, 58, 66
honey, 123
honeydew, 67
hummus, 55, 290
hunger signals of children
    by age, 129
    early signs of, 78
    and feeding on demand, 76, 77
    recognizing, 126–27
    and responsive feeding, 128
    and sign language for toddlers, 127–28, *127*
hydration. *See* water consumption and
        hydration
hypothyroidism, 99

Ice Cream Smoothie Bowl recipe, 249
indulgent feeding style, 154–55
infection risks, 80, 81, 99
inflammatory signaling molecules, 3
insulin-like growth factor (IGF-1), 144–45
insulin resistance, 3, 144
intelligence and IQ, 4, 31, 77, 81
intrinsic factor (IF), 34
iodine
    and brain development, 7, 31
    and breastfeeding, 30, 85, 287
    and goitrogens, 32

recommendations for, 30, 286, 287

sources of, 8, 31

for toddlers, 150-51

iron

    AAP recommendations on, 12, 13

    and brain development, 7

    and breastfeeding, 12, 23, 26, 86, 122

    and calcium, 25, 30, 58, 149

    cereal fortified with, 25, 27, 56, 57, 121, 148-49

    food pairings that optimize, 121-22

    foods inhibiting absorption of, 12

    and formula fed babies, 27

    heme vs. non-heme, 5, 24

    increasing absorption of, 24-25, 30, 54, 121-22

    iron deficiency, 5, 12-13, 23, 24, 149

    Iron-Optimized Oatmeal recipe, 57

    iron reserve of newborns, 26, 121

    legumes, nuts, seeds as sources of, 52, 54, 56

    and meat, 5, 23, 24, 120-21

    and milk consumption, 5, 24, 149

    and PB3 Plate, 56-57

    recommendations for, 23, 121-22, 286, 287

    in the second year, 148-49

    and skeptics' criticisms of plant-based diets, 2

    sources of, 23, 24, 25-26, 56, 121

    and spinach, 25

    supplementation of, 12, 26-27, 86, 90, 149

    and vitamin C, 24-25, 57-58, 121

isoflavones, 98

Italian Plate, PB3, *64*

juices, 68

kale, 29, 39, 48, 56, 59, 60

kidney beans, 26, 41, 294

kitchen participation of toddlers, 182-83

kombu, 31

LA (linoleic acid), 19, 55

Lactobacillus, 102

lactose, 16, 97, 143-44

leafy greens, 6, 57, 195, 227

Learning Towers, 183

legumes

    ALA in, 58

    and anti-nutrients, 54

    batch prepping, 62

    benefits of, 52

    as calcium source, 29

    as choline source, 41

    and composition of PB3 Plate, 46, *47*

    and gut microbiome, 6

    and iron, 24, 25-26

    multiple benefits of, 7

    pastas made of, 26, 56, 57

    as protein source, 17, 18, 52, 54

    serving sizes for, 53

    sprouting, 25, 54

    as zinc source, 28

Lemon Chia Waffles recipe, 233

lemon juice as vitamin C source, 57

lentils

    cooking, 294, 295

    as iron source, 25

    Lentil-A-Roni recipe, 261

    Lentil Sloppy Joes recipe, 270-71

    pastas made of, 56

    as protein source, 18

    Red Lentil Pizza Strips recipe, 216-17

    serving sizes for, 53

    as zinc source, 28

Le Petite Pizza recipe, 199

leptin, 81

life expectancy, 3, 144

liver function, 40

longest-lived populations, 8

Longo, Valter, 1

lysine, 17, 146

mac 'n' cheeze recipe, 250-51

macrobiotic diets, 14

macronutrients, 15

malnutrition, 6-7

mangoes, 39, 59, 60, 67, *110*

marinara, 57, 218-19

mastitis, 94-95

meals

    batch prepping/cooking, 61-62

    and kitchen participation of toddlers, 182-83

    and lack of appetite, 184

    missing, 161-62

    planning, 61-63

    sample meals, 297-98

    shared as a family, 179-81

    timing of, 126

    See also PB3 Plate

pea milk
    advantages of, 146
    as calcium source, 29, 58, 141
    and iron absorption, 58
    and PB3 Plate, 47
    recommendations for, 60
    as vitamin D source, 37
peanut butter
    as iron source, 58
    PB&J Smoothie recipe, 236
    saturated fats in, 22
    serving sizes for, 53
    in snack combos, 66
    as source of good fat, 55
    as zinc source, 28
peanuts, 52, 130, 131, 132
pea-protein formulas, 96
pears, 113
peas, 41, 50, 110, 239, 295
Peas Please recipe, 200
pecans, 53
pediatricians, 2, 12, 13
permissive feeding style, 154-55
persimmons, 59, 60
pescatarians, 9
pesticide residues, 66-67
phosvitin, 12
phytates/phytic acid, 24, 25, 54, 99
phytochemicals, 48, 66, 98, 124
picky eaters, 152-61
    and baby-led weaning, 106, 107
    and cooking techniques, 158-60
    and decreased appetite, 152-53
    and Division of Responsibility in Feeding, 153,
        155-56, 159
    and introducing new foods, 158-59
    and modeling healthy eating behaviors, 157,
        161
    and parenting styles, 153-55
    and promoting adventurous eating, 156-58
pineapple, 67
pinto beans, 29, 294
pita bread, 50
pizza recipes, 199, 216-17
plant-based diets
    benefits of, 3-4, 9-10
    and birthday parties, 175-76
    criticisms of, 2

and day cares, 174-75
and eating disorders, 185
family reactions to, 173, 184
fears and misconceptions about, 6-9
and modeling healthy eating behaviors,
    173-74
and omnivorous partners, 173-74
as a "restriction," 171-72
safety of, 2, 3, 173
Plant-Based Juniors (PBJs) online community, 1
plastic food storage, 63
plugged ducts, 93-94
polenta, 193, 295
polyunsaturated fatty acids, 7
pomegranates, 67
popsicle recipe, 256
porridge recipe, 234
portion sizes, 126
potatoes, 50, 57, 67, 112
pregnancy
    and alcohol consumption, 87
    and calcium, 86
    and choline, 40-41, 42
    and coffee consumption, 89
    and DHA, 19, 84
    and fenugreek, 92
    and iodine, 85
    and maternal smoking, 82
    and prenatal vitamins, 85, 87
    safety of plant-based diets during, 173
    and taste preferences of babies, 75
premature/preterm births, 19, 24, 27, 84, 99
prenatal vitamins, 85, 87
probiotics, 102
prolactin, 91
protein
    available in plants, 52
    and balancing macronutrients, 15
    grains as source of, 49-50
    legumes, nuts, seeds as sources of, 52, 54
    and milk consumption, 5
    myth of incomplete, 17-18
    recommendations for, 16, 18, 286
    role of, in early development, 7
    and skeptics' criticisms of plant-based
        diets, 2
    sources of, 16-17
    and soy intolerance, 101-2

prunes, 164, 211

pudding recipe, 243

puffs, snack, 65

pulses. *See* beans

pumpkin, 39, 40, 59, 60, 258-59

pumpkin seeds, 28, 52, 53

purees
  adding flavor to, 120
  offered in addition to baby-led weaning, 136
  portion sizes for, 126
  preparation and safety, 118-19
  recipes for, 191-203
  switching from, to baby-led weaning, 105
  traditional approach to weaning using, 105
  when to begin, 118

quesadillas recipe, 282-83

Quick Berry Syrup recipe, 222-23

quinoa
  and baby-led weaning, 114
  as choline source, 41
  cooking, 295
  Le Petite Pizza recipe, 199
  as protein source, 50
  Quinoa Prune Bars recipe, 211
  serving sizes for, 50
  Simple Breakfast Quinoa Porridge recipe, 234
  as zinc source, 28

raspberries, *109, 110,* 249

raw diets, 14, 54

raw foods, 123

recipe swaps, 292

Recommended Daily Allowance (RDA), 15

red beans, 29

Red Lentil Pizza Strips recipe, 216-17

reducetarians, 9

refined grains, 51, 52

respiratory infections, 38

responsive feeding, 128

restaurants, eating in, 178-79

restrictive feeding, 160, 167-68, 171-72

rewards, food as, 167

rice, 50, 72, 114, 195, 295

rice milk, 60, 146

rickets, 37

role modeling healthy eating behaviors, 157, 161, 171, 173-74, 179

round foods, avoiding, 123

routines, value of, 155

safe food storage, 63

safety of plant-based diets, 2, 3, 173

salt/sodium intake
  and baby-led weaning, 106
  and foods to avoid during weaning, 123-24
  and iodine, 31, 32, 85, 150-51
  recommendations for, 69-70

satiety cues of children, 129

Satter, Ellyn, 126, 136, 155

saturated fats, 4, 22, 84

Savory Corn Muffins recipe, 254-55

schools, meals at, 174-75

sea vegetables, 31, 150-51

seeds
  ALA in, 58
  and anti-nutrients, 54
  benefits of, 52, 54
  as iron source, 56
  and PB3 Plate, 46, *47*
  as protein source, 17, 18, 52
  serving sizes for, 53
  as source of good fat, 22
  sprouting, 54
  as zinc source, 28
  See also specific seeds

selenium, 33-34, 52, 286

self-regulation of food intake
  and avoiding pressuring children, 157
  and caloric requirements of children, 14
  and Division of Responsibility in Feeding, 126-27, 136, 155-56
  and feeding on demand, 76-79, 91
  and food restrictions, 160, 167-68
  and mindful eating, 181
  and obesity risks, 106
  and responsive feeding, 128
  with sweets and treats, 167
  See also baby-led weaning

sesame seeds, 52, 53, 58, 66

Sheet Pan BBQ Tofu Bowls recipe, 266-67

shellfish, 130, 132

SIDs (sudden infant death syndrome), 80, 82, 101

sign language for toddlers, 127-28, *127*

Simple Breakfast Quinoa Porridge recipe, 234